Renal Physiology
A Clinical Approach

John Danziger, MD
Instructor in Medicine
Division of Nephrology
Beth Israel Deaconess Medical Center
Harvard Medical School
Boston, MA

Mark Zeidel, MD
Herrman L. Blumgart Professor of Medicine
Harvard Medical School
Physician-in-Chief and Chair, Department of Medicine
Beth Israel Deaconess Medical Center
Boston, MA

Michael J. Parker, MD
Assistant Professor of Medicine
Division of Pulmonary, Critical Care, and Sleep Medicine
Beth Israel Deaconess Medical Center
Senior Interactive Media Architect
Center for Educational Technology
Harvard Medical School
Boston, MA

Series Editor
Richard M. Schwartzstein, MD
Ellen and Melvin Gordon Professor of Medicine and Medical Education
Director, Harvard Medical School Academy
Vice President for Education and Director, Carl J. Shapiro Institute for Education
Beth Israel Deaconess Medical Center
Boston, MA

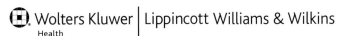
Wolters Kluwer | Lippincott Williams & Wilkins
Health
Philadelphia • Baltimore • New York • London
Buenos Aires • Hong Kong • Sydney • Tokyo

Acquisitions Editor: Crystal Taylor
Product Managers: Angela Collins and Jennifer Verbiar
Marketing Manager: Joy Fisher-Williams
Designer: Doug Smock
Compositor: Aptara, Inc.

351 West Camden Street
Baltimore, MD 21201

Two Commerce Square
2001 Market Street
Philadelphia, PA 19103

Printed in China

9 8 7 6 5 4 3 2 1

Library of Congress Cataloging-in-Publication Data
Danziger, John.
   Renal physiology : a clinical approach / John Danziger, Mark Zeidel,
Michael J. Parker. — 1st ed.
     p. ; cm. — (Integrated physiology series)
   Includes bibliographical references and index.
   ISBN 978-0-7817-9524-1
   I. Zeidel, Mark. II. Parker, Michael J. III. Title. IV. Series:
Integrated physiology series.
   [DNLM: 1. Kidney—physiology. WJ 301]
   616.614—dc23

2011050922

DISCLAIMER

Care has been taken to confirm the accuracy of the information present and to describe generally accepted practices. However, the authors, editors, and publisher are not responsible for errors or omissions or for any consequences from application of the information in this book and make no warranty, expressed or implied, with respect to the currency, completeness, or accuracy of the contents of the publication. Application of this information in a particular situation remains the professional responsibility of the practitioner; the clinical treatments described and recommended may not be considered absolute and universal recommendations.

The authors, editors, and publisher have exerted every effort to ensure that drug selection and dosage set forth in this text are in accordance with the current recommendations and practice at the time of publica-tion. However, in view of ongoing research, changes in government regulations, and the constant flow of information relating to drug therapy and drug reactions, the reader is urged to check the package insert for each drug for any change in indications and dosage and for added warnings and precautions. This is par-ticularly important when the recommended agent is a new or infrequently employed drug.

Some drugs and medical devices presented in this publication have Food and Drug Administration (FDA) clearance for limited use in restricted research settings. It is the responsibility of the health care pro-vider to ascertain the FDA status of each drug or device planned for use in their clinical practice.

To purchase additional copies of this book, call our customer service department at (800) 638-3030 or fax orders to (301) 223-2320. International customers should call (301) 223-2300.

Visit Lippincott Williams & Wilkins on the Internet: http://www.lww.com. Lippincott Williams & Wilkins customer service representatives are available from 8:30 am to 6:00 pm, EST.

To my parents, Avril and Julius, whose support enabled me to become a physician
—John Danziger

To my wife, Susan
—Mark Zeidel

To my wonderful wife, Yuanzhen, and my parents, Leonard and Gloria: for their boundless support, enthusiasm, inspiration, and love
—Michael Parker

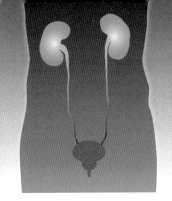

Preface

Introduction

The goal of *Renal Physiology: A Clinical Approach* is to provide a clear, clinically oriented exposition of the essentials of renal physiology for medical students, residents, nurses, and allied health professionals. We present the physiology in the context of a system to emphasize that the functions we associate with the renal system depend upon more than the kidney. This approach is essential for a complete understanding of the clinical problems that affect the elimination of toxic substances from the body and the fine-tuning, not only of our water status, but of our blood pressure as well.

This book is the third in *The Integrated Physiology Series,* a sequence of monographs on physiology. The first book, *Respiratory Physiology: A Clinical Approach,* describes the essential principles underlying breathing. The second book, *Cardiovascular Physiology: A Clinical Approach,* helps you navigate the complexities of the circulation. Each book is designed to meet the needs of the learners outlined below, and uses the same style and pedagogical tools. In addition, we have attempted to design common frameworks upon which the student can hang the large amounts of information confronting us in medicine today, and with which a foundation can be built to support the incorporation of new data in the future. In this book, for example, we describe the renal system in the context of filtration (the regulation of the factors that control how much and what kinds of substances are filtered by the glomerulus), reabsorption (the determinants of the selective reabsorption, and in some cases secretion, of key electrolytes and water in the different sections of the renal tubule), and the important renal-endocrine links that are essential for water handling and modulation of blood pressure, not only for the kidney but for the body as a whole.

The series addresses "integrated" physiology by its focus on systems rather than organs, and by making explicit links between systems. Understanding blood pressure control, for example, requires one to be conversant with the details of both cardiovascular and renal physiology. To provide care to a patient with an acid–base problem, one must be able to explain how the respiratory and renal systems combine to keep the pH in a range that enables enzymes to function normally.

Our goals are to present physiology in a clinically meaningful way, to emphasize that physiology is best understood within the context of an organ *system,* to demonstrate principles that are common to different systems, and to utilize an interactive style that engages and challenges the reader.

Level

The level of the book is intended to fit a range of needs from students who have had no previous exposure to physiology to residents who are now in the thick of patient care but feel the need to review relevant physiology in a clinical context. We have drawn upon many years of experience teaching students, residents, and fellows in making decisions with respect to the topics emphasized and the clinical examples used to illustrate key concepts. The book is not intended as a comprehensive review of renal physiology nor is it designed for the advanced, research oriented physiologist. Rather, we have focused on issues that are most relevant for the care of patients while, at the same time, we provide sufficient physiological detail to provide you with the foundation to examine and analyze new data on these topics in the future.

Most of the concepts presented in the book are well established, and we do not burden you with long reference lists for this information. When we present newer and, in some cases, more controversial issues, however, we do provide relevant primary source citations.

Content

The book begins with two chapters that serve to provide context for the study of renal physiology. In Chapter 1, we lay out the basic challenges confronting humans as land creatures who must conserve water but must also devise a system that filters from the blood potentially toxic byproducts of metabolism without losing all of the essential nutrients and electrolytes upon which we depend every minute of the day. We also introduce the concept of "steady state" conditions, which is critical to many aspects of physiology.

Chapter 2 begins an exploration of the compartments in the body that contain water, which makes up approximately 60% of our total body weight. Within this context, you will learn about the forces (osmotic and Starling forces) that control movement of water between the compartments. This chapter is an absolutely critical foundation for much of what will follow and we strongly urge you to spend as much time as is necessary to master these concepts.

Chapter 3 focuses on functional anatomy, linking the essential elements of the structure of the kidney, its vasculature and urinary collecting system to their physiological roles. In Chapter 4, we address the glomerulus, the portion of the kidney responsible for filtering 180 L of fluid each day from the blood. We will examine in detail the factors that regulate filtration and the mechanisms used by the body to preserve filtration even in the face of low blood pressure.

Since the human body deals with the problem of eliminating toxic metabolites, excess water, and electrolytes by essentially "filtering everything," it must then have a system to reabsorb selectively the water, glucose, and electrolytes that we must have to survive. Chapter 5 takes us on a journey through the renal tubule and examines the transporters essential for this work and the unique roles of each of the portions of the tubule.

Chapter 6 focuses specifically on the kidney's handling of sodium and water. Here you will be introduced to a number of hormones that are critical for helping us maintain our blood pressure and flow of blood to vital organs while simultaneously providing mechanisms to avoid flooding our lungs with excess fluid. In Chapters 7 and 8, we continue to examine how the body regulates water, with particular attention to the physiological principles underlying the ability to concentrate urine, without which we would have great difficulty surviving as land animals.

Every day, the human body makes thousands of millimoles of acid as a consequence of the metabolism of carbohydrates, protein, and fat. Much of the acid (carbonic acid) is excreted by the respiratory system in the form of carbon dioxide, but the kidney must eliminate approximately 70 meq of non-carbonic acid each day. Chapters 9 and 10 address the challenges of acid–base balance posed by normal metabolism and by common conditions such as vomiting, diarrhea, and dehydration.

Finally, in Chapter 11, we integrate many of the concepts you will learn throughout the book as you examine how the kidney responds to the difficulties encountered by a marathon runner. For those interested in a detailed look at the respiratory and cardiovascular systems during exercise so you can put together a complete picture of the physiology of exercise, we refer you to Chapter 9 of the first book in the series, *Respiratory Physiology: A Clinical Approach*. In that chapter, we examine exercise by taking an integrated approach to the adaptive responses of both the respiratory and cardiovascular systems.

Throughout this book we draw heavily upon clinical examples to emphasize concepts and to highlight how an understanding of normal physiological principles will help you understand pathological states. For the beginning student, you will see the relevance of the material presented. For the advanced student or resident, these examples will help you understand the signs and symptoms of your patients and the rationale for therapeutic interventions.

Pedagogy

The following teaching elements are common to all of the books in the *Integrated Physiology Series*.

- **Chapter Outline**. The outline at the beginning of each chapter gives a preview of the chapter and is a useful study aid.
- **Learning Objectives**. Each chapter starts with a short list of learning objectives. These objectives are intended to help you focus on the most critical concepts and physiological principles that will be presented in the chapter.
- **Text**. The text is written in a conversational style that is intended to recreate the sense of participating in an interactive lecture. Questions are posed periodically to offer you opportunities to reflect on information presented and to try your hand at synthesizing and applying your knowledge to novel situations.
- **Topic Headings**. Topic headings are used to delineate key concepts. Sections are arranged to present the material in easily digestible quantities as you move from simple to more complex physiology.
- **Boldfacing**. Key terms are boldfaced upon their first appearance in a chapter. Definitions for all boldfaced terms are found in the glossary.
- **Thought Questions**. Interposed within the text are *thought questions* that are designed to challenge you to use the material just presented in the text in a novel fashion. Many of these are posed in a clinical context to demonstrate the clinical relevance of the material as well.
- **Editor's Integration**. Periodically in the text you will notice a box that makes a link between concepts, as applied to one organ system, with the same or very similar concepts in another organ system. This information will help reinforce knowledge in both areas and illustrate further the ways in which physiology can be integrated.
- **Illustrations and Animated Figures**. The figures have been developed to demonstrate the relationship between physiological variables, to illustrate key concepts, and to integrate a number of principles enumerated in the text. To further help you integrate these principles, we offer interactive learning tools (called 'Animated Figures' in the text) that will provide you with an opportunity to view a physiological principle in motion or to manipulate variables and see the physiological consequences of the changes. These animations and computer simulations permit the reader to work with the concepts and to apply them in a range of circumstances. As you use these interactive animations,

proceeding through them at your own pace, our hope is that you will gain a deeper, more intuitive, understanding of the physiological principles discussed in each chapter.

- **'Putting It Together' Section.** At the end of each chapter is a clinical case presentation that poses questions about physical findings, laboratory values, or diagnostic and therapeutic issues that can be answered with the physiological information presented in the chapter. These cases are designed to integrate material, to demonstrate the clinical relevance of the physiology, and to provide you with an opportunity to test yourself by applying what you have just learned in a new situation.
- **Review Questions and Answers.** You can use the review questions at the end of each chapter to test whether you have mastered the material. For medical students, the USMLE-type questions should help you prepare for the Step 1 examination. Answers to the questions are presented at the end of the book, and include explanations that delineate why the choices are correct or incorrect.
- **Index.** A complete index allows you to easily find material in the text.

In the final analysis, most people study physiology because it offers great insights into the workings of the human body. We have organized and presented the material in this book in a way that we hope will allow you to achieve your individual goals while having some fun with a subject that continues to challenge and intrigue us.

Richard M. Schwartzstein, MD
Ellen and Melvin Gordon Professor of Medicine and Medical Education
Director, Harvard Medical School Academy
Vice President for Education and Director, Carl J. Shapiro Institute for Education
Beth Israel Deaconess Medical Center
Boston, MA
Editor, *The Integrated Physiology Series*

Acknowledgments

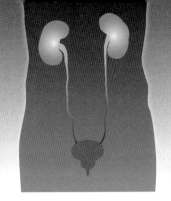

This project draws from the collective wisdom of many wonderful teachers who have inspired me (JD) along my path: Orson Moe, MD, whose thoughtful approaches to renal physiology stimulated my interest in nephrology as a medical student; Drs. Robert S. Brown and Franklin H. Epstein, who deepened my understanding of the field; and Dr. Stewart H. Lecker, mentor, colleague, and friend, who continues to provide support and insight. In addition, much of this work was completed as part of the Rabkin Fellowship in Medical Education within the Shapiro Institute for Education and Research at Harvard Medical School and Beth Israel Deaconess Medical Center under the outstanding guidance and tutelage of Dr. Christopher Smith and Lori Newman. The project would not have been possible without the wisdom of my fellow authors, Mark Zeidel and Michael Parker, and the masterful editorial skills of Rich Schwartzstein. Finally, a special appreciation to my wife and best friend, Emma, and to our son Quin.

I (MJP) am grateful to those who have inspired and supported me in my chosen path of teaching, writing, and creating interactive tools to help students visualize and understand difficult concepts in medicine. John Halamka, MD, has been a steadfast supporter of the development of animations and simulations in the Harvard curriculum, and his encouragement has been truly appreciated. For me, Rich Schwartzstein's influence extends beyond his role as an editor; our collaboration is a thread that has run through much of my career in medicine and teaching, and I look forward to more enjoyable hours working together. Liz Allison's guidance in navigating the publishing process has been invaluable throughout our work on the physiology series. I thank my co-authors John and Mark for spirited discussions of renal concepts; I think we all learned something new in the process. I would also like to warmly express gratitude to Tomas Berl, MD, for his supportive encouragement of my career and for furthering my love of renal physiology through his teaching.

Contents

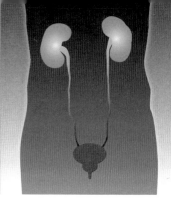

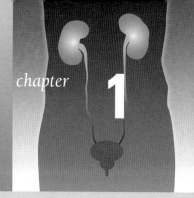

Getting Started

The Approach to Renal Physiology

CHAPTER OUTLINE

LEARNING OBJECTIVES

By the end of this chapter, you should be able to:

- **describe the basic functions of the renal system.**
- **define the concept of clearance and its relationship to body fluid.**
- **identify the role of the renal tubule in reclaiming fluid filtered by the kidney.**
- **describe the kidney's role in maintaining body homeostasis.**

Introduction

Every minute of every day, your body is faced with a number of challenges to maintain homeostasis. The metabolic processes necessary to keep us alive require fuel and result in the production of chemical waste products and acids. The pH of the blood and other bodily fluids that exist within and outside of cells must be carefully regulated to allow enzymatic reactions to proceed efficiently. Water and the concentration of key electrolytes, such as sodium and potassium, must be monitored and adjusted to maintain appropriate blood pressure and cellular function. The kidneys are vital organs that play a critical role to ensure that the body is able to successfully meet these challenges. When renal function is damaged, these processes are altered, homeostasis is disrupted and death may result.

Let us start with a simple example to give you a sense of magnitude of the job that the kidneys perform. You purchase a highly specialized fish, known to produce 10 particles of waste per hour. This fish survives well in the captivity of a fish tank, as long as the concentration of its own waste in the tank does not get above 2 particles/L. The shop owner

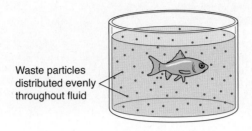

Waste particles distributed evenly throughout fluid

FIGURE 1-1 Waste accumulation in the tank. The fish is constantly producing waste. Waste distributes across all the fluid within the tank, and because there is no method for excretion, its concentration in the fluid continuously increases.

provides you with a special tank alarm that warns when the water waste concentration reaches 2 particles/L.

You bring the fish home from the fish store at 10 AM one morning, place him in a fresh 10-L tank, and marvel at your new purchase. Not thinking about waste removal for the moment, you are suddenly awakened from your morning nap at 12 noon by the tank's alarm system; the waste concentration has reached 2 particles/L. Since the fish makes 10 particles/hr and it has been in the 10-L tank for 2 hours, you are not really surprised (see *Figure 1-1*).

To correct the problem, you decide to try to strain the water in order to remove the waste material. A standard strainer with macroscopic holes does not work; the waste particles are too small to be caught within the strainer and pass right through. Your next idea is to use a particle filter with much smaller holes. You make a hole at the tank's base, place the filter in the hole, and drain the fluid into a fresh tank. The particulate matter remains within the original tank, and the fish is then placed into the freshly cleaned fluid (see *Figure 1-2*).

Because the fish is constantly making waste, however, the concentration within the tank begins to increase, and soon you will need to clean the tank fluid again. You calculate that you will need to clear the whole tank 12 times per day, exchanging 120 L of fluid per day! The fish probably will not tolerate being moved from one tank to another every 2 hr. In addition, you realize that each time you drain the tank, the fish's food also gets removed, and unless you constantly replace the food, the fish will starve.

Thinking further, you realize that you need a system that allows continuous cleaning of the tank's fluid while leaving the fish within the tank. The process must also preferentially eliminate waste products, but retain food products. As seen in *Figure 1-3*, you conceptualize two scenarios that allow continuous clearing of the tank.

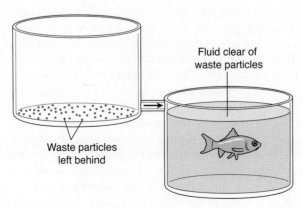

Fluid clear of waste particles

Waste particles left behind

FIGURE 1-2 Cleaning the tank fluid. By draining the waste-filled fluid through a specialized filter, cleaned fluid can be collected into a new tank, and the waste will accumulate at the tank's base. The fish will obviously need to be moved to the fresh tank.

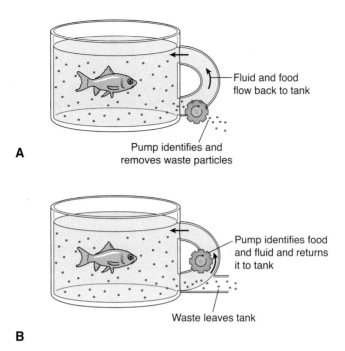

FIGURE 1-3 Continuous cleaning of tank fluid. In an idealized system, tank fluid can pass through a special-ized filter, allowing the removal of certain waste products but not affecting food particles, and then be continuously returned to the original tank. In this way, the fish does not need to be moved from tank to tank; instead, there is a continuous cleaning of the original tank. In **(A)**, this is achieved by allowing constant recycling of fluid through a tube, with a specialized pump selecting the waste products for elimination. Of course, the pump must somehow be able to recognize all types of waste products. For example, if the fish eats something unusual and toxic, the pump might not recognize the substance as waste, and thus, would not choose to excrete it, leading to continuous toxin accumulation. In **(B)**, the default is excretion. Here, tank fluid is destined for excretion. The pump's role is to reclaim necessary par-ticles (food) and water. Obviously, however, if the pump breaks, the tank will quickly be emptied of fluid!

In *Figure 1-3A*, a tube is placed into the side of the tank allowing fluid to continuously re-circulate. A pump is placed in the tube that identifies and removes particles of waste. In *Figure 1-3B*, a tube allows drainage of the waste-filled fluid. The pump, instead of remov-ing waste particles, must focus on, identify, and reclaim drained water and needed particles (such as food); it allows the waste to continue along the elimination tube. In the first sce-nario, waste is selectively filtered and removed from the container. In the second example, everything leaves the container, and clean water and essential particles are reclaimed and put back into the container. Although both scenarios will be able to continuously recycle the tank's fluid, each has certain advantages and disadvantages.

In *Figure 1-3A*, if the pump breaks down, the waste particles will not be excreted. In addition, the pump must recognize every type of waste product that the fish either con-sumes or creates. In *Figure 1-3B*, the default position is waste excretion; i.e., if the pump breaks down, the tank fluid (water and food) will not be reclaimed, and everything will be excreted. Thus, *Figure 1-3B* is perhaps a more efficient/hardy system for removing waste, but it requires a pump that can reclaim all types of needed particles (food), and must be avid in reclaiming water, otherwise, the tank will quickly be emptied.

In many ways, the simple fish tank example replicates what occurs in our body. Through cellular metabolism, we are constantly making waste, which diffuses throughout our body fluid (equivalent to the tank). This fluid flows through the kidneys many times per day and, in a process that is somewhere between *Figure 1-3B* and *1-3A*, there is some selective filtration (based on the charge and size of particles—large particles are not removed from the blood) but there is a need to reclaim many small essential particles and water that are filtered with the waste. Most of the filtered fluid is returned to our body.

The kidneys clear our waste products by passing fluid through a filter, which is located anatomically in the **glomerulus**. This filtered fluid is then largely reclaimed by the portion of the **nephron** known as the **renal tubule**; electrolytes, minerals, and other critical particles are reabsorbed while leaving waste and excess fluid for excretion. By altering both the amount and the composition of what is reclaimed, the kidney determines the body's net balance, which can be defined as follows:

Net balance = (amount ingested + amount created) − amount eliminated

Note: For some substances, there is no creation of the material within the body and net balance reflects only the amount ingested minus the amount eliminated.

The kidney has the ability to determine water and electrolyte balance, while simultaneously assuring the removal of our body's waste. In response to important stimuli from elsewhere in the body, the kidney is able to regulate the absorption process to account for changes in the amount of a substance ingested or produced by the individual. Hormones from the brain, heart, adrenal gland, and other organs, which are constantly monitoring the internal state of the body, regulate this process. Ultimately, in a beautifully orchestrated and coordinated manner, the combination of stimuli from these organs and the kidney's ability to respond to these stimuli enable our bodies to maintain net balance of water and particles. Thus, even on days when we ingest or lose large amounts of water, sodium, potassium, or other electrolytes, our kidneys excrete just enough to maintain a **steady state** (in steady state conditions, we eliminate as much of a substance as we ingest and produce; the result is that the concentration of that substance in the body remains constant).

In this chapter, we will explore how the organization of the renal system supports these important functions, and give you an overview of how this book is designed to help you develop a deep understanding of renal physiology.

Excreting the Body's Waste

In the example above, the fish constantly produces waste. We do too. Our diet consists of protein, which is broken down to amino acids and is used to build tissues throughout our bodies. The breakdown of these amino acids, either directly from the dietary source or from catabolism of our tissue sources, leads to the production of nitrogenous waste, in the form of **urea**. In addition, the process of cell metabolism leads to various other waste products as well as acids (such as sulfuric and phosphoric acids). If these waste products were to accumulate, they would be toxic to the body. Thus, their excretion must be efficient and must occur continuously.

Just as the fish's waste particles distribute throughout all the water in the tank, our waste distributes throughout all the water in our body. Urea, as an uncharged particle, can pass freely across most cell membranes, and its **volume of distribution**, i.e., the amount of fluid in the body into which a substance disseminates, is equal to our **total body water**. Total body water includes water found inside and outside of cells. Since about 40% of our body weight is made up of non-aqueous substances, such as bone, 60% of our body weight is water. Women's bodies, which typically have a higher proportion of fat than men for any given weight, tend to have slightly less water than men. Nevertheless, the average 70-kg person consists of approximately 42 kilograms or liters of water. Chapter 2 will be dedicated to describing the fluid compartments within our bodies.

On average, a volume equal to our total body water is cleaned of waste four times daily. In other words, our body's water is filtered through our kidney approximately four times a day. For a 70-kg person, this equates to 180 L of filtrate passed through his/her kidneys! Since only a fraction of the blood that perfuses the kidney is filtered, i.e., leaves the vascular space and enters the renal tubule, the **renal blood flow** is actually much greater than this. Approximately 20% of the body's cardiac output, or 1 L of blood per minute, is sent to the kidney under resting (non-exercise) conditions; this amounts to 1,440 L daily, which far exceeds the blood flow needed to meet the metabolic needs of the kidney. Under conditions of significant loss of body fluids or low blood pressure, or in response to significant changes in the volume of filtrate in the renal tubule, the blood flow and/or pressure within the glomerular capillaries may be altered, which allows the body to regulate filtration. Chapter 3 will focus on the anatomic structures that support these functions.

As noted above, 180 L of fluid are filtered across the renal capillaries in the glomerulus and exit the vasculature into the renal tubules. Blood cells and large molecules such as proteins do not pass across the walls of the glomerular capillaries. This high capacity system, which is able to handle these large volumes of fluid, allows for the constant clearance of waste products, and keeps our body's urea levels nice and low. Chapter 4 will be dedicated to delineating how our body excretes waste.

> **?** **THOUGHT QUESTION 1-1** Two men undergo specific testing to quantify exactly how much fluid is filtered through their kidneys per day. Each is found to have a normal glomerular filtration rate of 125 mL/min, or 180 L/day. The first man weighs 80 kg; the second is larger at 120 kg. How many times a day is the total body water in each man cleared of waste?

Reclaiming Filtered Fluid

Although this system of filtering large quantities of fluid across the renal capillaries into the tubules provides an efficient mechanism for clearing the body's waste, it creates an obvious challenge for the body. Unless that filtered fluid (and essential electrolytes and other small molecules contained therein) is immediately and continuously returned to the body, we would die from massive fluid loss and/or electrolyte depletion. Indeed, our kidneys are constantly returning filtered fluid and small molecules to the bloodstream. This reclamation process occurs via the system of renal tubules. Of the 180 L filtered daily through the glomeruli, 178 L are reclaimed by the tubules under typical conditions. In this manner, the body recaptures particles—such as sodium, potassium, and other electrolytes—as well as water. Clearly, this is a high flow system in both directions!

As filtrate passes across the endothelium of the capillary loops into the lumen of the tubule, called the **urinary space**, it has actually passed to the "outside" of the body (there is a continuous path from the renal tubule to the collecting system of the kidney, to the ureters, which empty into the bladder, and then to the urethra and the outside world). The tubules, like skin, provide a barrier between the "outside" urinary space and the "inside" renal interstitium. Like skin, the tubules are composed of epithelial cells. These are not inherently permeable to water and electrolytes, and thus, mechanisms of transportation, either through or between these epithelial cells, are needed to facilitate filtrate reclamation. Furthermore, as we will discuss in a moment, these mechanisms must be subject to regulation so that the body can determine how much water, electrolytes, and other filtered molecules will be recaptured, depending on the internal and external environment of the body.

There are other important examples of structures "within" our body that, like the urinary space, actually represent extensions of the outside world. The respiratory tract, from the nasal and oral openings down to the alveoli, and the gastrointestinal tract, from the mouth to the anus, consist of a tube, the lumen of which is separated from the *real* "inside" of the body by a relatively impermeable epithelial lining, which must protect the body from excessive fluid losses and the movement of infectious agents into the bloodstream.

We will learn more about the unique structure of the renal tubule in Chapter 2, and about the importance of cell membrane proteins as facilitators for tubular reclamation in Chapter 5.

Fine-Tuning the Filtrate

Finally, the third important function of the renal system is to determine the exact amounts of particles and water it chooses to retain rather than excrete. In the fish tank example, we could postulate that such a filter might "sense" how much food or nutrients had been added to the tank water and alter its retention or excretion of food in order to maintain a food homeostasis. If the system were successful, the tank would be protected from excess food as well as from deficiency. At times of overfeeding, the filter would choose not to reabsorb filtered nutrient particles, and thereby excrete more. At times of underfeeding, the filter would choose to reabsorb just about every nutrient particle and, thus, protect the fish from starvation.

In order for the filter to adjust its function to prevent unnecessary loss of nutrients in the waste, it would have to meet three requirements. First, it must be able to sense the overall food level within the tank. Second, the sensing mechanism must have a way to communicate to the filter, that is, the system must have an **effector mechanism**, which allows it to make changes to sustain the internal balance of the body. Finally, in response to the sensor's input to the filter, the filter must have the ability to alter the way in which it manages the nutrient particles.

The kidney uses a combination of selective filtering at the level of the glomerulus and selective reabsorption at the level of the renal tubule to achieve homeostasis with respect to water and electrolytes. For instance, if we eat too much potassium one day, the renal system will excrete more potassium so that our serum levels remain normal. If we eat a lot of sodium, the renal system puts out more sodium. Conversely, if we drink very little water, the renal system is able to respond by making very concentrated urine, i.e., it retains as much water as possible. In these ways, the renal system establishes and maintains balance despite a wide array of dietary and metabolic challenges.

?

THOUGHT QUESTION 1-2 We have described a system in which the fluid is filtered in a fairly unselective manner only to be selectively reclaimed in the tubule. Why did the body evolve in this manner as opposed to developing the capacity to filter selectively in the first place, thereby avoiding the need to reabsorb or reclaim water and electrolytes in the renal tubule? What advantages can you imagine that would favor the evolution of this model?

The processes that enable our body to maintain homeostasis are complex. The body must have mechanisms to sense changes in body composition. In addition, there must be effector pathways that the body can stimulate to direct the kidney to modify its excretion of particular substances. The majority of this book, Chapters 5 to 10, is dedicated to describing how this is accomplished for a variety of important substances. Chapter 5 includes a section on the handling of potassium. Chapter 6 focuses on sodium regulation, Chapters 7 and 8 address how the body regulates water, and Chapters 9 and 10 discuss the mechanisms by which we maintain a normal pH in the body (acid–base balance). All of these chapters will focus on a theme—homeostasis—and will describe the mechanisms by which the kidney contributes to sustaining balance within the body. Finally, in Chapter 11, we provide you with a clinical example that will challenge you to integrate and apply many of the concepts you will be learning throughout the book.

THE KEYS TO THE VAULT: HELPING YOU MASTER THE MATERIAL

Renal physiology is not complex. In fact, despite its reputation, it is simple, straightforward, and functions in a beautifully integrated and orchestrated manner. The key to learning nephrology is to understand each and every concept within a framework that helps you understand how things fit together. Simple memorization of terms and rules may help you pass the test, but it will do nothing to help you learn how the kidney works.

Most importantly, gaining a thorough and complete understanding of the basic principles is critical. In order to move forward in your comprehension, you must master the basics. Proceeding one step at a time, while building on the basics and not taking any concepts for granted, is key.

In order to help you master the basics, we have provided a number of learning tools throughout all the chapters. These will reinforce your understanding of the concepts, and allow you to think like a renal physiologist. No matter what type of practitioner you ultimately become, you will always need to understand renal physiology. We hope that the concepts that you learn in this book will stay with you throughout your career. Take the time and effort to learn them thoroughly now, as the rewards will be rich. Make the concepts your own.

Animated Figures: To give you a chance to work on the concepts developed in the text, you will be able to employ a variety of computer based animations and simulations. These Animated Figures can be accessed via a website with the password provided at the front of the book. The interactive nature of these animations and simulations will allow you to manipulate different aspects of the physiology and watch how changes produce different results. By altering the parameters, and by attempting to predict the consequences of these changes, you can test your understanding of the principles at hand. The first animation is located at the end of this chapter under the section "Putting It Together" (see below).

Thought Questions: Throughout the chapters, Thought Questions are posed (you should have seen two of these earlier in this chapter). These often place the concepts into a clinical context, and challenge you to think about issues from a different perspective. The thought questions are strategically placed to reinforce the concepts in the accompanying text. If you are having trouble answering a thought question, it may be an indication that you did not thoroughly understand the concepts in the text that preceded the question; this is an opportunity to go back and review the material to see where you may have gone off track.

Putting It Together and Review Questions: At the end of each chapter, there will be a clinical vignette, titled "Putting it Together." This section will integrate many of the concepts learned within the previous chapter. In addition, review questions, accompanied by answers (found in an appendix at the end of the book) will allow additional self-assessment. Finally, a glossary of terms is included within the index to help facilitate your learning of the vocabulary of renal physiology.

PUTTING IT TOGETHER

While reading this first chapter, you become hungry and decide to eat a hamburger and fries, and you wash it down with a large glass of orange juice. Your body uses these foodstuffs as energy. As part of the process of digestion, the amino acids of the hamburger become nitrogenous waste, which are potentially toxic when in large concentrations in the blood. The fries are full of salt, and the orange juice has lots of potassium (which can be lethal if its levels accumulate).

Despite this ingestion of large amounts of potentially toxic particles, as well as 2.2 lbs of water, your body's composition of these substances barely changes. How is this body homeostasis maintained?

Using Animated Figure 1-1 (Homeostasis), initiate ingestion of the hamburger, fries, and beverage meal. Notice how the body handles each component of the meal such that homeostasis is maintained. The body's sensors (more on these sensors in later chapters), shown lighting up in the animation, indirectly detect the ingestion of substances such as sodium and water and trigger effector mechanisms that alter the kidney's reabsorption or excretion of those substances. You can observe the changes in the colored reabsorption/excretion arrows as the components of the meal make their way through the body.

The ability to maintain balance of the body's composition is the defining function of the kidneys. Despite a wide variety of dietary and environmental influences, the kidneys are able to excrete just the right amount of water, electrolytes, and metabolic byproducts to maintain a "steady state." The amount excreted is affected by many factors. If you happen to read this book while lying on a hot beach in Mexico, you will likely be losing lots of water via sweat. Thus, your kidneys will know to make concentrated urine by reabsorbing filtered water from the tubule. If you happen to be a person who likes to be well hydrated, and so you have consumed many glasses of water in the last few hours, your kidneys will know to rid your body of excess water. Similarly, after eating all that salt in the hamburger and fries, the kidney will excrete excess sodium. Rest assured, after such a meal, you would soon feel the urge to urinate, a sign that your kidneys are doing the work of body homeostasis. Try out these scenarios (sweating, drinking a lot of fluid, or eating a sodium-rich meal) using Animated Figure 1-1 and see how the body reacts.

The concept of "steady state" describes the balance between net intake, predominantly through dietary ingestion plus, for some substances, internal production of the substance, and net loss, through a variety of pathways including sweat, respiration, gastrointestinal, and renal mechanisms. Despite wide fluctuations in both intake and loss, the body is able to maintain an appropriate net balance. By integrating various stimuli and by altering the kidney's avidity for water and electrolytes, the levels of total body fluid and the composition of that fluid are held constant.

Summary Points

- Our body is constantly making waste products, which are toxic to the body if they accumulate in high concentrations.
- The kidneys allow continuous excretion of metabolic waste, preventing toxicity.
- Most waste products distribute across all the water in the body.
- A volume of water equal to total body water is filtered through the kidney across capillaries in the glomeruli several times per day.
- Filtered water and molecules pass out of the body into the renal tubules, from which they are then almost completely reabsorbed.
- Waste products generally remain within the tubule and are eventually excreted in the urine.
- The process of reclamation of water, electrolytes, and nutrients by the tubules is critical if the body is to maintain homeostatic conditions.
- Within the renal tubule, the kidneys can "fine tune" the filtrate, deciding exactly how much water and filtered molecules should be reabsorbed or eliminated in the urine; to a lesser degree, the kidneys can adjust the blood flow and pressure within the glomerular capillaries, thereby providing some regulation of filtration.
- The regulatory capacity of the kidneys governs fluid and particle balance within the body, despite a wide variety of environmental factors that may challenge homeostasis.
- There are sensing mechanisms throughout the body that allow us to detect changes in fluid and particle levels within the body.
- These sensing mechanisms set in motion processes that stimulate the kidney to either excrete or retain substances.
- At times of deficiency, the kidneys are avid (reabsorb most of what is filtered); at times of excess, the kidneys excrete (allow filtered water and molecules to be eliminated in the urine).

Answers TO THOUGHT QUESTIONS

1-1. The kidneys of both men have the same filtration rate of 180 L/day. The smaller man, weighing 80 kg, has a total body water of about 48 kg. Thus, his total body water filters through the kidneys nearly 3.75 times daily. Such a constant recycling of his body water is important, since waste is constantly being produced by the body, and thus, must be constantly excreted.

The larger man's total body water is about 72 kg. It is filtered 2.5 times per day. Thus, although both men have the exact same level of renal function (i.e., they filter the same number of milliliters of blood per minute), their volume of distribution of waste differs; consequently, the relative efficiency at clearing body waste differs as well. We shall learn more about this concept in Chapter 4.

1-2. First, we should clarify what we mean by "unselective filtration" in this thought question. As we will learn in future chapters, larger particles, such as cells and proteins, are not filtered. Water and smaller particles, such as urea and electrolytes, however, are freely filtered. Thus, renal filtration is indeed selective. However, the conceptual question remains, why not filter only the waste products (i.e., be very selective)?

The answer relies on the efficiency of the system. In the process of unselective filtration of water and small particles, the rate of flow across the glomerulus multiplied by the concentration of particles within that fluid determines the amount filtered. So, increasing concentration within body fluid will automatically lead to increasing filtration. This is useful for us; if our bodies were to make more waste than usual (for instance, after eating a large steak, which has a high protein content) and our serum urea levels rise, our kidneys are easily able to filter out this additional load. If we relied primarily on selective filtration, we would need a process to identify and then transport the large number of molecules associated with the increasing urea concentration. This would require time and energy and, overall, would make the system less efficient.

Review Questions

DIRECTIONS: *Each of the numbered items or incomplete statements in this section is followed by answers or by completions of the statement. Select the ONE lettered answer or completion that is BEST in each case.*

1. A 20-year-old college athlete has been in training for several months. As part of his regimen, he drinks milkshakes into which he adds protein supplements. The body metabolizes the protein to make muscle and in the process produces urea. You predict:

    A. The kidney will filter more urea.
    B. The kidney will filter less urea.
    C. There will be increased absorption of urea from the renal tubule.
    D. The amount of urea in the urine will decrease.

2. Two Olympic marathoners are training together on a hot, summer afternoon. They decide to run for 15 miles today. Bob has taken salt tablets during the run whereas John has not. Assuming the two athletes are the same size and have the same total body water at the beginning of the run, and that both sweat the same amount and drink the same amount of water during the run, you predict:

    A. John will filter more Na via his glomerulus than Bob.
    B. Bob will filter more Na via his glomerulus than John.
    C. They will filter the same amount of Na.
    D. John will reabsorb more Na than Bob.

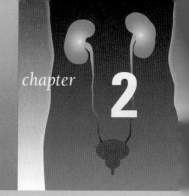

The Body's Compartments
The Distribution of Fluid

LEARNING OBJECTIVES

By the end of this chapter, you should be able to:

- **describe the body's fluid compartments.**
- **define the unique membrane characteristics separating each compartment.**
- **delineate the forces that determine the size of each compartment.**
- **define the general processes by which water and particles cross barriers between compartments.**
- **determine how ingestion of salt and water change the size and/or composition of the body's fluid compartments.**
- **characterize the unique characteristics of the kidney that allow the movement of particles to be separated from the movement of water.**

Introduction

Our bodies are primarily composed of water; approximately 60% of our total body weight is attributable to water. Of course, there are important substances within that water, including cells, proteins, and minerals. This body fluid, composed of water and all the substances within it, circulates within the body continuously among three major compartments: the **intracellular space (IC)**, the **intravascular space (IV)** (within arteries, veins, and capillaries), and the **interstitial space (IT)** (outside of the cell and outside of the vasculature). These compartments are defined by two important barriers: the cell membrane,

Total Body Water

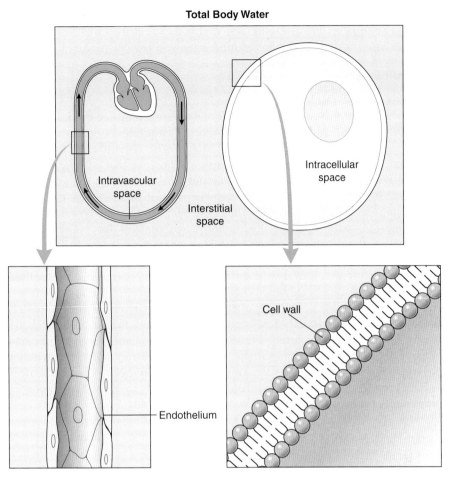

FIGURE 2-1 **The major fluid compartments in the body.** The intravascular space is defined by the endothelial layer of the blood vessels. The intracellular space is defined by the cell membrane. The interstitial space surrounds these two compartments.

which separates the IC from the interstitium, and the thin layer of endothelial cells, which lines blood vessels and divides the IV from the surrounding interstitium. This is illustrated in *Figure 2-1*.

Driven by important physiologic forces, body fluid moves both within and across these compartments. For example, the contractions of the heart muscle pump intravascular fluid around and around the vasculature. Important electrical and chemical forces move charged particles across cell membranes; this movement generates osmotic forces that lead to shifts in water between compartments. Yet, there are important differences between the barriers that ultimately determine just how much fluid will remain in each body compartment. Knowledge of the properties of the cell membrane and the endothelial lining of the vasculature is essential to understanding how body fluid is distributed across our body compartments. Barrier permeability, and the driving forces across these barriers, will be the focus of this chapter; with this information in hand, we can understand exactly what determines the size of our body compartments.

Because of the critical role of the kidney in the body's regulation of fluid and electrolytes, it is important that you comprehend the basic principles that govern movement of water and solutes within the body. While many of the principles discussed in this chapter will be a review of concepts you first encountered in chemistry and cell biology courses, you must be sufficiently facile with them that you can calculate changes in body composition with ease, a skill that will be required when you have responsibility for patients.

THE THREE BODY COMPARTMENTS

As we just noted, 60% of our total body weight is attributable to water. Of that body water, approximately two-thirds lie within the cells. Of the remaining one-third, approximately two-thirds are within the interstitium, and one-third is within the IV. So, for a 70-kg person, his or her **total body water (TBW)** is about 42 kg, or 42 L. Twenty-eight liters are within the cells, and 14 L are in the **extracellular space**. Thus, for that a 70-kg individual, about 9.5 L of water are within the interstitium and 4.5 L are within the IV. Of course, these are gross estimations, with wide variations between men and women; part of the variation among individuals is because of the percentage of their body weight comprising fat versus muscle—fat is relatively hydrophobic and contains less water than lean tissue. Nevertheless, these estimations can be used to provide some clue as to how much fluid can be found within each compartment.

The fluid within each compartment has a special function. Intravascular fluid, the liquid part of blood, carries red blood cells and nutrient molecules that support metabolism, and removes the waste byproducts of cellular activity. Driven by the pumping heart, this fluid circulates approximately 1,500 times daily to ensure that aerobic metabolism is sustained. In addition, the volume of fluid within the vasculature is one of the major determinants of blood pressure; for example, if you sever an artery and start bleeding profusely, the volume of fluid within the vascular space declines and your blood pressure will begin to fall. The IT, separating the vast majority of our cells from the IV, is a conduit for the movement of nutrients to cells and waste away from cells. Finally, the intracellular fluid supports cell function, and is a major factor in determining cell size.

Our survival depends on moving TBW, and the solutes it contain, effectively among these body compartments. Homeostasis also requires that our body's physiological systems regulate the size of each of these compartments. If the vascular compartment becomes overly filled with fluid, blood pressure will rise; if the volume in the vascular compartment falls too low, hypotension or shock may occur, and the body may be unable to perfuse vital organs. If fluid accumulates excessively in the IT, **edema** develops. Accumulation of fluid within brain cells, leading to cellular swelling within a rigid skull, can lead to severe neurological consequences, including seizure, coma, and death. Thus, appropriate regulation of the movement of fluid within these compartments is critical to life.

THE IMPORTANCE OF MEMBRANE PERMEABILITY

The two barriers that define the body compartments are the cell membrane and the endothelial lining of the vasculature. These barriers are entirely different biological entities. The cell membrane is a component of a single cell; in contrast, the endothelium is composed of millions of cells joined together by intercellular junctions. It is not surprising that the permeability of these two barriers is very different. We shall describe these barriers in detail in a moment; first, let us review why the presence of barriers with differing permeability is critical to the determination of compartment size and composition.

We will begin the discussion with a few simple physics concepts and an experiment. As seen in *Figure* 2-2A, we begin with a large tank of fluid separated by a totally permeable membrane. By totally permeable, we mean that both water and particles can cross freely. If you were to add 10 particles to one side of the membrane, random movement of the particles would eventually lead to the equal distribution of particles to each side; at equilibrium, there are five particles on each side of the membrane.

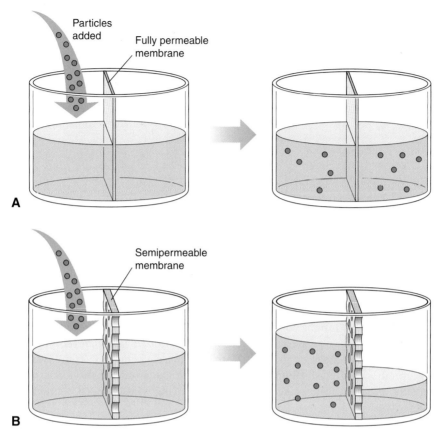

A

B

FIGURE 2-2 Osmotic forces. The characteristics of the membrane separating two fluid compartments determine how the addition of particles and water affect the respective compartments. In **(A)**, the membrane is fully permeable. Thus, the added particles diffuse across the barrier and occupy both compartments, the concentration of both increase, and the level of the water on each side does not change. In **(B)**, the membrane is semipermeable, so that fluid can cross, but particles, cannot. Now the addition of particles leads to changes in the level of water on each side.

   Use Animated Figure 2-1 (Membrane Permeability) to choose a totally permeable membrane and add 10 particles to the tank. Observe how over time, particle movement leads to an average of five particles on each side.

You now change the character of the membrane dividing the tank, making it semipermeable; water, but not particles, can cross. This time addition of 10 particles to one side would have a different effect. The added particles, restricted to one side of the membrane, would cause water to move towards the particle-laden side, as illustrated in *Figure 2-2B*. The net effect would be an increase of volume of fluid on one side of the membrane, with a loss of fluid on the other side.

Now choose the semipermeable membrane in Animated Figure 2-1, and try the experiment by adding 10 particles to the tank. You can observe how, in this case, the movement of water leads to an increase in volume on the side of the tank that contains the particles.

Depending on the type of membrane, the addition of particles can have vastly different effects. The addition of particles to a tank divided by a fully permeable membrane leads to an increased particle concentration shared equally across the total tank fluid, with no change in fluid volume on either side; in contrast, the addition of particles to a tank

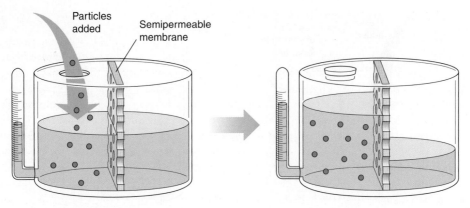

FIGURE 2-3 Measuring osmotic pressure. The ability of particles to pull fluid across a semipermeable membrane is measured by the height of the water column that rises against atmospheric pressure.

divided by a semipermeable membrane leads to water movement from one side to the other, with consequent changes in volume.

The movement of water across a semipermeable membrane, what we call **osmosis**, is due to the greater number of water-to-membrane collisions on the side of the membrane with pure water as compared to the side with a mixture of water and solute. Water is moving along its concentration gradient from a higher concentration (pure water) to a lower concentration (water + solute). To measure the magnitude of the force, or the osmotic pressure, it is best to imagine the process occurring within closed containers with fixed walls.

In *Figure 2-3*, a closed tank is separated into two compartments by a semipermeable membrane, and has a small opening at its base. The addition of particles to side A will induce water movement into compartment A. As the height of water rises, the hydrostatic pressure near the bottom of the tank on that side rises (assessed by the height of the column of water in the adjacent tube). This pressure rises until the force exerted by the height of the water (which would tend to move water to the other, less deep, side of the membrane) is equal and opposite to the osmotic force exerted by the different concentrations of water on either side of the membrane. At that point, the hydrostatic pressure in compartment A is such that there is no net movement of water across the membrane; the tank has reached equilibrium.

To determine the osmotic pressure of the solution, you can measure the hydrostatic pressure in compartment A, i.e., assess the height of the column of water. The **osmotic pressure** of a solution is defined to be equivalent to the hydrostatic pressure required to counter the movement of water molecules across the membrane. A perhaps more intuitive, albeit less precise, way of thinking about osmotic pressure is as the "pulling" force of particles dissolved in solution; the water is pulled across the semipermeable membrane by the osmotic force. When discussing the circulatory system, the osmotic pressure exerted by proteins and other particles unable to move across the membrane is typically referred to as **oncotic pressure**.

The Cell Barrier

The cell membrane is the barrier that defines the IC. It has several unique structural characteristics that allow it to be a semipermeable membrane, thereby allowing the passage of water and small solutes but preventing movement of many other molecules.

THE ARCHITECTURE OF THE CELL MEMBRANE

The cell membrane is composed of a lipid bilayer. Phospholipids, combining polar, phosphoglycerol headgroups with long aliphatic carbon chains, form the lipid bilayer. The polarity of the headgroups and the hydrophobic properties of the aliphatic chains are responsible for the formation of the bilayer. Gases, such as carbon dioxide and oxygen, cross lipid bilayers extremely rapidly. Water also crosses most lipid bilayers rapidly, although, as we will describe below, there are a few important exceptions. Small noncharged molecules, such as urea and glycerol, can also cross the bilayer, albeit slowly. Charged electrolytes, such as sodium, chloride, and potassium, however, cannot cross cell membranes. They are so highly charged that the energy required to dissolve them in the extremely hydrophobic core lipid bilayer precludes their passage across it.

 Use Animated Figure 2-2 (Barriers—Cell Membrane and Endothelium) to zoom in on the cell membrane and observe the differences in the abilities of water, gases, non-charged molecules and electrolytes to cross the membrane. The membrane, in the absence of the transport mechanisms, which we will discuss in a moment, forms an effective barrier to charged particles.

For charged particles to enter or exit a cell, transport mechanisms must exist. Specific proteins must be embedded within the lipid bilayer to facilitate the movement of these particles across an otherwise impermeable barrier. There are many types of **transport proteins**. Some allow movement of particles down concentration or electrical gradients, and are typically called **channels**; the process is passive, i.e., no additional energy is needed to effect movement of the particle, and is called **passive transport**. Others, however, require energy to move particles against their electrochemical gradients, and are typically called **transporters**. The energy for this process, called **active transport**, is usually provided by coupling the cleavage of an ATP molecule to the movement of the particle. In addition to active and passive transport, there is a process called **secondary active transport** in which a transporter capitalizes on a concentration gradient generated by active transport of one solute to facilitate the movement of another solute down its electrochemical gradient. Most cell membranes have many transporter proteins. As we shall learn, their presence or absence ultimately determines the permeability of cells to charged solutes.

 Animated Figure 2-3 (Transport Mechanisms) shows animated representations of the transport mechanisms; play the animation for each to observe how that protein facilitates movement of certain particles across the cell membrane. You will see these same representations of the various transporters in other animated figures throughout the book.

GIBBS–DONNAN EFFECT AND Na/K ATPases

Just as cell membranes do not allow the passage of charged electrolytes, they are also impermeable to proteins. With ongoing cellular protein transcription and translation, the cell has an abundance of intracellular proteins, most of which are negatively charged. The presence of these anionic particles, which cannot cross the cell membrane, has two effects on the cell. The protein particles themselves create an oncotic gradient favoring the movement of water into the cell. The presence of the negative charges on the proteins creates an electrical gradient, favoring the movement of positive charges into the cell.

The cumulative effect of these forces has been called the **Gibbs–Donnan Effect**, which describes how the presence of a negatively charged protein on one side of a semipermeable membrane generates both osmotic and electrochemical gradients across the membrane. The membrane is *permeable* to charged ions, but *impermeable* to larger proteins. At equilibrium, there are equal numbers of ions and water molecules on each side of the membrane. If one were to add negatively charged protein to the left side of a container divided by a semipermeable membrane, the negatively charged proteins will provide an electrical attraction for positively charged particles, ultimately resulting in more positively charged particles on the left side than the right. In addition, since the sum of all the charges on each side of the membrane must equal zero, the presence of the negatively charged protein will lead to fewer negatively charged ions on the left side. Upon reaching equilibrium, there will be relatively more positive charges on the left than the right, and more diffusible negative charges (small anions) on the right than the left. However, because of the large protein particles, which cannot cross the membrane, there will be more total particles on the left. These will exert an osmotic force, and cause water to flow to that side of the beaker. The combination of these electrochemical and oncotic gradients is called the Gibbs–Donnan Effect.

If the Gibbs–Donnan Effect were not countered by another force, the presence of intracellular protein would induce an inflow of water, leading to cell swelling and eventual death. How do cells, which have an abundance of intracellular negatively charged proteins, protect themselves?

The presence of an ion exchange pump on most cell membranes provides such protection. The Na/K ATPase, an energy dependent cellular pump, defends against the inward force created by the Gibbs–Donnan Effect by pumping 3Na$^+$ ions out in exchange for each 2K$^+$ ions pumped in. Although most cell membranes are filled with ion channels, which make them structurally permeable to ions, the presence of continuously pumping Na/K ATPases makes the membrane functionally impermeable to sodium ion flow. By maintaining a high sodium concentration outside the cell to counter the Gibbs–Donnan Effect, the Na/K ATPases protect the cell from swelling and rupturing. This is illustrated in *Figure 2-4*; the oncotic force created by a high concentration of protein within the cell is offset by the osmotic force generated by the movement of sodium outside the cell.

In summary, the cell membrane is permeable to water, but relatively impermeable to proteins and sodium ions. Negatively charged intracellular proteins provide a Gibbs–Donnan Effect that leads to inward flow of ions, while Na/K ATPase supported extrusion of positively charged sodium ions provides a compensatory outward flow; the net balance prevents excessive inward movement of water and stabilizes cell volume.

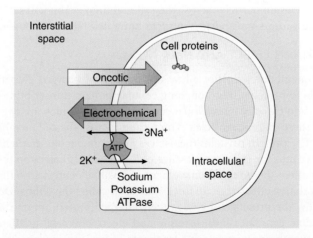

FIGURE 2-4 Summary of pressures across the cell membrane. The cell membrane is semipermeable, so that water can cross freely, but charged particles such as sodium and chloride cannot. The negatively charged proteins within the cell create an inward force, that is balanced by the outward force of the osmotic or electrochemical gradient generated by the Na/K ATPases.

? **THOUGHT QUESTION 2-1** **If a cell were deprived of its energy source, thus losing its ability to run its ATP dependent Na/K pumps, how would the cell size and intracellular concentration change?**

The Vascular Barrier

ONCOTIC AND HYDROSTATIC FORCES

The endothelium creates the barrier between the intravascular and interstitial compartments. The endothelial cells link up with each other via relatively loose junctions that allow the free passage of water and small charged particles such as sodium and other electrolytes. Large proteins, however, such as albumin, cannot cross these endothelial junctions. Thus, just as the intracellular proteins provide an inward osmotic force favoring movement of water from interstitium to cell, the intravascular proteins provide an inward force, to which we refer as oncotic pressure, from the interstitial to the intravascular compartment.

 Return to Animated Figure 2-2 (Barriers—Cell Membrane and Endothelium) and use it to zoom in on the endothelial barrier; observe the differences in the abilities of water, electrolytes, and large proteins to cross. The endothelium forms an effective barrier to large proteins but not water or electrolytes; this restriction of proteins leads to the inward (directed toward the vascular lumen) oncotic force discussed further below.

A hydrostatic force, represented by the mechanical pressure exerted by the fluid within the blood vessel, predisposes to the movement of fluid from the vascular to the interstitial compartment. The energy that creates this force is supplied by the pumping heart, as well as the elastic and muscular properties of the vasculature. The hydrostatic force opposes the inward oncotic force generated by lumen bound proteins (see *Figure 2-5*).

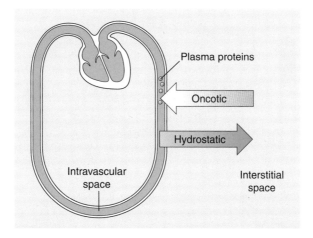

FIGURE 2-5 **Summary of pressures across the vascular wall.** The loose junctions of the vascular endothelium allow water and small charged particles to cross, but not large proteins such as albumin. The proteins create an inward oncotic pressure. This is balanced by the outward hydrostatic pressure generated by the pumping heart and the intrinsic contractile properties of the vasculature.

The balance between the inward oncotic force and the outward electrochemical force determines cell volume. Similarly, the balance between the vascular protein oncotic force (acting to move fluid into the vessels) and the hydrostatic force (acting to move fluid out of the vessels) governs movement of fluid between the intravascular and interstitial compartments. The differences in the characteristics of the barriers that separate the compartments lead to different types of gradients. Concentration gradients between particles develop across cell membranes. In contrast, hydrostatic gradients develop across the vascular endothelium. Oncotic pressures exist across both barriers.

STARLING FORCES

The summation of the oncotic and hydrostatic forces across the vascular endothelial wall determines fluid balance between the IV compartment and the IT compartment. Poignantly described in the late 19th century by Starling, there are four elements, termed **Starling forces**, that must be considered to determine how fluid will move across the vascular endothelium. The outward hydrostatic force, generated by cardiac contraction and vascular elasticity, the inward hydrostatic force, represented by the pressure resulting from interstitial water, the inward oncotic force, generated by plasma proteins and, finally, the outward oncotic force generated by interstitial proteins. In the tissue surrounding most capillaries in a healthy individual, the IT compartment is constantly drained by lymphatic vessels; therefore, the interstitial fluid has little hydrostatic pressure and is relatively free of protein. Consequently, the inward hydrostatic and the outward oncotic force provided by the interstitial fluid are negligible. Thus, flow of water across the vascular endothelium is largely determined by the balance between the plasma hydrostatic pressure and the plasma oncotic pressure.

This process is illustrated in *Figure 2-6* for a typical capillary within the skeletal muscle. At the beginning of the capillary, outward hydrostatic forces are at their highest, reflecting the tone of the proximal smooth muscle that encircles the arterioles; hydrostatic pressure

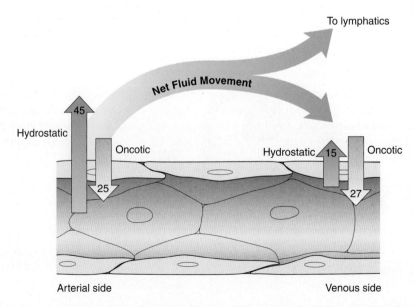

FIGURE 2-6 Summary of pressures in a peripheral capillary. The combination of the outward hydrostatic pressure and the inward oncotic pressure set up a microcirculation, where the fluid flows out at the beginning of the capillary but flows in toward the end of the capillary. Some of it is drained by lymphatics; the rest returns into the capillary as the hydrostatic pressure falls and the oncotic pressure increases.

typically reaches 45 mm Hg. The inward oncotic force of protein within the lumen of the vessel is quantitatively less at about 25 mm Hg and, thus, fluid flows outwards into the interstitium. The contributions of interstitial hydrostatic and oncotic pressures to fluid movement are minimal, as explained above.

As plasma moves along the capillary and protein free filtrate moves from the vessel into the interstitium, several changes occur within the capillary. First, the concentration of protein actually increases slightly, thereby increasing the plasma oncotic pressure. Second, as the distance from the contractile arteriole to any given point in the capillary increases and as additional fluid moves out of the lumen into the interstitial compartment, the plasma hydrostatic pressure falls. With these changes, a net inward gradient arises, reclaiming some of the initially filtered fluid. This balance of forces along the capillary wall creates a circulation of plasma fluid (vascular space to IT space and back to vascular space) that leads to mixing of plasma and interstitial fluid.

Animated Figure 2-4 (Starling Forces) shows a typical skeletal muscle capillary, along with the hydrostatic and oncotic forces (represented by arrows) and a graph of those forces along the length of the capillary. In the figure, drag the point of interest along the capillary and observe the changing balance of forces and the resultant (net) force favoring filtration (movement out of the capillary) or reabsorption (fluid movement into the capillary).

EDITOR'S INTEGRATION

The drop in hydrostatic pressure as fluid flows through a tube is due, in part, to the work that must be done to overcome the resistance of the tube. The change in pressure between any two points in the tube is equal to the product of the flow and the resistance.

$$\Delta P = \text{Flow} \times \text{Resistance}$$

This principle holds for the flow of a liquid (blood through a capillary) as well as for a gas (air in the bronchi of the lungs) and is an important concept applicable to renal, cardiovascular, and respiratory physiology.

This classic description of fluid movement across the capillary wall holds true for those vessels that are impermeable to protein, which results in the oncotic gradient between the protein-laden plasma and the protein-poor interstitium. In an upcoming chapter we will describe how Starling forces regulate filtration across a specialized capillary bed, the glomerulus.

EDITOR'S INTEGRATION

In cardiovascular physiology, diseases that lead to an increase in the hydrostatic pressure of capillaries in the lung increase the likelihood that a patient will develop "pulmonary edema," a term that denotes the accumulation of water in the interstitium and alveoli of the lung. With greater hydrostatic force (equal in this example to the blood pressure in a capillary), there is a greater tendency for water to move across the capillary wall and into the interstitium of the lung. Pulmonary edema impairs the movement of oxygen from the lungs into the blood and causes shortness of breath. In severe cases, it can lead to death.

THOUGHT QUESTION 2-2 Individuals with hypertension may have marked elevations in their systemic blood pressure, yet do not necessarily develop edema. However, individuals with small changes in pulmonary capillary pressures, say from left ventricle failure, quickly go into pulmonary edema. Can you provide a physiologic explanation for these different effects of changes in hydrostatic pressure?

 THOUGHT QUESTION 2-3 Some renal diseases lead to severe proteinuria (loss of protein in the urine), resulting in marked hypoalbuminemia. These individuals develop anasarca (swelling of the face, arms, and legs), but not pulmonary edema. Can you explain why the loss of oncotic pressure resulting from hypoalbuminemia affects the lungs differently from the remainder of the body? (Hint: Compare the hydrostatic pressures of the systemic versus the pulmonary circulation.)

    Use Animated Figure 2-4 (Starling Forces) to choose the hypoalbuminemia (hypoproteinemia) condition and observe how the balance of forces along the typical skeletal muscle capillary changes. Drag the point of interest along the capillary to see how the forces favor filtration in this case and can lead to edema (in the legs, for example, but not the lungs as mentioned above).

Changing the Compartments

THE ADDITION OF PARTICLES VERSUS WATER

On any given day, we ingest sodium and water, often in different proportions. As you begin to treat patients, you will have opportunities to administer sodium and water as intravenous fluids. Because of the differences in barrier permeability between the vascular wall and the cell membrane, the addition of sodium and water has important and unique effects on each compartment; you must understand these effects.

The process of adding sodium, water, or a combination of sodium and water, and the effects of each upon the different compartment sizes and composition are illustrated in the simple diagram (*Figure 2-7*).

The initial balloon sizes reflect typical body compartments; thus, a 5 L balloon signifies the IV space, a 10 L balloon the IT space, and a 25 L balloon the IC space. The "barriers" separating the balloons reflect the cell membrane and vascular endothelium. Thus, the membrane between balloons IV and IT is permeable to sodium and water, whereas the membrane between IT and IC is impermeable to sodium, but permeable to water.

We will begin with a normal concentration, or **osmolality**, within each balloon (*Figure 2-7A*). For the ease of calculations, we will start with an osmolality of 300 mOsm/kg (recognizing that it is a bit higher than our normal body osmolarity of about 280 mOsm/kg). Remember, all the compartments are permeable to water. Thus, in steady state conditions, no concentration gradient exists among the compartments; water will flow across all the barriers to keep the osmolality even. In addition, since you know the volume of each compartment and the concentration of particles within each compartment, you can easily calculate the actual number of particles contained by them. The intravascular balloon has approximately 1,500 mOsms, the interstitial balloon about 3,000 mOsms, and the intracellular balloon about 7,500 mOsms. The composition of these particles is different between compartments; sodium and chloride are the most important intravascular

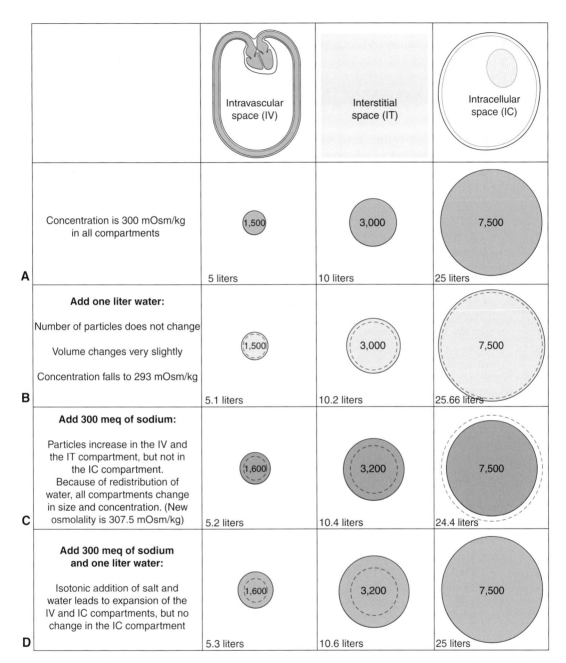

	Intravascular space (IV)	Interstitial space (IT)	Intracellular space (IC)
A Concentration is 300 mOsm/kg in all compartments	1,500 5 liters	3,000 10 liters	7,500 25 liters
B Add one liter water: Number of particles does not change Volume changes very slightly Concentration falls to 293 mOsm/kg	1,500 5.1 liters	3,000 10.2 liters	7,500 25.66 liters
C Add 300 meq of sodium: Particles increase in the IV and the IT compartment, but not in the IC compartment. Because of redistribution of water, all compartments change in size and concentration. (New osmolality is 307.5 mOsm/kg)	1,600 5.2 liters	3,200 10.4 liters	7,500 24.4 liters
D Add 300 meq of sodium and one liter water: Isotonic addition of salt and water leads to expansion of the IV and IC compartments, but no change in the IC compartment	1,600 5.3 liters	3,200 10.6 liters	7,500 25 liters

FIGURE 2-7 The effect of adding sodium, water, and a combination of sodium and water to the distribution of fluid among the body's compartments.

and interstitial particles, and potassium is the most abundant intracellular particle. With the model defined, we begin our first experiment.

In *Figure 2-7B*, you begin the experiment by adding 1 L of water to the IV space. Because all membranes are permeable to water, the added fluid will distribute among all three compartments to maintain the same ratio of particles to water in all three spaces (i.e., generating no concentration differences). Thus, about one-ninth (11%) of the water will remain in the IV compartment, two-ninths (22%) will remain in the IT space, and two-thirds (66%) of the added liter of water will distribute to the IC space. The concentration of particles in all the compartments will decrease equally. The IV space will now have 1,500 particles in 5.1 L of water, the IT will have 3,000 particles in 10.2 L of water, and IC will have 7,500 particles in 25.66 L of water. Consequently, the concentration in all compartments will fall equally to approximately 293 mOsm/kg. After equilibrium is reached, the net effect of adding 1 L of water to the IV space is a decrease in *concentration of particles* among all compartments. The *volume* of each compartment changed minimally.

 Use Animated Figure 2-5 (Body Compartments) to try adding 1 L of water; observe how the volume and particle concentration of each of the compartments change.

In the second part of the experiment (*Figure 2-7C*), you choose to add 300 meq of sodium. Since the vascular wall is permeable to sodium, but the cell membrane (with the constant activity of Na/K ATPase) is effectively not permeable, these 300 particles will distribute only between the IV and the IT space, but not into the IC space. The particles will distribute according to the initial compartment volumes. Since the IT space is twice as large as the IV space, two-thirds of the added sodium will end up in the IT space and one-third in the IV space. Thus, of the added 300 particles of sodium, 200 will be in the interstitium and 100 within the vascular lumen. None will go into cells.

 Now use Animated Figure 2-5 (Body Compartments) to reset the experiment and try adding 300 meq of sodium; observe how added sodium leads to changes in the volume and particle concentration of each of the compartments.

These added particles will increase the total number of particles in the IV and IT compartments. Thus, a concentration gradient across the cell membrane will arise (the system is no longer in a steady state) and, consequently, water will flow across the permeable cell membrane into the extracellular space until the osmolarity has equalized across all compartments (restore steady state or equilibrium conditions).

How much water will leave the IC space? Since both membranes are permeable to water, the osmolality will be the same across all compartments. Thus, the new osmolality will be defined by the total number of particles (1,500 IV, 3,000 IT, and 7,500 IC, plus the 300 newly added particles of sodium, to total 12,300 particles); the total volume of water has not changed. Thus, the new concentration will be 307.5 mOsm/kg. Using this new concentration, you can now figure out how much water will be distributed from the IC space to the other compartments.

There has been no change in the total number of particles in the IC space. In order to have a concentration of 307.5 mOsm/kg, the IC space must shrink to a volume of 24.4 L (7,500/24.4 = 307.4). Thus, 600 mL of water will flow out of the cells and will be distributed as follows: 200 mL will end up in the IV space, and approximately 400 mL in the IT space. In this experiment, the addition of sodium caused an increase in concentration shared equally among all compartments. The IC space, however, decreased in volume, whereas the IV and IT spaces both increased in volume.

Although we frequently ingest water by itself (coffee, tea, juice, water, beer, etc.), it is rare to eat sodium in isolation. Typically, we eat sodium, and then wash it down with a beverage of choice. How these processes are regulated will be discussed in later chapters. However, let us look briefly now at how the addition of salt and water changes the body's compartments.

In this experiment (*Figure 2-7D*), add 300 mmol of sodium and 1 L of water to the system. The sodium particles will again be restricted to the IV and IT spaces, in the same one-third to two-thirds distribution as above. The addition of these particles to the IV and IT spaces will keep the added water within the IV and IT spaces in the same distribution. Thus, the net effect of adding sodium and water in this example is an isotonic (no disproportionate shifts of water between compartments) expansion of the IV and IT *volumes*, with no increase in the IC volume, and with no change in *concentration of the particles* within each compartment.

In summary, because of the differences in the membrane permeability of the vascular endothelium and the cell membrane, adding sodium alone or the combination of sodium and water, leads to an expansion of the IV and the IT volume. Adding water without solute leads to changes in total body concentration shared equally among all compartments, with little change in the IV volume and a relatively large change in the IC volume. The important concept illustrated is as follows: sodium leads to changes in volume within the IV space whereas water leads to changes in body concentration.

The Unique Physiology of the Renal Epithelium

We have just seen how the addition of sodium, water, or a combination of the two affects our body compartments. There are two ways for sodium and water to enter the body: the gastrointestinal (GI) tract and the kidneys. Ingested food and water enters our body across the epithelial cells of the intestine. In a similar manner, fluid that has been filtered across the glomerulus "re-enters" our body across the epithelial cells of the renal tubule. Because of anatomical differences in the epithelial cells, however, this absorptive process differs markedly in the GI tract and the kidneys, and leads to profound differences in the way our body handles sodium and water.

Because we absorb all of the sodium we eat, the amount of sodium and water entering the body from the GI tract is determined by what we ingest. Sodium in our diet is transported across the intestinal epithelium in a manner similar to that in the kidney. Sodium pumps and channels within the gastrointestinal epithelium facilitate the movement of sodium from the lumen of the intestine into the portal circulation. As sodium is absorbed, osmotic gradients are created between the lumen and the basolateral surface of the epithelium (more concentrated in the basolateral region). Because these gastrointestinal epithelial cells are permeable to water, water then flows along the concentration gradient; "water follows salt" is a common way to describe this phenomenon. Fluid absorption occurs isotonically, meaning no concentration gradient is generated once equilibrium has been re-established. Since it is rare for humans to ingest sodium without water, sodium and water are absorbed together.

In the distal part of the renal tubule, sodium is reabsorbed in a similar manner to the GI tract; the body makes use of pumps, transporters, and channels. There are two very important structural differences, however, between the kidney and the gastrointestinal epithelium. First, the renal tubule has the unique ability to alter the amount of filtered sodium it reclaims. By regulating the number of transporter proteins within its cell membrane, the tubules can greatly alter the amount of sodium that re-enters the blood. In addition, as will be discussed in detail in later chapters, unique modifications of the renal tubule make sections of it impermeable to water. In our previous discussion of membranes, either between the cell and the interstitium or between the vasculature and the interstitium, the compartmental barriers were inherently water permeable. Thus, water flowed passively towards areas of higher osmolarity. However, the distal tubule of the kidney is one of the few epithelial barriers in the body that can be fully impermeable to water. Particles, therefore, can be absorbed without water "following" and concentration gradients can be established; "water does *not* 'always' follow salt" in parts of the renal tubule.

As we will see in later chapters, the kidney can regulate or "handle" water and sodium independently of each other. Sodium regulation is dependent on the presence and activity of sodium channels and pumps in the cells of the tubule. Given the unique barrier membranes of the renal tubule, water handling is dependent on the presence or absence of specialized water channels called **aquaporins** found in the cells of the distal tubule. The independence of water and particle handling is one of the most important concepts of renal physiology. This principle allows the kidneys to regulate particle reclamation without affecting water reclamation, and creates two separate physiologic axes, one that regulates the body's water content (covered in Chapters 7 and 8), and one that regulates the body's particle content (covered in Chapter 6).

PUTTING IT TOGETHER

A young man is brought into the emergency room after being involved in a car accident. He has suffered multiple lacerations, and has lost a lot of blood. On arrival, he has a weak pulse and his blood pressure is low at 80 mm Hg/40 mm Hg (normal is 120/80). He is able to tell you that he weighs 70 kg.

You immediately order intravenous fluids to help improve his blood pressure. The nurse asks if you want "normal saline" or "D5W". Upon reading the labeling of each bag, you discover that saline contains approximately 150 meq of sodium and 150 meq of chloride, that results in a total osmolarity of around 300 mOsm/L. The solution called D5W, in contrast, contains no sodium or chloride, but instead has about 50 grams dextrose/liter, which translates to about 278 mOsm/kg.

If you want to improve his blood pressure, which type of fluid would you choose? How much of each solution will remain in the IV space?

Since blood pressure depends, in part, on the amount of fluid in the vascular space, you should begin thinking about this question by determining whether the 1 L of each solution will be distributed in the same or different ways among the three compartments. You know that water moves easily among the compartments, so the key issue to address is: how will the particles within the solutions be distributed and will they change the relative particle concentrations of each compartment?

Test your hypothesis by using Animated Figure 2-6 (Body Compartments—Intravenous Fluids) to try this out; choose and administer 1 L of normal saline or D5W and see the effect on the body's compartments.

The bag of normal saline has approximately the same amount of particles/liter as serum, thus it is isotonic. Since the cell membrane is functionally impermeable to sodium (and chloride), the 300 particles will distribute across the intravascular and interstitial compartments. One-third of the particles, or approximately 50 particles of sodium and 50 particles of chloride, will remain intravascular, and the remaining 200 particles will distribute into the interstitium. The liter of infused water into which the sodium chloride is dissolved will shadow the particle distribution; it will distribute as follows: One-third will remain in the vascular space, whereas the other two-thirds will go into the IT space. It should not affect the intra-cellular space at all.

Although the D5W solution has nearly the same numbers of particles per unit volume (and therefore a similar osmolality), the dextrose in the D5W solution will be metabolized rapidly (it is taken up and used by cells as a source of energy), leaving only **free water** (water without particles) behind. Thus, the 278 mOsm/L of solution are transient; they disappear as the cells consume dextrose. Since all the barriers between the body's compartments are permeable to water, the remaining water, now devoid of particles, will distribute evenly across the whole body. Thus, of the 1 L of D5W, 667 mL will go into the body's cells, 222 mL into the interstitium, and only 111 mL will remain in the IV compartment.

In summary, normal saline is a superior choice to improve intravascular volume and blood pressure. On the basis of your analysis, 333 mL of a liter of normal saline will remain in the vasculature, compared to only 111 mL of a liter of D5W.

Summary Points

- The human body is composed primarily of water, which distributes into three major compartments: the IC, the IT, and the IV.
- The compartments of the body are separated from each other by unique barriers. The vessel wall (capillary endothelium) separates the vascular space from the interstitium. The cell membrane separates the cell's interior from the surrounding interstitium.
- Each barrier has unique characteristics. The vessel wall is permeable to water and electrolytes, but not protein. The cell membrane is permeable to water, but not to either electrolytes or protein.
- Because of the different permeabilities of the barriers separating the different body compartments, different forces arise across the barriers.
- The negatively charged protein present in cells generates an inward oncotic and electrochemical force. Cell membrane Na/K ATPases generate a compensating outward electrochemical force by moving three sodium ions outside the cell in exchange for two potassium ions. The balance of forces (oncotic and electrochemical) maintains cell volume.
- The intravascular protein generates an inward oncotic force. Since the endothelial junctions provide no barrier to electrolyte movements, a compensatory outward electrochemical gradient cannot be generated. Rather, an outward hydrostatic force, produced by cardiac contraction and the intrinsic tone of the vessel wall, balances the oncotic force.
- The balance of the oncotic and hydrostatic forces across the capillary wall changes along its length, and ultimately determines net movement of fluid from lumen, into interstitium, and then back into lumen. These forces are termed Starling forces.
- Molecules cross membranes via different mechanisms, including diffusion across the lipid bilayer, facilitated diffusion through channels, active transport, and secondary active transport.
- Because of the different permeabilities to electrolytes of the barriers between the compartments, the addition of sodium affects the compartments in different ways. Adding sodium to the vascular space causes an increase of volume within the intravascular and interstitial compartments, yet a decrease in intracellular volume.
- Water distributes equally among all compartments. Thus, adding water to the vascular space leads to a decrease in the concentration of particles among all compartments, with little change in volume of the IV.
- Water and sodium enter our body through two portals: the GI tract and the renal tubule.
- GI absorption of sodium occurs isotonically, which means that water follows sodium as the sodium is absorbed across the intestinal epithelium.
- Because of its potential to become impermeable to water, the renal tubule has the ability to generate large concentration gradients across the lumen wall. This property of the tubular epithelium allows for sodium absorption without necessitating water absorption. Unlike the GI tract, water does not necessarily follow sodium in the renal tubule.
- The separation of water and sodium handling in the kidneys allows sodium regulation and water regulation to occur independently of each other.

Answers TO THOUGHT QUESTIONS

2-1. The intramembrane ATPases generate an outward electrochemical force that opposes the inward force generated by the intracellular negatively charged proteins, as described by the Gibbs–Donnan equilibrium. Loss of the ATPases would leave the oncotic forces unopposed, resulting in osmotically driven inflow of fluid; in addition, because of the negatively charged proteins in the cell, there would be an electrical gradient favoring inflow of sodium particles, which would also result in water coming into the cell (remember, the ATPases maintain a high concentration of sodium outside relative to inside the cell). Thus, the cell would have a higher sodium concentration than the interstitium that surrounds it and would begin to swell. This process could lead to cell rupture.

2-2. The structural difference between the pulmonary vasculature and tissue blood vessels is at the root of this thought question. The pulmonary capillaries are relatively "leaky" to protein, whereas the tissue capillaries are mostly impermeable. Thus, the inward oncotic gradient is much higher for tissue capillaries than pulmonary capillaries. Consequently, both hydrostatic and oncotic gradients are important in tissue capillaries, whereas the pulmonary vasculature is subject primarily to hydrostatic forces. With this as a background, let us answer the thought questions.

The etiology of systemic hypertension is often multifactorial, and arterial vasoconstriction may in fact protect the more distal capillary beds from "seeing" higher hydrostatic pressures (remember, $\Delta P = \text{Flow} \times \text{Resistance}$; a constricted vessel increases resistance, which leads to a drop in the pressure within the vessel distal to the resistance). However, with that as a caveat, it is likely that the capillary hydrostatic pressure increases. The large inward oncotic gradient, however, is protective, dampening the effect of the hydrostatic change. Whatever fluid does extravasate into the interstitium is likely absorbed by the lymphatic system.

Changes in hydrostatic pressure in the pulmonary capillary system have dramatically different results. Since they have little oncotic gradient "buffer", small changes in hydrostatic pressure drive fluid extravasation, and pulmonary edema results.

2-3. Let us discuss the effects of changes in serum protein, as in the case with marked proteinuria and resulting hypoalbuminemia. Because of the loss of the protective inward oncotic force, peripheral capillaries are exposed to unbalanced outward hydrostatic pressure, and interstitial edema occurs. This can be seen in all tissue beds. Often patients will notice this around their eyes first, likely because of the lack of periorbital connective tissue and consequent low tissue elasticity, which probably diminishes interstitial hydrostatic pressure.

However, because the capillaries in the lungs are relatively leaky to protein, the oncotic pressure will fall equally on both sides of the capillary, and the gradient will remain the same. As a result, the pulmonary capillaries are not affected by changes in serum protein levels. Thus, as long as hydrostatic pressure does not change, pulmonary edema will not ensue. Whereas fluid movement across peripheral vessels is a balance between oncotic and hydrostatic pressure, hydrostatic forces largely determine fluid movement across the pulmonary capillaries. This important physiologic fact cannot be overstated. Said another way, if a patient develops pulmonary edema, the pulmonary hydrostatic pressures are too high!

Review Questions

DIRECTIONS: *Each of the numbered items or incomplete statements in this section is followed by answers or by completions of the statement. Select the ONE lettered answer or completion that is BEST in each case.*

1. An unfortunate animal eats a pesticide that poisons the cell membrane Na/K ATPases. What will happen to the animal's cells?

    A. They will shrink
    B. They will swell
    C. No change in cell size

2. A 25-year-old man returns from vacation with profuse diarrhea for 2 days in duration. Due to the fluid loss, his weight decreases by 3 pounds. Which of his body compartments change in size?

    A. IV
    B. IC
    C. IT
    D. A and B
    E. A and C

3. A young woman develops frothy urine, and is found to be spilling large amounts of protein in her urine. (Protein is usually not filtered across the glomerulus in any appreciable amount.) Consequently, her serum protein levels are very low. What would you expect her blood pressure to be?

    A. Higher than normal
    B. Lower than normal
    C. No different than normal

4. For the same patient in question 4, what (if any) abnormality might you find on chest x-ray?

    A. Pulmonary edema
    B. Pleural effusions
    C. Edema of her ankles
    D. A and B
    E. B and C

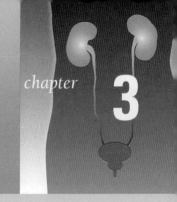

chapter **3**

Form Determines Function
The Uniqueness of Renal Anatomy

LEARNING OBJECTIVES

By the end of this chapter, you should be able to:

- define the basic anatomic features of the kidney.
- delineate the vascular network supplying the kidney and the differences in the vascular structures as one goes from the superficial cortex to the medulla.
- describe the structural alterations of the afferent arteriole that enable it to regulate filtration pressure in the glomerulus.
- describe the importance of granular cells and their ability to secrete renin.
- describe the location of the juxtaglomerular apparatus (JGA) and the importance of its position relative to the afferent arteriole.
- describe the structural alterations of the glomerular capillary loop that facilitate filtration.
- define the significance of the "hairpin" loop architecture of the descending vasa recta.
- define the concepts of "inside" and "outside" the body with respect to renal anatomy.
- describe the unique structural modifications of the basement membrane and podocyte that determine glomerular permeability.
- describe the importance of the structural modifications that make the tubular epithelium an impermeable barrier.
- define the concept of cell polarity and describe the structural importance of the unique apical and basolateral membranes of the tubular epithelium.
- describe how the kidney senses water and particle balance in the body.

Introduction

On average, approximately one quarter of the cardiac output reaches the kidneys; approximately 1.0 L of blood per minute, or 1,440 L, passes through the kidneys daily. The blood moves from the aorta through the renal arteries and then percolates through smaller and smaller vessels, eventually making its way into a "cul-de-sac" of a capillary loop. Under normal circumstances, fluid is then filtered out of this capillary loop into the renal tubule. The tubule initially acts as a "drain," catching all the filtered fluid. As we will learn in Chapter 4, the constant pumping motion of the heart, by generating pressure within the capillary loop, drives this filtration of fluid out of the capillary loop into the tubule in a *nonselective* manner (recall the Starling forces described in Chapter 2). For normal individuals, approximately 120 to 125 mL/min, or about 180 L/day, is filtered from the capillary loops into the tubules. On the one hand, this provides an efficient manner for excreting the body waste. On the other hand, however, a filtration rate of this magnitude creates several challenges.

In passing from the glomerular capillary loop into the tubule, filtered fluid has essentially passed from inside the body to outside of the body. The renal tubule is a long epithelial cell-lined tube that connects the capillary loop to the collecting system. One could theoretically place a small tube from the urethra, through the bladder and ureters, into the renal pelvis, and along the length of the tubules, without crossing any epithelial barriers. Thus, one can see the challenge. If 120 mL/min of fluid is constantly being filtered out of the body, considerable liquid must be reclaimed; otherwise, rapid death due to fluid loss would occur. This process of fluid reclamation happens along the length of the tubule.

The tubule has unique structural modifications that allow this process of reclamation to occur in a coordinated and precise manner. As we will discuss in Chapter 5, hormonal stimuli alter the tubule's permeability to both particles and water. The tubule has the capacity to be fully impermeable or permeable to both particles and water.

In this chapter, we will review the critical features of the anatomy of the kidney that enable it to filter large quantities of toxins along with fluid and essential molecules in a regulated manner that accommodates hemodynamic changes and then selectively reabsorb the necessary fluid and electrolytes to maintain homeostasis.

Basic Anatomy Overview

The most basic structural and functional unit of the kidney is called the **nephron**, which is illustrated in *Figure 3-1*. It is composed of a **glomerulus**, which is the filtering part of the nephron, and a tubule, which is responsible for reclaiming the majority of filtered fluid and eliminating what must be excreted. The glomerulus is composed of a network of capillary loops; each capillary is lined by a single endothelial layer, which is supported by a basement membrane and capped by a uniquely modified epithelial cell, known as the **podocyte**. Structurally, the renal tubule is a long tube-like structure of interconnecting epithelial cells. As the tubule approaches the collecting system of the kidney, the epithelial lining cells change, and it is then called the **collecting duct**. The collecting duct subsequently opens into the renal collecting system and eventually into the **urogenital system**.

The nephron and the more proximal parts of the collecting tubule are derived from a different embryological source than the renal pelvis and the urogenital system. In early development, the ureteric bud, which arises from the mesonephric duct, grows into the metanephric cap. The ureteric bud ultimately forms the **ureters**, the **renal pelvis**, and the more distal parts of the collecting duct, whereas the metanephric cap will form the nephron and the proximal tubule. This is quite important as the tissue derived from the ureteric bud is highly enervated (and hurts when injured), whereas much of the metanephric cap is not.

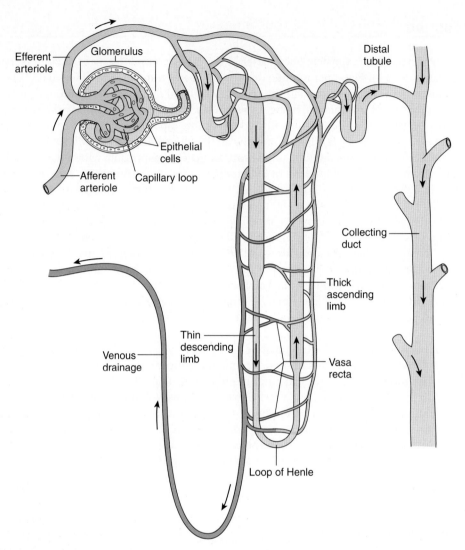

FIGURE 3-1 The anatomy of the nephron. Note the intricate relationship between the glomerulus, the tubule, and the vasculature.

The gross anatomy of the kidney is represented in *Figure 3-2*. The outer layer is termed the **cortex**, which is filled with glomeruli, their associated blood vessels, and their attached tubules.

As the tubules move toward the collecting system, they descend into the **medulla**. The medulla lacks glomeruli and is primarily composed of different tubule types. Much of the medullary tissue is arranged in segments termed renal pyramids. The tubules, as they become collecting ducts, descend through the pyramids, draining into the renal pelvis via an open pouch, termed the **renal calyx**.

The calyx is a part of the urogenital system and actually grasps the most distal point of the pyramid. This interface between pyramid and calyx is called the papilla; it is composed of the most distal aspects of the collecting tubules surrounded by urogenital-derived epithelial and muscular layers. The muscular layer allows for contractions that occur sequentially to provide peristalsis, a process that "milks" filtrate down the collecting tubules into the pelvis.

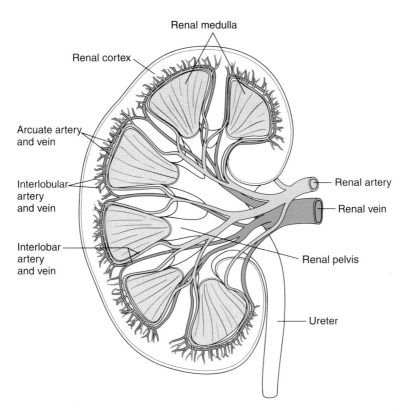

FIGURE 3-2 Anatomical structure of the kidney. The renal cortex contains the glomeruli. Parts of the renal tubule and the collecting duct course through the deeper parts of the renal parenchyma, known as the medulla, before draining into the renal pelvis.

Renal Vasculature

The renal vessels must provide three key functions: 1) supply oxygen and nutrients to the kidney's tissue, 2) sustain adequate pressure in specialized capillaries for filtering the blood, and 3) maintain a gradient of osmolarity (which is critical for the absorption of water and electrolytes from the tubule) in the renal medulla.

The renal artery arises from the abdominal aorta, just below the superior mesenteric artery. Near the hilum of the kidney, the renal artery divides into several segmental branches, entering the renal parenchyma and progressing up between the lobes and the pyramids. There they turn into arcuates, which run horizontally along the surface of the kidney, along the junction between the cortex and the medulla. From the arcuates, penetrating interlobular arteries ascend into the cortex, branching off into afferent arteries that supply glomeruli. Similar to other arterioles elsewhere in the body, the proximal portions of the afferent arteriole are composed of a thin endothelial layer surrounded by smooth muscle cells. This muscular layer, enervated by sympathetic nerves, allows for contraction and relaxation of the afferent arteriole, which permits regulation of the perfusion pressure of the glomerulus, as will be discussed in greater detail later in this chapter.

In the later or more distal section of the afferent arteriole, as it approaches the glomerulus, the smooth muscle cells are replaced by granular cells. These cells contain the machinery to produce **renin**, a regulatory peptide important in sodium regulation. In humans, the average afferent arteriole is around 20 μm in diameter.

Immediately upon entering the glomerulus, as seen in *Figure 3-1*, the **afferent arteriole** splits into a lace-like network of capillaries. Unlike the afferent arterioles, which are enclosed by either smooth muscle or granular cells, the capillary loops are made of thin endothelium with no surrounding structure. This capillary is the site of filtration of blood and the point of entry of filtered fluid into the renal tubule.

Upon return to the region of the glomerulus, the capillary loops drain into the **efferent arterioles**, which then exit the glomerulus. Efferent arterioles vary widely in diameter, depending on their location within the kidney, and can have relatively large amounts of smooth muscle support. It is important to note that this segment—afferent arteriole to capillary loop to efferent arteriole—is quite unique in the human body; elsewhere, capillaries empty into veins. In the glomerulus, a somewhat flimsy capillary plexus, lacking vascular smooth muscle cell support, is sandwiched between two muscular arteries. The vascular smooth muscle cells of both afferent and efferent arterioles are enervated and thus can respond to a wide range of neurohormonal stimuli. Consequently, the balance between afferent and efferent constriction and dilatation regulates the pressure within the capillary loop; the interaction between the afferent and the efferent arterioles helps to sustain a relatively consistent filtration pressure in the glomerulus despite changes in the body's blood pressure. This is an important concept that we will discuss in greater detail later.

The efferent arteriole branches into a second capillary loop, the **vasa recta**. These capillaries are composed of flat endothelium with extensive fenestrations and have no smooth muscle elements that would permit contraction; the fenestrations and low hydrostatic pressure within these vessels make the vasa recta ideally suited to absorb fluid and vital molecules from the renal interstitium. Unlike the glomerular capillary loop, the vasa recta comprise a low-pressure capillary plexus, like those in other parts of the body, and drain directly into a venous system. The vasa recta have several important roles. On the one hand, they provide oxygen and nutrients to many structures of the renal parenchyma, and on the other hand, they provide a conduit for reabsorption of approximately 180 L of filtrate formed each day.

The relationship of the two capillary beds is important to understand. If we discuss this relationship in electrical terms, the glomerular tuft and the vasa recta are capillary beds in "series." The vasa recta are dependent on blood flow coming from the glomerulus. As we will discuss in future chapters, glomerular blood flow is highly regulated, and in many circumstances, the muscular efferent artery will constrict to maintain a certain pressure within the glomerular tuft. Although this may protect glomerular filtration, the downstream effect is to limit flow to the vasa recta, a change that may alter reabsorption of the filtered material from the tubule.

For an average individual, the initial pressure within the afferent arteriole is approximately 100 mm Hg. Arterial resistance dampens the systemic pressure, reducing pressure in the afferent arteriole to approximately 60 mm Hg. The pressure across the efferent arteriole fluctuates between 60 and 20 mm Hg, and the balance between these two arteriole systems ultimately determines the pressure within the capillary loop. Once the blood flows into the vasa recta, pressure remains quite low and falls to approximately 10 mm Hg as it reaches the renal vein.

The vasa recta must provide oxygen and nutrients to the tubules, which are highly active and energy-dependent structures; absorption of electrolytes and water from the tubular fluid often requires significant amounts of ATP as we will discuss below. Certain conditions create a "double-hit" phenomenon, in which the vasa recta's capillary flow is undermined by more proximal constriction of the efferent arteriole, and at the same time, energy requirements of the tubules are increased; thus, blood flow and oxygen delivery to the tubules is reduced at a time that oxygen consumption is increased. This can be seen in the setting of hemorrhage or relative hypotension, when the glomerular loop attempts to maintain glomerular filtration and the tubules are stimulated to reabsorb more sodium particles. Such situations, and the physiologic response of the kidney to hypotension, may lead to tubular injury (this clinical condition is termed acute tubular necrosis or ATN).

In some sections of the kidney, after the vasa recta, the renal vasculature turns into a hairpin loop, which descends into deeper parts of the medulla before returning to the renal vein and exiting the kidney. This aspect of the vascular structure is critical for the maintenance of an osmolar gradient within the renal medulla; the importance of this hairpin loop will be discussed in detail in Chapter 7.

So far, we have discussed the vascular supply of a single nephron unit. In reality, the vascular architecture shows great heterogeneity, with three major vascular pathways, defined by the direction of the vasa recta flow, as seen in *Figure 3-3.*

The vasa recta, after leaving the efferent arteriole of a superficial glomerulus, flow outward toward the renal capsule. They supply nutrients to, and reclaim filtrate from, the proximal tubules and distal convoluted tubules of these superficial glomeruli. The vasa recta exiting the efferent arteriole of midcortical glomeruli flow down toward the arcuate veins at the corticomedullary junction, without descending into the medulla. They supply and drain both the midcortical nephrons as well as the deeper tubular parts of the more superficial nephrons. The third vascular pathway supplies the deepest juxtamedullary nephrons. Unlike the other two pathways, these vasa recta descend deep into the medulla. They have a unique structural organization, in which a loop-like turn provides a mechanism to prevent the dissipation of the concentration of the interstitial fluid of the medulla (necessary for the reabsorption of water from the collecting duct); at the same time, the vessels provide blood to the deepest structures of the kidney.

Among these three different pathways, the vasa recta that supply the superficial and midcortical glomeruli are the most abundant in the kidney; it is in this region that we find most of the proximal tubules from which much of the fluid and electrolytes filtered in the glomerulus are reabsorbed. Many fewer vasa recta descend into the medulla, as reflected by the distribution of blood flow within the kidney. Of the total renal blood flow, almost 90% circulates through the superficial or midcortical glomeruli vasa recta, with the other 10% reaching the medulla. Only 1% to 2% of the total renal blood flow reaches the deepest parts of the medulla; this organization of the vasculature is important in protecting the medullary concentration gradient and also results in relative hypoxia in this region of the kidney. The importance of the anatomic structure of the blood supply within the kidney will be detailed in Chapter 7.

The Glomerulus

The interface between the flow of blood pulsating though the kidneys and the fluid filling the lumen of the tubules, which we have noted are outside the body, is the glomerulus, as seen in *Figure 3-4.*

The increased pressure within the capillary loop produces a hydrostatic pressure gradient that leads to a filtrate, free of cells and protein, which enters the urinary space. The urinary space is a potential space; it serves as a receptacle for the filtrate and leads into the tubular system. Filtrate is constantly flowing across the glomerulus. On average, approximately 120 mL of filtrate is formed each minute, or almost 180 L per day. The rate at which this fluid is generated is termed the **glomerular filtration rate (GFR)**.

The glomerulus, which separates the circulating blood from the urinary space, is composed of three layers, as seen in *Figure 3-5.*

The capillary endothelial cell forms the innermost layer, a collagenous basement membrane forms the middle layer, and an outer modified epithelial cell, called the podocyte, forms the third layer. These three layers—the endothelial cell, the basement membrane,

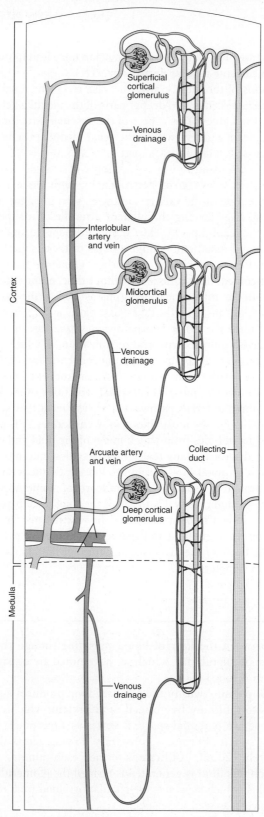

FIGURE 3-3 Three major pathways of renal blood supply. Most renal blood flow proceeds through the superficial and midcortical glomeruli. Vasa recta from these glomeruli exit the kidney without descending into the medulla. A much smaller portion of blood flow feeds the deep glomeruli. Vasa recta from the deep glomeruli descend into the medulla before returning to the renal vein.

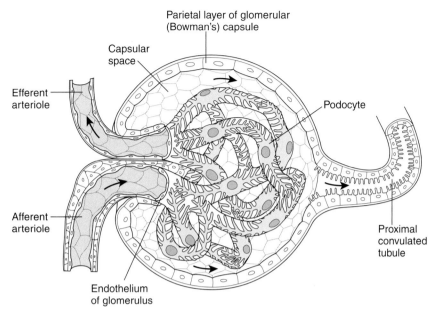

FIGURE 3-4 Anatomical structure of the glomerulus. The glomerulus is comprised of a tuft of loop-like capillary offshoots from the afferent arteriole. Pressure within the capillary loop pushes protein and cell free filtrate into the capsular space, which drains into the renal tubule. The loops reconvene to become the efferent arteriole.

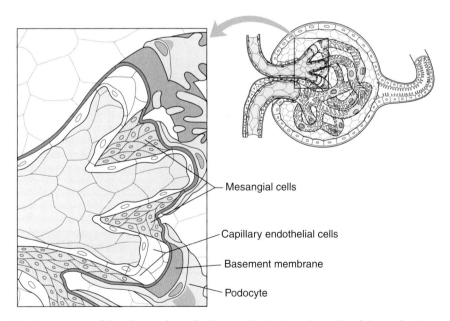

FIGURE 3-5 The three layers of the glomerular tuft. The endothelium lines the inside of the capillary loops. The basement membrane is a thin layer of collagen that sits on the endothelial layer, separating it from the urinary space. The basement membrane is the "skin" of the kidney, separating the inside (endothelium and blood vessels) from the outside (epithelial cells and urinary space). Blood pulsates into these capillary loops under high pressure, which is maintained by the variable tone of the afferent and the efferent arterioles as they constrict and relax according to the needs of the body. To prevent these loops from unraveling like a flexible hose under high water pressure, the podocytes anchor the loops in place and keep the structure intact.

and the podocyte—collectively make up the filtration barrier that keeps blood cells and protein within the body, yet allow fluid and small molecules to pass into the urinary space. There are supporting cells nestled between the capillary loops, known as the mesangial cells; the exact role of these cells is unclear. The relationships between these three layers are areas of ongoing research among renal physiologists. An understanding of the basic relationship between these structures is critical to your ability to evaluate normal physiology and diseases of the kidney.

A single endothelial cell layer makes up the capillary loop. Many capillary loops branch off a single afferent arteriole to form the glomerular tuft, a collection of these fine lace-like structures. At the base of tuft, where each capillary is attached to its respective arteriole, a supporting matrix and cells surround the capillary loops. This area is called the mesangium. It is important to note that only a thin layer of endothelium separates the mesangium from the rest of the body, i.e., it is not separated from the body by an epithelial layer and thus is considered to be on the "inside" of the body.

As discussed above, the constant vasoactivity of the afferent and efferent arterioles adjusts the pressure within the capillary loop to sustain effective filtration; typically, this pressure is fairly high compared to a typical capillary in other parts of the body. You might imagine that the capillary loop, given its simple and delicate endothelial structures, would unravel under high pressure, like a hose that uncoils when the water is turned on. To add stability to the loop, a basement membrane sits upon the capillary to which it is anchored by the finger-like projections of the podocytes. The basement membrane and podocytes are like the "skin" of the glomerulus; filtrate that crosses these layers is now considered to be "outside" of the body.

The basement membrane is an interesting and complex scaffolding structure. It is made of type IV collagen. The basement membrane is primarily composed of alpha chains 3, 4, and 5, which are arranged in a triple helix structure, connected end to end, and folded upon each other by connecting disulfide bonds. The unique structure of this basement membrane enables it to act as "filter paper," preventing some particles from passing, yet allowing others, along with water, to move freely through it.

The extent to which the basement membrane acts as a barrier to particle movement is determined primarily by particle size and charge (*Table 3-1*). Larger particles, typically greater than 10 nm in diameter, are usually prevented from passing. The charge of the particle, however, can affect this permeability; negatively charged particles, for example, are unable to pass through the basement membrane. Because of this charge and size selectivity, cells and larger proteins remain within the capillary, whereas water and small ions pass freely. It is generally accepted that proteins such as albumin, because of their size and negative charge, are not filtered, although this explanation is contested by some and remains an area of debate among physiologists.

TABLE 3-1 PARTICLE DIAMETER

PARTICLE	DIAMETER (nm)
Red blood cell	8,000
Hemoglobin	6.5
Albumin	7
Sodium	0.4
Chloride	0.35
Glucose	0.7
Water	0.2

The last cell layer of the glomerulus is composed of podocytes, which are modified epithelial cells that form an interlacing network. Podocytes have finger-like projections that interdigitate upon the basement membrane, thereby providing structural support. In a manner analogous to the mechanism by which the ends of a flexible tube such as a hose must be held down to prevent it from unwinding and flailing about when the water is turned on, the podocytes anchor the high-pressure capillary loops. Openings between the finger projections are termed **filtration slits,** and the glomerular filtrate passes through these gaps on its way into the urinary space. The podocyte plays an important role in determining the characteristics of the filtration barrier of the glomerulus, but the exact nature of the interaction between the podocyte and the basement membrane structure remains uncertain. Disease processes that primarily affect the podocyte, however, can greatly affect glomerular permeability, allowing passage of large proteins such as albumin. Thus, it is likely that both the basement membrane and the podocyte have important roles in determining the ultimate permeability of the glomerulus, particularly with respect to protein.

?

THOUGHT QUESTION 3-1 **There are many disease processes that affect the glomerulus. Inflammatory processes, such as systemic lupus erythematous (an auto-immune disease) or pyelonephritis (an infection involving the kidney), can cause accumulation of white blood cells within the glomerulus. These cells may cluster inside the capillary loop and the mesangium; in some cases this can cause disruption of the glomerular architecture.**

When there is inflammation of the glomerular capillaries, the basement membrane may be damaged and the barrier function compromised; cells and protein may leak into the urinary space. Since cells are not reclaimed by the renal tubules, these inflammatory cells might be seen in the patient's urine. Because the inflammatory process can damage the capillary loops, clogging them with cells and cellular debris, glomerular filtration can be severely decreased in these conditions. These patients often present with renal failure, or more specifically, with an inability to adequately filter their blood.

Other disease processes, however, can directly damage the podocyte, yet they are not associated with inflammation. What molecules or cells do you predict you would see in the urine of these patients? Why?

The Tubule

As we discussed above, approximately 120 cc/min (180 L/day) of filtrate moves across the glomerulus into the tubular system. The great majority (on average, all but 2 L) of this fluid is reclaimed and moved back into the body. Thus, the tubules are constantly moving particles and fluid from the lumen back into the interstitial space of the kidney from where it is returned to the vascular space.

The tubule is a hollow tube lined by epithelial cells. Filtrate flows along this tube, from glomerulus downstream toward the urinary collecting system. The tubule is traditionally subdivided for the sake of discussion into segments, based on structural differences in the anatomy and consequent varying functional roles over the length of the tubule. The first part of the tubule is called the **proximal tubule**. It reclaims approximately 75% to 80% of the filtered fluid and has important structural features to facilitate this process. Its many in-foldings along the basement membrane increase the surface area for reclamation. In addition, since reclamation of particles is an energy-dependent process, the proximal tubule cells are full of mitochondria.

Use Animated Figure 3-1 (Nephron Map) to zoom in on the cells of the proximal tubule. Observe the mitochondria and basal in-foldings of the cell membrane; both of these features are crucial to the role of the proximal tubule in the reclamation of particles. You can also use the pull-down menu to show the percentage of total fluid reabsorption along each segment of the nephron; the main thing to note here is that the proximal tubule is responsible for the majority of fluid reclamation, as mentioned above.

The proximal tubule connects to the **Loop of Henle**, which is called a "Loop" because of its hairpin anatomic structure. The loop comprises a **thin descending limb** and a thicker ascending limb. The **thick ascending limb** has an important role in pumping ions against a concentration gradient, and thus, its cells also have a high concentration of mitochondria. As we will learn in Chapter 7, the Loop of Henle plays an important role in water conservation. In addition, it reclaims about 5% to 10% of the filtrate. The later sections of the tubule include the **distal tubule** and, finally, the **collecting duct**. The collecting duct absorbs a very small percentage of the filtered load. However, as we will learn in future chapters, it has a unique sensitivity to a wide range of hormonal stimuli, which alter its permeability to water and particles. The collecting duct is like the "fine tuner" of the body's composition; here, the body decides how much sodium, potassium, and water to keep and how much to let pass as waste for excretion as urine.

Return to Animated Figure 3-1 (Nephron Map) and use the pull-down menu to turn on the "fluid reabsorption percentage" overlay. You can see from the relative percentages of fluid reabsorption along the tubule that the later segments absorb only a small fraction of the total filtered fluid; given the large volume of fluid passing through the tubules, however, even these small percentages represent a significant absolute volume, which can play a crucial role in fine-tuning the body's fluid status.

The epithelial cells of the tubule are unique and have several important modifications that ultimately affect their function. Unlike other epithelial cells of the body, those within the tubule are relatively impermeable. Thus, water and particles cannot freely cross the tubule's surface; they must be carried via a transporter or pass through a channel or move between neighboring cells. These two important concepts, the natural impermeability of the renal tubule and the modifications that enable fluid and small molecules to cross the barrier selectively, are the topics of the next two sections.

TUBULAR IMPERMEABILITY—CELL MEMBRANE COMPOSITION AND TIGHT JUNCTIONS

All cell membranes are composed of lipid bilayers, embedded with proteins and cholesterol; the relative amounts of these substances determine the permeability of the bilayer. Long carbon chains within the lipid bilayer resist water (recall the old saying that oil will not mix with water). Thus, tight packing of lipids into a bilayer reduces water permeability. The presence of embedded cholesterol molecules within the bilayer has the opposite effect, possibly by disrupting the structural integrity of the membrane. Although increasing lipid concentration within a bilayer makes the membrane less permeable, increasing the number of cholesterol molecules increases the permeability.

The renal tubule's epithelium is unique in the richness of its lipid bilayer, tightly packed with phospholipid particles. This architectural design makes the cell membrane impermeable to water. Of course, the membrane is also impermeable to small molecules. In addition to the modifications of the membranes of the tubule cells, the junctions between the cells are unique too. Tubular epithelial cells are connected via a branching network of sealing strands, which join the membranes together in a tightly approximated lattice-work. This **tight junction complex** is composed of several proteins, including zonula occludens-1 (ZO-1), the occludin family, and the claudin family. By creating overlapping connections between neighboring cells, these proteins prevent ions and water from moving around cells via the paracellular route.

Since the cell membrane of the tubules is impermeable, the distribution of tight junction proteins determines each segment's intrinsic permeability by controlling the paracellular route for movement of water. The thick ascending limb and the collecting duct have the highest concentration of such proteins. The thin descending limb has the lowest concentration. Consequently, from a functional perspective, the movement of water and small solute is least likely to occur via the paracellular route in the thick ascending limb and the collecting duct.

Once again, return to Animated Figure 3-1 (Nephron Map) and use the pull-down menu to turn on the permeability overlay. Observe how the tight junction proteins (shown between cells) are distributed along the tubule. These tight junctions, along with the impermeable lipid bilayer of the cell membrane, determine the baseline or intrinsic level of permeability of each segment of the tubule; other factors also contribute to the overall permeability of each segment, as discussed below.

The combination of the impermeability of the cell membrane and the presence of tight junctions between neighboring cells gives the renal tubule the potential to be impermeable in some sections. In those segments, water and particles cannot flow across or around the epithelial cells. How then is it possible for the tubules to so efficiently reclaim almost all of the glomerular filtrate? The answer to this question is found in the cell membrane proteins that allow particle and water movement across the tubule back into the body.

TUBULAR PERMEABILITY—MEMBRANE PROTEINS THAT FACILITATE PARTICLE AND WATER RECLAMATION

Important proteins, which we will discuss in great detail in future chapters, reside in the cell membrane of the tubular epithelium and have the potential to change its permeability. Membrane proteins have unique affinity for particular substrates. A **transporter** is a protein that requires energy, usually in the form of ATP, to move particles against their concentration gradient. A **channel** is a protein that simply provides a pathway for particles to move passively down their electrochemical gradient; no energy is required.

To move particles from the tubule's lumen back into the body, the transport proteins must be organized in a way that facilitates a vector of movement, i.e., movement that has a particular direction. For instance, if transporter proteins were haphazardly inserted into all sides of a cell, there would be frequent movement of particles, but without net direction. To facilitate vectored flow, all the transport proteins must be "lined up" to orchestrate one direction of movement.

To achieve this spatial organization, the renal tubule has a "front and back" side, which provides a sense of topographical direction. This concept is known as **polarity**. Furthermore, the membranes on each side of the cell are unique. The **apical membrane** of the cell, which faces the lumen, and the **basolateral membrane** of the cell, which faces the interstitium, have distinct features. Polarity allows the cell to direct certain proteins to the apical membrane and others to the basolateral membrane. The apical and basolateral membranes are labeled in the cellular zoom images shown in Animated Figure 3-1.

The functionality of transport proteins determines cell polarity. The correct positioning of these proteins is the consequence of dynamic cellular processes that either maintain the proteins within the membrane or reclaim them back into the cytosol. **Exocytosis** is the process of shuttling synthesized proteins from nucleus into the cell membrane, whereas **endocytosis** is the process of engulfing these membrane proteins back into the cell cytosol, often followed by cellular degradation. Collectively, these processes are termed **protein trafficking**, reflecting the dynamic nature of protein biology. At all points of protein synthesis, from the DNA transcription to the posttranslational trafficking described above, there is great potential for regulation. In this manner, the functionality of the renal tubule transporter can be exaggerated or diminished, thereby allowing large variations in the reclamation of particles from the tubular lumen.

There are two major types of membrane proteins: those that facilitate particle reclamation and those that facilitate water reclamation. As we will learn in future chapters, proteins are specific for particular particles. For example, there are glucose transporters, sodium transporters, and phosphate transporters. Each one has a specific affinity for its particular particle. Water, however, cannot move through these protein transporters. In order for water to be reclaimed from the tubule's lumen, it must either pass along the paracellular route or through water-specific channels in the cell membranes. These channels are called **aquaporins**. Aquaporins, covered in more detail in Chapter 5, are specific to water molecules and do not provide access for other small particles.

In summary, although the tubule is intrinsically impermeable, it has the ability to synthesize and insert specialized proteins into the cell membranes facing the lumen. These proteins, by creating passageways for either particle or water movement, greatly alter the tubule's permeability. As we will learn in later chapters, this process of protein trafficking can be controlled by various external stimuli, thereby allowing the tubule to alter its permeability according to a variety of situations and bodily needs. Under certain conditions, for example, the tubule is stimulated to avidly absorb sodium. In other situations, it reclaims water. Despite the huge amount of filtrate that is delivered to it daily, the tubules have the unique ability to selectively reclaim specific filtrate components and, ultimately, determine the body's fluid composition.

THE ENERGY SOURCE FOR PARTICLE RECLAMATION—THE Na/K ATPase

Although membrane proteins help overcome the impermeability of the tubular epithelium, many of these processes are energy dependent. Glomerular filtrate flows from the capillary loop into the tubular lumen driven in large part by the high hydrostatic pressure of the capillary loop. In contrast, the lumen of the tubule is an extremely low-pressure system. Although the venous complex of the draining renal veins, which collect reclaimed filtrate, is also a low-pressure system, the filtrate must be moved from tubular lumen, across the epithelial barrier, into the interstitium. Since gradients of hydrostatic pressure cannot provide the force for this movement, an alternative energy source must be present.

Cell membrane pumps along the basolateral membrane of the tubule's epithelium provide the energy for reclamation of filtrate. These pumps, well known as Na/K ATPases, are ubiquitous on all cell membranes. In many places throughout the body, these pumps balance electrolytes between the inside and outside of the cell, thereby preventing the cell from swelling. In the kidney, however, the Na/K ATPases perform an additional important role. In keeping with the cell's polarity, the Na/K ATPases line up on the basolateral side of all tubule cells, creating a directional vector of particle movement. Since these particles are charged, the net effect of moving the molecules is the creation of an electrochemical gradient across the cell membrane; when the effects of the individual cells are combined, an electrochemical gradient is created across the whole tubule. This gradient is the driving force for filtrate reclamation.

We will study the unique structure of the tubules, and how this process of reclamation occurs, in Chapter 5.

THOUGHT QUESTION 3-2 A patient suffers a heart attack, which leads to a drop in cardiac output and blood pressure. Oxygen delivery to the tissues, including the kidney, is significantly decreased. Since the tubules are energy dependent, requiring considerable Na/K ATPase activity for tubular reclamation, what do you think the clinical result of the patient's hypotension will be? Will his urine output be increased or decreased? Why?

THE JUXTAGLOMERULAR APPARATUS

We have now seen how huge amounts of fluid are filtered across the glomerulus and then reclaimed along the length of the tubule. Although this high flow system is efficient for clearing the body's waste, tubular reclamation must be carefully regulated and coordinated. Small abnormalities in tubular function could have disastrous consequences, leading to rapid body fluid loss and death.

Fortunately, the kidney has a local "watchdog" of this process, carefully weighing the rate of filtration to the rate of reclamation. Termed JGA (the juxtaglomerular apparatus), this collection of cells sits sandwiched between the glomerular arteries and the tubules. *Figure 3-5* is drawn to show the structural proximity of the JGA to the afferent arteriole. This proximity of the JGA to both the blood supply and the tubular flow allows it to monitor and regulate both glomerular filtration and tubular reclamation.

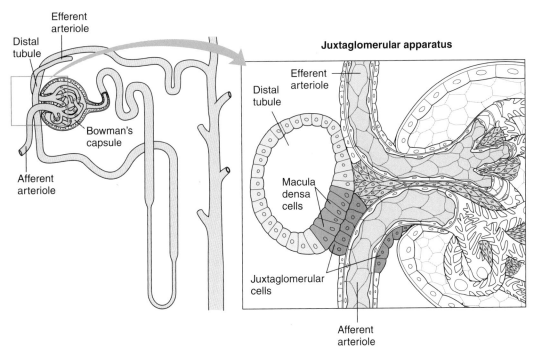

FIGURE 3-6 **The juxtaglomerular apparatus.** The juxtaglomerular apparatus (JGA) of each nephron sits between the artery and the tubule of that particular nephron. The tubule of each nephron curves back on itself, ultimately inserting between the afferent and the efferent arterioles that supply that nephron. Thus, the JGA has the ability to sense and respond to changes in both arterial and tubular flows and coordinate the processes of reabsorption and glomerular filtration. Two types of specialized cells are located in this region of the kidney to help regulate filtration. First, cells in the distal tubule, called the macula densa, can sense flow within the tubule. Second, cells along the afferent arteriole produce renin, a hormone with widespread physiologic effects resulting in conservation of body fluid volume, i.e., sodium and water.

The JGA is composed of two different types of cells: the **macula densa** and juxtaglomerular cells. The macula densa, further discussed in Chapter 6, is a specialized tubular epithelial cell with the ability to detect flow within the tubule's lumen. Juxtaglomerular cells line the afferent arteriole. They have unique modifications that allow them to produce and release **renin**. The role of renin will be discussed in greater detail in Chapter 5; for now, we will note that the release of renin leads to the formation and release of a series of other chemicals including angiotensin and aldosterone, which play critical roles in the regulation of sodium (and, hence, total body water), blood pressure, and renal blood flow. The juxtaglomerular cells, sitting next to the macula densa and on top of the afferent arteriole, provide a communication link between the tubules and the afferent arteriole; a decrease in tubular flow, for example, which occurs as glomerular filtration falls, might suggest a decrease in body fluid volume and can stimulate renin release. In addition, nerve fibers that supply the juxtaglomerular cells provide a link to the rest of the body; activation of the sympathetic nervous system stimulates renin release. In this manner, changes in blood pressure, tubular flow, or nervous system activity can all stimulate renin release. The ability to both sense and modulate filtration and reclamation makes the JGA particularly important in coordinating afferent arteriole and tubular flow, thereby protecting the body's ultimate fluid volume.

We have now described the major structures of the kidney. Let us return to Figure 2-1 presented in Chapter 2 and superimpose a schematic representation of fluid movement across the kidneys in relation to the body's fluid compartments. We will return to this figure many times; so it is important to understand.

Figure 3-7 shows that the glomerular capillary loop is an extension of the intravascular compartment. The afferent arteriole leads into the glomerular capillary loop and then

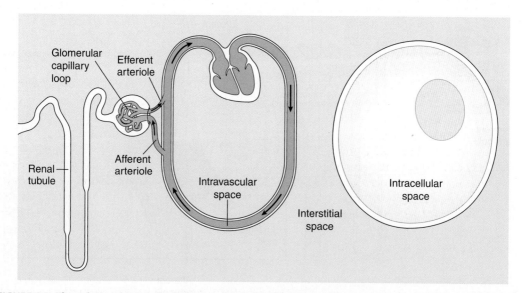

FIGURE 3-7 The relationship of the kidney to the body fluid compartments. We have now added a schematic representation to the body compartment sketch introduced in Chapter 2. The glomerular capillary loops are an extension of the intravascular compartment, connected via the afferent and the efferent arterioles. Note that in this very conceptual schematic sketch; we have represented one glomerulus and its afferent and efferent arterioles, not the whole kidney. Thus, the renal artery and vein, the major connection from the kidney to the aorta and inferior vena cava, are not represented. In addition, there is no distinction between the arterial and venous sections of the intravascular compartment. Because of the combination of pressures within the capillary loop, fluid is filtered across the glomerulus into the tubule. Although the tubule is actually contiguous with the interstitial compartment, its unique structural modifications make it a conduit to the outside of the body, allowing excretion of waste products.

proceeds to the efferent arteriole. As we will discuss in the next chapter, various forces within the capillary loop determine how much fluid is filtered out of the loop into the renal tubular system.

Maintaining Homeostasis—the Balance of Input Versus Output

In this chapter, we have outlined the anatomical modifications of the kidney that allow it to filter the blood, excrete waste, and then reclaim the exact amount of particles and water necessary to keep the body in net balance. In order for this to happen, there must be mechanisms to sense the net amount of particles and water, i.e., the balance between what is ingested across the gastroinstestinal (GI) tract and what is lost from various organs including the respiratory system secondary to evaporation, across the skin via sweat, and from the GI tract in the stool. The kidney must be able to assess these different amounts and respond appropriately. Water, along with some particles, such as sodium and potassium, are highly regulated (requiring a sensing mechanism and a response mechanism). Others, such as creatinine, are not regulated.

Consider the example of what happens after eating a meal. Let us build on *Figure 3-7*, adding a schematic representation of the GI tract, and consider three examples: eating a carbohydrate meal, ingestion of sodium, and ingestion of water. These are represented in *Figure 3-8A, B,* and *C,* respectively.

As seen in *Figure 3-8A*, protein and carbohydrates contained in the meal will be ingested across the GI tract, metabolized, and delivered to the cells, where they will be catabolized into energy and essential amino acids. Protein catabolism will create nitrogenous waste products, which will be converted into soluble urea. Urea is permeable across all cell compartments and represented by the arrows showing movement freely across the capillary endothelium and the cell membrane. Urea is also freely filtered into the tubular space, from where it is eventually excreted as waste. (Some urea is reclaimed along the tubule, which we have not represented.)

Although we have a sensation of hunger, which affects our intake of protein and carbohydrates, no receptor has been identified as the sensing mechanism that would assess the relative amounts of each substrate we have or need within our body. Thus, intake of these substances is determined by how much we eat while excretion is mostly determined by renal filtration. Neither of these processes is tightly regulated.

Sodium metabolism, however, is quite different, as illustrated in *Figure 3-8B.*

Ingested sodium is transported across the intestinal epithelium into the interstitial and vascular spaces. Because of the action of the cellular Na/K ATPase, sodium will not remain in the cellular space even if it enters the cell. Depending on how much water is ingested during the meal, the sodium intake may lead to an isotonic expansion of the vascular and the interstitial space, or if water is not ingested (which almost never happens as we are usually driven by thirst when we eat sodium), water will shift from the intracellular to the interstitial/vascular spaces. Ultimately, the circulation will carry sodium to the kidney, where it will be filtered into the tubular space. Because such a large amount of sodium is filtered, the great majority is reclaimed. However, net sodium homeostasis is determined by balancing just how much was ingested versus what is lost in sweat, respiration, and the GI tract.

Using a wide range of receptors and stimuli, the body directs the kidney to reclaim exactly the right amount of filtered sodium to maintain sodium balance. Since the ingestion of sodium primarily affects the intravascular and the interstitial space, it makes conceptual sense that the sensing mechanisms for sodium balance would be located in one of these compartments. As we will learn in Chapter 6, the sensors that ultimately orchestrate sodium avidity are found within the vasculature and within the JGA.

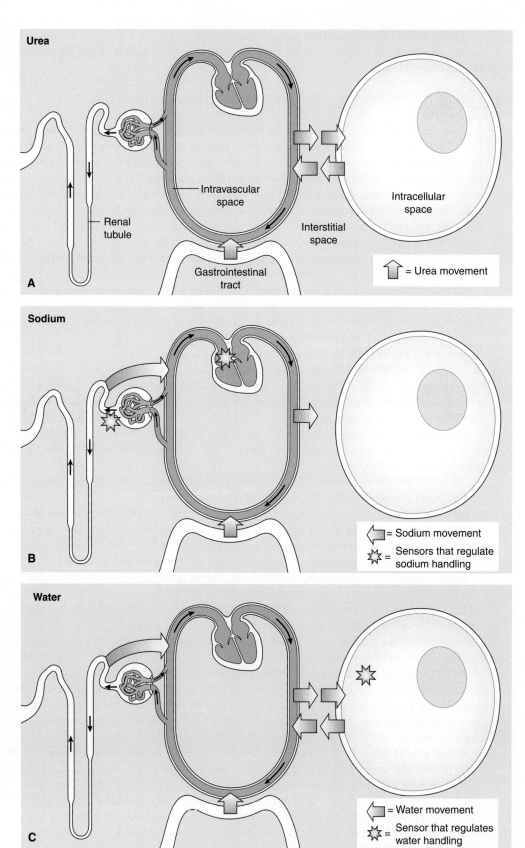

Urea

Intravascular space

Renal tubule

Interstitial space

Intracellular space

Gastrointestinal tract

⬆ = Urea movement

A

Sodium

⬅ = Sodium movement

✸ = Sensors that regulate sodium handling

B

Water

⬅ = Water movement

✸ = Sensor that regulates water handling

C

The fate of water is different, as seen in *Figure 3-8C*.

Ingested water passively moves across the permeable GI tract, being pulled along by particle absorption. Because most cell membranes are permeable, ingested water diffuses into all the body compartments. Upon arriving at the glomerulus, water is filtered into the tubule in keeping with the Starling forces. In the tubule, the fate of water depends on the tubule's avidity of water. Just like sodium, the tubule has the ability to either excrete water (in times of excess) or reclaim almost all ingested water (in times of water deficit). This process, however, can occur independently of sodium and other particle reclamation, thereby allowing the body to regulate water homeostasis without affecting particle homeostasis. Because water distributes across all compartments equally, the receptor for water homeostasis is situated within the cellular space. The change in concentration within the cell reflects the change of concentration elsewhere in the body. This sensing mechanism will be detailed further in Chapter 8.

PUTTING IT TOGETHER

Jed Nicholson is a 70-year-old golfer who developed an infected blister on his left hand. He is prescribed an antibiotic, the metabolic products of which are filtered by the kidney. Because of the high cost of the antibiotic, Jed takes an antibiotic that his 25-year-old grandson had at home after being treated for a recent infection. One week later, having played golf in 90-degree temperature on a daily basis, Jed comes to the emergency department. His blood pressure is 80/60 mm Hg and his heart rate is 120 beats/minute. His mucus membranes are dry and he is confused. Laboratory studies show that the concentration of the antibiotic in his blood is elevated, as is the serum sodium level. Analysis of his urine shows that it is very concentrated and it contains no sodium. Why has he developed elevated blood levels of the antibiotic? How would you explain the elevated serum sodium level and the absence of sodium in the urine?

As individuals age, the GFR declines, even in healthy people. Consequently, the dosage of drugs that are excreted by the kidneys via filtration must be reduced in older patients to avoid the accumulation of toxic metabolites. Volume depletion, which reduces blood pressure and leads to tachycardia (a compensatory mechanism to try to increase cardiac output and restore blood pressure), may exacerbate this

---

FIGURE 3-8 **The metabolism of urea, sodium, and water.** In Figure 3-8, a schematic gastrointestinal GI) tract has been added to illustrate how different particles are metabolized. There is little regulation of what is absorbed across the small intestine; to a large degree, whatever is ingested is absorbed (after intraluminal digestion of course). In **(A)**, the fate of a protein meal is represented. Ingested protein is metabolized, forming its breakdown product, urea. Urea is freely permeable to all body spaces. Urea that is dissolved in the serum is filtered into the tubules and excreted, allowing excretion of the waste and preventing toxicity. There is little regulation of this process. In **(B)**, the fate of sodium is outlined. Ingested sodium distributes between the vascular and the interstitial space, but does not enter the cell. Because it is dissolved in serum, it is filtered into the renal tubule. The exact amount of sodium reclaimed across the tubule is determined by a wide range of stimuli, balancing what is absorbed from the intestines against losses from the respiratory tract, skin, and bowel. The sensing receptors that actually make these decisions are located within the vascular space as well as in the juxtaglomerular apparatus. In **(C)**, the course of ingested water is outlined. Water enters across the GI tract and distributes across all body compartments, including the intracellular space. It too is filtered across the glomerulus into the tubular system, where much of it is reclaimed. The exact amount of water reclaimed along the tubule is determined by the overall balance between ingested water and water lost across the respiratory mucosa, skin, and GI tract. The sensing receptor (osmoreceptor) that determines just how much water is needed is placed within the cellular compartment. This conceptually makes sense, since water enters all spaces equally, and thus the concentration is the same throughout. As initially mentioned in Chapter 1, and as we will continue to learn in future chapters, the regulation of sodium and water are independent of each other.

problem by further reducing filtration. There is evidence on physical examination that the patient is total body fluid depleted. In addition, the serum sodium is elevated, which indicates that he has lost more water than sodium from his body in recent days; consequently, there will be shifts of fluid from the intracellular compartment to the vascular and interstitial compartments. This shift in fluid reduces the volume of the cells and increases intracellular osmolarity, which may cause altered brain activity manifested as confusion. The kidney is attempting to compensate for this problem by reabsorbing as much sodium and water as possible from the renal tubule, which explains the absence of sodium in the urine and the high urine concentration.

Summary Points

- The basic functional unit of the kidney is termed the nephron. It is composed of a glomerulus, its supporting vasculature, and its draining tubular system.
- The glomerulus is made up of a capillary loop, a basement membrane, and a podocyte.
- The tubule is composed of modified epithelial cells.
- Tightly packed lipid within the cell membrane and tight junctions between neighboring cells of the tubular epithelium can make the tubule impermeable.
- Sections of the renal tubule have different names that relate to their anatomic position, and they are distinguished by underlying structural differences.
- Filtrate flows from the capillary loop into the tubular lumen at a rate of approximately 120 cc/min.
- Most of the filtrate in the renal tubule is reclaimed as it passes along the length of the tubule.
- Although much of the tubule is inherently impermeable, important transporter proteins in the cell membranes of the tubular epithelial cells permit movement of specific particles or water across the tubular epithelium, i.e., there is selective permeability, which facilitates filtrate reclamation.
- The relative distribution and function of these transporter proteins ultimately determine how the tubules reclaim filtrate.
- Aquaporins are water channels found in tubular cells in those regions of the tubule responsible for absorption of water.
- High-energy pumps along the basolateral side of tubular epithelial cells provide the energy necessary for transport of filtrate across the impermeable epithelium.
- The JGA is the integration center of the kidney; it monitors tubular flow and it can alter afferent arteriole pressure and provoke renin release, both of which will lead to changes in glomerular filtration.
- The body has receptors that sense sodium and water balance and, consequently, can direct the kidney to excrete or retain sodium or water. Regulation of these two substances occurs independently of each other.

Answers TO THOUGHT QUESTIONS

3-1. Unlike the disorders that cause inflammation within the capillary loop, disorders that primarily affect the podocyte usually do not cause renal failure, at least not initially. Instead, the damage to the podocyte disrupts the delicate relationship between the podocyte and the basement membrane, resulting in loss of the structural support usually supplied by the podocyte. Consequently, integrity of the basement membrane is undermined, and it loses its size and charge selectivity, allowing larger molecules, such as proteins, to pass into the urinary space. Such patients usually present with large amounts of protein in their urine, termed proteinuria. Typically, the syndrome of renal inflammation is termed "nephritis," whereas podocyte damage is termed "nephrosis."

3-2. Hypotension starves the kidney of blood. The tubules are particularly susceptible to injury for two reasons. First, the tubules receive blood in "series," meaning that the tubule is supplied by the second capillary network after the glomerulus. As the kidney attempts to maintain pressure within the glomerulus, by causing efferent arteriole constriction, filtration is sustained but perfusion to the tubule is compromised. Second, the tubules are highly energy dependent due to their role in reclaiming filtrate; they have a high concentration of Na/K ATPases.

This thought question focuses on the relationship between tubular damage and the ability of the tubule to reclaim filtrate. In this case, although the tubules will be damaged, the patient will not lose large amounts of tubular filtrate. In fact, his urine output will likely fall to nothing, at least for a few days. The explanation for this phenomenon is quite complex. The major point to consider is that damage to the tubules almost always causes loss of filtration in that particular nephron; the response of a tubule to damage is to turn off the filtration of its own glomerulus. Thus, tubular damage almost always presents as lack of glomerular filtration, otherwise known as renal failure, and almost never as an inability to reclaim filtrate.

Review Questions

DIRECTIONS: *Each of the numbered items or incomplete statements in this section is followed by answers or by completion of the statement. Select the ONE lettered answer or completion that is BEST in each case.*

1. A patient presents to the emergency room with a large gastrointestinal bleed and very low blood pressure. Which part of the kidney is most likely to be affected?

   A. Endothelial cell
   B. Basement membrane
   C. Podocyte
   D. Tubule

2. A young woman develops an auto-immune disease and develops antigen–antibody complexes. Upon flowing into the glomerular capillary, these complexes deposit within the mesangium and within the capillary lumen. Because of their size, they do not pass through the basement membrane into the urinary space of the tubule. Which of the following findings is least likely to be present?

   A. Renal failure
   B. Low serum albumin due to protein loss in the urine
   C. Hypertension
   D. Signs of inflammation in her urine

3. As part of an experimental therapy regimen, a cancer patient is given an investigative drug that damages specifically the podocyte within the glomerulus. Which of the following is the patient most likely to develop?

   A. Renal failure
   B. Low serum albumin due to protein loss in the urine
   C. Hypertension
   D. Signs of inflammation in her urine

4. A patient receives cancer therapeutic agent, which has damaged the renal tubule. Which of the following is least likely to develop?

   A. Low serum phosphorus
   B. High serum sodium
   C. Proteinuria
   D. Renal failure.

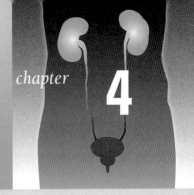

Clearing Waste
Glomerular Filtration

CHAPTER OUTLINE

INTRODUCTION
THE GLOMERULAR FILTRATION RATE
DETERMINANTS OF THE GFR
- Hydrostatic Pressure
- Oncotic Pressure
REGULATING THE GFR
- Autoregulation
- External regulation

MEASURING THE GFR
- The relationship of clearance to GFR
- Adequacy of clearance
- Using the serum creatinine concentration as a marker of the GFR
PUTTING IT TOGETHER
SUMMARY POINTS

LEARNING OBJECTIVES

By the end of this chapter, you should be able to:

- describe the importance of the kidney's role in removing the body's waste products.
- define the glomerular filtration rate (GFR).
- describe the unique characteristics of the glomerulus which determine the pressure within the capillary loop.
- enumerate and explain the mechanisms that control the GFR.
- delineate the autoregulatory processes by which the renal blood vessels control their intrinsic resistance, thereby maintaining appropriate renal blood flow over a wide range of physiological conditions.
- describe the importance of angiotensin II in controlling the GFR.
- define the concepts "clearance" and "work" with respect to the kidney.
- describe the relationship of serum creatinine to renal clearance.

Introduction

In Chapter 1, we discussed how a fish constantly makes waste which, if not removed (or excreted from the tank), would lead to increasing concentrations of solutes within the tank. In a similar manner, our cells constantly make waste, such as urea, via the process of cellular metabolism. If these waste products were to accumulate, we would become increasingly sick, and eventually would die. Thus, efficient excretion of our metabolic waste products is essential to maintaining homeostasis and to our well-being.

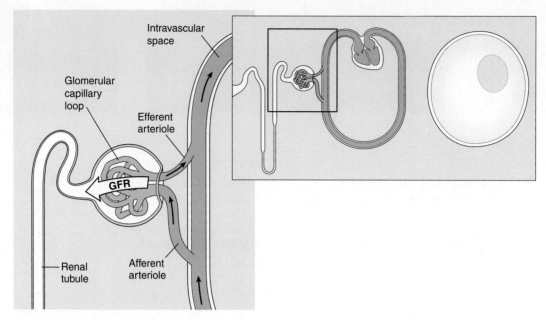

FIGURE 4-1 **The glomerular filtration rate.** The glomerular filtration rate is the term used to describe the flow of filtrate across the glomerular capillary into the tubule. The rate of flow is determined primarily by the pressure within the capillary loop. Filtration is the major method for eliminating waste products that accumulate via ingestion and cell metabolism.

Most cell membranes, as well as our vascular endothelium, are permeable to urea, one of the major byproducts of protein metabolism. Thus, urea easily moves into all of our three body compartments, distributing across our total body fluid. To prevent waste accumulation, this body fluid must be cleansed many times per day. The process by which our total body fluid is cleaned of these metabolic byproducts is the focus of this chapter.

Approximately 120 mL/min, or 7.2 L/hr, of body fluid flows across the glomerular capillaries into the urinary space. This fluid contains a certain amount of waste product dissolved within it. The great majority of this filtered fluid is reclaimed along the tubular system in a manner that excludes much of the filtered waste. In Chapter 5, we will outline the mechanisms by which selective reabsorption of the filtrate occurs.

The Glomerular Filtration Rate

The rate at which filtrate flows out of the glomerular capillary loop, across the basement membrane, into the tubule, is termed the **glomerular filtration rate (GFR)**. This is conceptually illustrated in *Figure 4-1*, which depicts the fluid compartments of the body and shows, schematically, how the vascular fluid is filtered by the glomerulus; the resulting filtrate enters the tubule. Since the GFR is a rate, its units are volume per unit time (mL/min or L/day). It describes how quickly the body is filtering out fluid and, thus, gives an estimation of how efficiently the body can excrete waste.

Knowing an individual's GFR is very important, since it tells us how well the kidneys are working. The process of filtration is important not only for excretion of the body's own waste but also for the excretion of exogenous substances, such as ingested potassium or phosphorus, and some medications. An impaired GFR can result in the accumulation of all types of substances and has the potential to disrupt many of the body's homeostatic mechanisms. Consequently, maintaining a normal GFR is one of the most important physiological tasks of the body; when we think of "renal function," we are usually describing the GFR. As we will discuss, there are many factors that determine the GFR, and many ways of regulating these processes.

Determinants of the GFR

As outlined in Chapter 2, movement of fluid across a membrane is determined by the intrinsic permeability of the membrane and the driving force. In the setting of cell membranes, the driving force is generated predominantly by differences in solute concentration, whereas movement of fluid across the vascular endothelium is determined by the balance of hydrostatic and oncotic pressure. We will now explore how fluid moves across the capillary loops of the glomeruli. This rate of movement is likewise determined by the permeability of the capillary loop, which is affected by the unique structure of these capillaries, and the driving force.

HYDROSTATIC PRESSURE

The glomerular basement membrane, in conjunction with the supporting structure of the podocyte, determines glomerular capillary permeability. The size and charge of a particle are the major factors that determine whether a solute will cross the capillary. Particles that are large (>5000 Daltons) and/or negatively charged cannot cross the capillary loop; small particles like sodium, potassium, and other electrolytes, as well as creatinine, urea, glucose, and of course, water, pass freely.

Given the capillary's high permeability for these smaller particles, the predominant factor determining the GFR is the pressure gradient between the capillary lumen and the urinary space. This gradient consists of the balance between hydrostatic and oncotic pressures, similar to what we described for a peripheral capillary, such as one might see in skeletal muscle. The GFR is best explained by the following formula:

$$GFR = Lp(S) \text{ (change in hydrostatic pressure − change in oncotic pressure)}$$

In this equation, Lp is the unit for permeability of the capillary wall and S is the surface area available for filtration.

There are unique features of the glomerular capillary, however, that distinguish it from all other capillaries in the rest of the body. First, although the glomerular capillary is composed of thin endothelial cells without a muscular layer, it connects an afferent and an efferent arteriole, both of which have supporting muscular layers, rather than an arteriole and a venule, the latter of which has limited ability to constrict. Thus, since the afferent and the efferent arteriole muscular layer can contract or relax (leading to vasoconstriction or vasodilatation), they have the capacity to change hydrostatic pressure within the glomerular capillary. The combination of afferent arteriole dilation and efferent arteriole vasoconstriction increases pressure within the glomerulus, whereas the combination of afferent arteriole vasoconstriction and efferent arteriole dilatation decreases pressure. Typically, the afferent and the efferent arterioles work in concert to maintain a relatively constant hydrostatic pressure throughout the capillary loop.

Whereas the typical hydrostatic pressure in a peripheral capillary bed may fall from 40 mm Hg at its beginning, to less than 15 mm Hg at its end, there is little change in hydrostatic pressure across the glomerular capillary loop. The ability of the afferent and the efferent arterioles to modulate pressure within the capillary loop, and the intrinsic low resistance within the vast capillary plexus, combine to maintain a relatively constant and robust hydrostatic pressure. On an average, the typical hydrostatic pressure within a glomerular capillary loop is approximately 45 mm Hg, notably higher than other capillaries of the body. Furthermore, whereas the hydrostatic pressure within a typical peripheral capillary bed drops off due to the resistance along its length, high hydrostatic pressure is sustained along the length of the glomerular capillary.

EDITOR'S INTEGRATION

The very low resistance seen in the glomerular capillary loop reflects the fact that the capillaries act as multiple tubes in parallel. The laws of physics tell us that the total resistance of tubes in series is equal to the sum of the resistance of each tube ($R_T = R_1 + R_2 + R_3$). In contrast, for tubes in parallel, the total resistance is less than the resistance of any single tube ($1/R_T = 1/R_1 + 1/R_2 + 1/R_3$). This principle holds in the lungs as well. The resistance of the airways diminishes as air moves from the trachea (single tube) to the small airways in the periphery of the lung (millions of tubes in parallel). See *Respiratory Physiology: A Clinical Approach* for a more complete discussion of the factors that affect resistance in the airways.

The high hydrostatic pressure within the capillary loop is a strong force that favors filtration. In contrast, the urinary space, on the other side of the glomerular capillary wall, has very low pressure, often in the range of 10 mm Hg. Thus, there is a high gradient favoring filtration from plasma to urinary space. On an average, approximately 120 mL/min or nearly 180 L/day of fluid cross the capillary. Compare this to the typical renal plasma flow of 625 mL/min; about 20% of fluid that is delivered to the kidney is filtered across the glomerulus into the urinary space. Plasma is simply blood without the cellular component. The relationship of GFR to renal plasma flow is termed **filtration fraction**.

It is defined by the following equation.

$$\text{Filtration Fraction} = \text{GFR}/[(1 - \text{hematocrit})(\text{renal blood flow})]$$

? **THOUGHT QUESTION 4-1** **Vasoconstriction of either the afferent or the efferent arteriole increases resistance within the capillary plexus. Vasoconstriction of the afferent arteriole increases the resistance within the circuit, thus decreasing renal blood flow. The efferent arteriole follows in series (returning to our electrical analysis). For circuits, in which resistors are arranged in series, the resistance is additive. Why then does the vasoconstriction of the efferent arteriole not lead to decreased renal perfusion?**

? **THOUGHT QUESTION 4-2** **In the setting of renal injury, in which some but not all of the glomerular capillary loops are injured, how might the relationship between renal blood flow, capillary pressure, and glomerular filtration change?**

ONCOTIC PRESSURE

Oncotic pressure is the second determinant of the driving pressure for filtration. In the glomerular capillary, however, changes in oncotic pressure assume an even more prominent role than in other capillary beds. Let us explore why this is true.

In peripheral vessels, relatively small amounts of fluid pass across the capillary wall since hydrostatic pressure drops fairly quickly. In contrast, glomerular hydrostatic pressure remains robust and relatively constant along the length of the capillary loop, leading to loss of fluid across the endothelium. Approximately 20% of renal plasma flow is filtered out of the capillary in the glomerulus. Despite the high hydrostatic pressures, plasma proteins, particularly albumin, are not filtered due to their large size and negative charge. In addition,

Chapter 4 | CLEARING WASTE   **55**

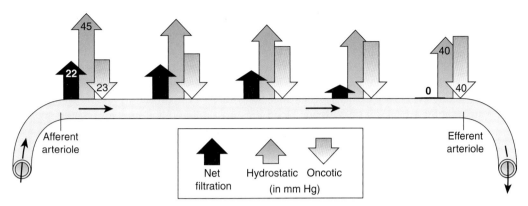

FIGURE 4-2 The balance of oncotic and hydrostatic pressures determines filtration. The afferent and the efferent arterioles alter their diameter (and, consequently, resistance) to maintain a relatively constant hydrostatic pressure within the capillary loop, despite changes in cardiac output and systemic blood pressure. Oncotic pressure at the beginning of the capillary loop is the same as in blood, and thus, filtrate moves rapidly out of the capillary loop (hydrostatic pressure exceeds oncotic pressure). However, as water and charged particles increasingly vacate the capillary, the remaining cells and protein become increasingly concentrated, and the osmotic pressure increases. Toward the end of the capillary loop, the outward hydrostatic pressure is matched by an inward oncotic pressure, and filtration equilibrium is reached. In a peripheral capillary (Chapter 2, Figure 6), the reduction of the net outward gradient (hydrostatic minus oncotic pressure) is due primarily to the fall in hydrostatic pressure. In the glomerular capillary, the reduction of the net outward gradient is due to a marked increase in inward oncotic pressure.

cells are not filtered. The combination of filtration of a high percentage of plasma and retention of serum proteins and cells within the capillary leads to an increasingly concentrated capillary fluid; consequently, there is a strong oncotic force favoring reabsorption of fluid toward the terminal end of the capillary. Oncotic pressure increases from approximately 23 mm Hg in the afferent arteriole to about 40 mm Hg in the efferent arteriole.

The increasing inward force of the plasma protein ultimately rises to the level of the outward hydrostatic force described above. Equilibrium is reached, and further filtration ceases. This point is termed **filtration equilibrium.**

As seen in other capillaries, the balance of outward hydrostatic pressure and inward oncotic pressure determines filtration across the glomerulus. The structure of the glomerulus, however, makes this relationship unique. Within the glomerular capillary loop, hydrostatic pressure is high and can be sustained at these levels, despite changes in the body's blood pressure, by altering the tone of the afferent and the efferent arterioles. The inward oncotic pressure increases dramatically over the length of the capillary due to the large amount of fluid that is filtered and to the inability of large molecules to cross the capillary membrane. The hydrostatic and oncotic forces in a typical glomerular capillary are illustrated in *Figure 4-2.*

 Use Animated Figure 4-1 (Glomerular Capillary Forces) to compare the hydrostatic and oncotic pressures, and their effect on fluid movement, for glomerular capillaries and capillaries elsewhere in the body. Use the slider to move the point of interest along the capillary and observe how the net force for filtration or reabsorption changes along the length of the capillary. Do this for both the glomerular capillary and the skeletal muscle capillary to see how the forces differ.

Regulating the GFR

Since glomerular filtration is the pathway for excretion of the body's waste, maintaining the GFR is important. We discussed above how the balance of hydrostatic and oncotic forces determines GFR. In most scenarios, serum protein levels do not fluctuate; thus, the body cannot regulate filtration by altering the oncotic pressure of the blood that enters the capillary loop. Instead, we alter the hydrostatic pressure as the major method of regulating GFR. The kidney has two major types of hydrostatic regulation, some intrinsic to the kidney, and some that depend on a wide range of neurohumoral stimuli.

Without these regulatory mechanisms, the glomerular hydrostatic pressure would be fully and wholly dependent on systemic blood pressure; falling blood pressures would automatically lead to a decrement of the GFR. The kidney, however, has a remarkable ability to maintain its glomerular hydrostatic pressure despite wide fluctuations of systemic blood pressure.

AUTOREGULATION

Basic principles of physics (Ohm's law) govern flow through tubes. Flow is determined by both the driving pressure (the difference between the pressures at each end of the tube) and the resistance within the tube:

$$Flow = Pressure/Resistance$$

Thus, if the driving pressure and the resistance are reduced in proportion, flow will not be affected. This ability of a vessel to modify its own resistance in response to changes of pressure is termed **autoregulation**, and is common to many types of blood vessels. Blood vessels have a baseline "tone," which is affected by a multitude of factors, including the intrinsic pliability of the vessel wall, the activity of the sympathetic nervous system, and a host of neurohumoral mediators, including epinephrine, angiotensin, and vasopressin. In addition, however, some vessels have an intrinsic ability to respond to changes in pressure. This is termed **myogenic stretch**. The term myogenic refers to the fact that muscle cells (i.e., myocytes) around the artery are able to induce their own contraction (or relaxation), without depending on an external stimulus such as electrical activity from a nerve or biochemical activation from a hormone.

EDITOR'S INTEGRATION

Other organs that are particularly sensitive to changes in blood pressure also demonstrate the phenomenon of autoregulation within their vascular beds. Brain function, for example, can be adversely affected by even transient changes (either up or down) in the systemic blood pressure. Consequently, the cerebral circulation has the capacity to regulate resistance (and flow and pressure) on a minute-by-minute basis. See *Cardiovascular Physiology: A Clinical Approach* for a description of the mechanisms by which this regulation is achieved.

In kidneys, afferent arterioles respond to changes in pressure by either constricting or dilating. Specifically, in the setting of decreased perfusion pressure, the muscles of the afferent arterioles relax, which reduces tension within the vessel wall and increases the radius of the vessel, which decreases the resistance, thereby maintaining the flow. Conversely, in the settings of increased perfusion pressure, the muscles of the afferent arterioles will contract, leading to decreased radius of the vessel and increased resistance, thereby preventing the systemic pressure from inducing a large change in the GFR.

Use Animated Figure 4-2 (Vascular Autoregulation) to explore the concept of autoregulation. Use the slider to adjust the pressure in the vessel and observe the resulting constriction or dilation and its effect on the flow. As mentioned, changes in resistance of the vessel can compensate for changes in pressure, maintaining relatively constant flow over a range of pressures.

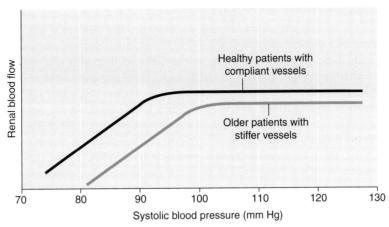

FIGURE 4-3 The relationship of renal blood flow to systemic blood pressure. Since most healthy individuals have pliant renal blood vessels that can dilate in response to hypotension, thereby reducing glomerular resistance and maintaining renal perfusion, changes in systemic blood pressure do not necessarily lead to decreases in renal blood flow. In fact most individuals can maintain a constant renal blood flow until the systolic pressures fall to around 90 mm Hg. In individuals with less compliant blood vessels, however, much milder decrements in systemic blood pressure can lead to reduction in renal blood flow.

As seen in *Figure 4-3*, renal blood flow is typically maintained in young healthy individuals as the systemic systolic pressure falls to about 90 mm Hg. Further reductions in pressure are associated with a decrement in renal blood flow. In individuals who have lost the ability to modulate the vasoactivity of the afferent and the efferent arterioles, however, renal perfusion may fall at much higher (or less severe drops in) systolic blood pressure. Older individuals often develop increasingly stiff or rigid arteries, which are unable to dilate significantly. In such individuals, renal perfusion is much more sensitive to changes in systemic blood pressure, and a marked decrease in renal blood flow can occur at relatively high systemic blood pressures compared to what is seen in a young, healthy individual.

The benefits of the myogenic stretch response are relatively limited with respect to persistent changes in systemic blood pressure. Although this response is important in preventing changes in GFR associated with the frequent transient fluctuations in blood pressure that are common throughout the day, it probably does not play an important role in responding to more sustained blood pressure alterations.

EXTERNAL REGULATION

In addition to this intrinsic myogenic driven autoregulation, external mechanisms also regulate intraglomerular hydrostatic pressure, and hence GFR. These mechanisms are likely more important in maintaining the GFR under conditions in which the blood pressure changes are more persistent, e.g., clinical conditions such as congestive heart failure or volume depletion from blood loss.

As discussed above, decreasing systemic blood pressure will lead to afferent arteriole vasodilatation via autoregulation in an attempt to preserve renal blood flow. In addition, the decrement of blood pressure stimulates vascular receptors (to be discussed in Chapter 6), which results in stimulation of the sympathetic system and release of epinephrine and norepinehrine. These peptides stimulate efferent arteriole constriction (and, to a lesser degree, afferent arteriole constriction).

Use Animated Figure 4-3 (Renal Glomerulus—Vascular Tone) to vary the tone of the afferent and the efferent arterioles and observe the effect on renal blood flow and GFR. This figure uses a lawn sprinkler analogy for the glomerulus, with the height of the sprinkler stream indicating the magnitude of the GFR, to help you gain an intuition for the effect of changes in glomerular vascular tone. You can demonstrate, for example, that afferent arteriolar dilation will positively affect renal blood flow and GFR.

In addition, as described in Chapter 2, the juxtaglomerular apparatus (JGA) has an important role in regulating the GFR. In the setting of either a decrease in afferent arteriole pressure (as may happen with systemic hypotension) or in response to a decrease in tubular flow, the JGA secretes **renin**. Upon its release, renin stimulates the formation of angiotensin I, which is converted to the biologically active angiotensin II by angiotensin converting enzyme. As we will learn about in Chapter 6, one of angiotensin II's major effects is to stimulate the production of aldosterone, a hormone that plays a major role in regulating sodium in the body. In addition, angiotensin II has important vasoconstrictive effects systemically as well as on the kidney. Vasoconstriction of systemic vessels maintains blood pressure when the volume of the vascular compartment is reduced or the force of contraction of the left ventricle is diminished. Within the kidney, angiotensin II leads to constriction of both afferent and efferent arterioles. The predominant effect, however, is upon the efferent arteriole. Preferential efferent arteriole vasoconstriction leads to an increase of intraglomerular hydrostatic pressure, and is one of the most important mechanisms for maintaining the GFR despite changes in systemic blood pressure. In addition, prostaglandins are released, which cause afferent arteriole dilation, and further protect the GFR.

EDITOR'S INTEGRATION

The systemic blood pressure (the pressure you measure in a person's arm with a blood pressure cuff) reflects the force of contraction of the left ventricle and the resistance of the blood vessels averaged over the entire circulation. Stimulation of the sympathetic nervous system, in addition to producing vasoconstriction, as described above, leads to an increase in the force of contraction of the heart (a phenomenon referred to as increased inotropy) and the amount of blood pumped by the heart each minute, i.e., the cardiac output. See *Cardiovascular Physiology: A Clinical Approach* for a more complete discussion of the cardiac contributions to blood pressure control.

Decreased renal perfusion pressure is one of the factors that stimulates renin release. For instance, if a decrement in systemic blood pressure is sustained, thereby overwhelming the ability of myogenic autoregulation to maintain capillary pressure, a transient decrease in glomerular hydrostatic pressure and, hence, GFR will occur. With less fluid filtered in the glomerulus, the volume of fluid moving through the tubule will also diminish. The subsequent decrease in tubular flow, as perceived by the macula densa, stimulates juxtaglomerular release of renin. Renin, leading to the formation of angiotensin II, leads to preferential efferent vasoconstriction, which re-establishes glomerular hydrostatic pressure and brings the GFR back toward normal despite the change in systemic blood pressure.

Whereas vasodilatation of the afferent arteriole maintains renal blood flow in the setting of hypotension or decreased cardiac output, the unique placement of the efferent arteriole makes it a more important protector of the GFR. In the setting of falling systolic pressure, as afferent dilatation attempts to protect renal blood flow, efferent constriction attempts to maintain hydrostatic pressure within the capillary loop, thereby maintaining glomerular

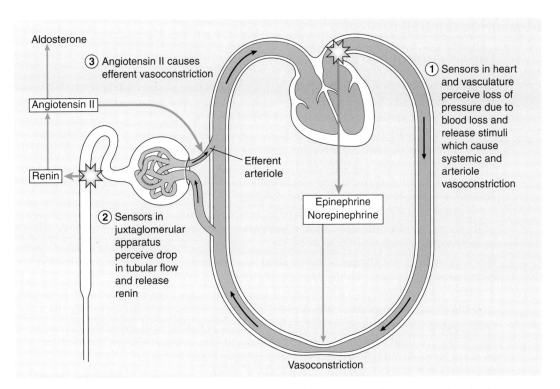

FIGURE 4-4 **External regulation of the GFR in the setting of hypotension.** There are several mechanisms whereby the GFR is preserved in the setting of decreased renal perfusion. (1) In the setting of decreased blood pressure, the sympathetic nervous system releases epinephrine and norepinephrine and other vasoconstrictive peptides. These chemicals cause constriction of the systemic vasculature, a compensatory response to stabilize blood pressure. In addition, these peptides can result in preferential efferent arteriole constriction (not illustrated). (2) The juxtaglomerular apparatus, responding to a decrease in tubular flow (less filtration when glomerular pressure is down) and afferent arteriole pressure, stimulates the activation of the renin–angiotensin system. (3) The renin–angiotensin system causes preferential efferent arteriole constriction, which helps to re-establish a near-normal glomerular pressure. Finally, local prostaglandins are released, which result in afferent arteriole dilation (not illustrated). The combination of afferent arteriole dilatation and efferent arteriole constriction preserves intraglomerular pressure, thereby sustaining the GFR.

filtration. Efferent constriction acts by creating the equivalence of a "bottleneck" obstruction; the outflow track is narrowed, flow decreases, and pressure rises. In the kidney, the result is that glomerular pressure is maintained despite falling renal perfusion pressure.

The process of protecting the GFR in the settings of low blood pressure is illustrated in *Figure 4-4*.

In this figure, the pressure within the vascular component has fallen due to blood loss. Receptors (which will be discussed in Chapter 6) within the vasculature release a variety of substances, which cause systemic vasoconstriction and efferent arteriole vasoconstriction. The decrease of tubular flow is detected by the JGA, which stimulates the renin–angiotensin–aldosterone axis. As noted above, angiotensin is a potent vasoconstrictor (preferentially affecting the efferent arteriole). Aldosterone causes sodium reclamation from the tubule and, as we will learn in Chapter 6, helps return filtered fluid back to the body.

Use Animated Figure 4-4 (External Regulation of GFR) to explore some of the factors mentioned above that help the kidney maintain renal blood flow and GFR. For example, choose "Decreased renal arterial pressure" to see the chain of events involving renin, angiotensin II, and prostaglandin release; you can see on the graph that renal blood flow and GFR are relatively preserved despite the fall in pressure.

Measuring the GFR

THE RELATIONSHIP OF CLEARANCE TO GFR

In the previous section, we have described the importance of the GFR in removing waste products produced during metabolism. In the following sections we will learn about how we quantify the amount of waste removed, and how this calculation relates to the GFR. Let us start with an example.

Imagine that you have a beaker that contains fluid in which a number of small particles is dissolved. You make a small hole at its base, allowing the fluid to drain. How could you calculate how many particles were removed as the fluid leaves the beaker? Obviously, the answer is to simply count the number of particles.

To describe the relationship of particles removed, relative to the initial concentration of fluid, we use the term clearance. **Clearance** is defined as the amount of fluid cleared completely of a certain substance. Instead of focusing on the amount of particles actually removed, we use the particle-free fluid as a "mirror image," a reflection of what has been removed. We focus on the amount of cleared fluid rather than the amount of actual particles removed. Imagine a tank with a small hole in its base, outfitted with a specialized filter that removes particles. As seen in *Figure 4-5*, as fluid passes across the filter, eight particles are removed, and the cleared fluid is returned to the tank. Clearance is the amount of fluid completely cleared of the particles; it is defined by the total amount of particles removed (8) divided by the starting concentration of fluid within the tank (4 particles/L). In this example, 2 L has been cleared completely of particles. Note that the total amount of fluid in the tank does not enter into this equation. Rather, clearance reflects the relationship of removed particles to the starting concentration of that particle in the tank.

Obviously, the clearance of particles will be determined by how quickly fluid moves through the hole (i.e., the rate or flow), as well as how freely the particles are able to transit through the hole. For instance, if the particles are too big to pass, no particles will exit the beaker, and the clearance will be zero.

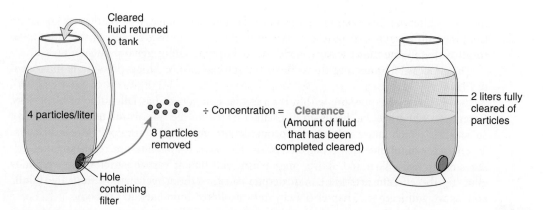

FIGURE 4-5 Clearance. Clearance is defined as the amount of fluid completely cleared of a particle. In this example, a hole containing a filter is made in the bottom of a tank. The fluid within the tank has an unknown volume, but a known concentration of 4 particles/L. As fluid flows out of the hole, particles are removed, and the filtered fluid is returned to the tank. Conceptually, the amount of particles removed (8), divided by the starting concentration in the tank (4 particles/L), is the amount of fluid that has been completely cleared of particles (2 L).

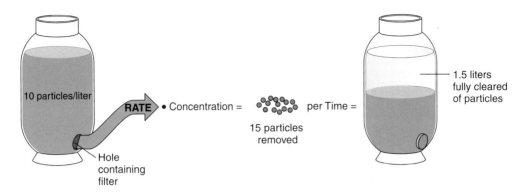

Rate (liters per time) = Clearance (liters per time)

FIGURE 4-6 **The relationship of clearance to rate of flow.** In Figure 4-5, we knew nothing about the rate of flow across the hole. Under certain conditions (when particles are freely filtered), the clearance of a particle can be used to measure the rate of flow across the hole per unit time. In this example, fluid flows at a known rate of 1.5 L/hr. After 1 hr, assuming fluid flows freely across the tank's filter, the rate times the concentration (1.5 L/hr × 10 particles/L) equals the total amount of particles removed (15 particles) per unit time. Since clearance is defined by the amount of particles removed (15), divided by the starting concentration within the tank (10 particles/L), then clearance per time equals the flow rate (both 1.5 L/hr).

Figure 4-6 illustrates how clearance of a particle can be used to calculate the rate of fluid movement across the hole (R). In this scenario, you have an unknown sized tank, which has fluid with the concentration of 10 particles/L. You make a small hole in the base. If the particles flow freely across the hole, then the following formula is true.

R (liter/min) × concentration of particle (particles/liter) × time (minutes)
= amount of particles that are drained in time

Rate, therefore, is defined by the total amount of particles drained divided by the particle concentration. This is the same definition for clearance that we just derived in Figure 4-5. Thus, in the setting where particles freely flow across the filter, the flow rate across the filter is the same as the clearance of that particle, per unit time.

In this example, you collect all the excreted waste (15 particles) over a time period (say 1 hr as an example), divided by the starting concentration (10 particles/L), to give you a rate of 1.5 L/hr. In this example, clearance (1.5 L/hr), and flow (1.5 L/hr) are the same. In summary, we have used the amount of removed particles (divided by the starting concentration) to estimate the rate of flow of fluid across the tank's filter.

Let us try another example to further illustrate, as seen in *Figure 4-7*. A tank has a concentration of four particles of A/liter and four particles of B/liter. Again you make a small hole outfitted with a specialized filter, and then attempt to measure exactly what the rate of fluid flow through the hole. How would you do it?

As before, you measure the total amount of drained particles. Surprisingly, despite similar concentrations in the tank, fewer particles of B are removed (4) compared to A (8). It turns out that the filter has various size pores, and since B is a larger particle, only half as many particles of B are filtered as A, despite the same flow rate. Consequently, the clearance of A will be twice as much as the clearance of B. The clearance (per time) is the same as the flow of fluid across the hole for particle A, whereas this is not true for particle B. Thus, only if the particle moves freely through the hole, can clearance of a particle be used to measure the flow of fluid across the hole.

We measure the GFR in a similar manner by assessing the clearance of a particle. As seen in *Figure 4-8*, the kidney can be represented by the beaker. Fluid is filtered out of the

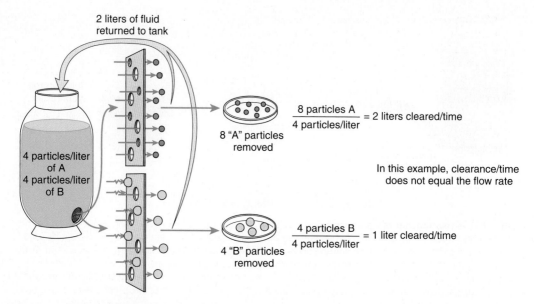

FIGURE 4-7 **The importance of particle size.** Under conditions in which particles are not freely filtered, the rate of flow across the tank's filter is not equal to the clearance of particles per time. In this example, fluid flows out of the tank, but particle B passes less easily than particle A due to its larger size. Thus, despite the same flow rate of fluid across the beaker hole, the clearance for particle B is half that of particle A.

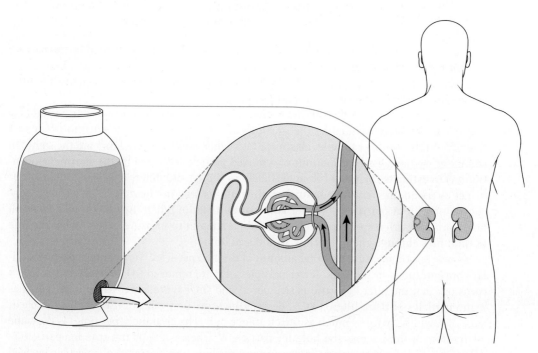

FIGURE 4-8 **Using particle clearance as a marker of glomerular flow.** Clearance of creatinine is used to measure the rate of flow across the collective glomeruli. Since creatinine is filtered freely across the glomerulus, and not handled (i.e., neither secreted nor absorbed) along the length of tubule, a measurement of creatinine clearance can be used to estimate the glomerular filtration rate GFR).

body, across the glomerulus (akin to the hole in the beaker), passing into the tubule. Some particles (albumin, phosphate, calcium) are not filtered freely. Other particles are altered (added or removed) by the tubule (sodium, potassium, bicarbonate).

Thus, although the clearance of all these particles can be measured, that clearance cannot be used to estimate the flow of liquid unless you knew exactly how the particles moved across the glomerular capillary and whether they were reabsorbed or secreted by the tubule. Particles such as creatinine and urea, however, partially meet the above criteria. Both are freely filtered across the glomerulus and are not modified significantly by the tubule under normal conditions. Thus, the clearance of these particles can be used to measure the GFR.

Since the amount of creatinine filtered is not modified as it passes along the tubule, the amount of filtered creatinine is equal to the excreted creatinine in a timed urine collection. Since creatinine is freely filtered, the excreted amount is equal to the GFR multiplied by the serum concentration.

$$\text{Filtered creatinine} = \text{excreted creatinine}$$

$$\text{GFR} \times \text{Serum creatinine concentration} = \text{Urine concentration of creatinine} \times \text{urine Volume}$$

$$\text{GFR} = \frac{\text{Urine concentration of substance} \times \text{urine Volume}}{\text{Plasma concentration of substance}}$$

This formula is the same formula for clearance described above. In the situation where a substance is freely filtered, and not modulated (i.e., not absorbed or secreted) on its passage through the tubules, clearance of that substance is the same as the GFR. Inulin is the classic substance used to measure GFR, because it is freely filtered and not affected by the tubules. However, urea and creatinine are used more often clinically. They are both freely filtered, and although they are slightly modulated by the tubules, the changes in the quantities of these substances are small.

To measure an individual's GFR, a 24-hr urine collection is required. By collecting all the urine over a 24-hr period, one can calculate the amount of filtered creatinine or urea per day. Dividing this amount by the serum creatinine (or urea) concentration gives the individual's daily GFR.

There is another condition that must be present for this calculation to represent GFR accurately—the individual must be in "steady state." This means that the renal function is stable and that the amount of substance (i.e., creatinine) being produced is the same as the amount of substance being eliminated. If this is not true (i.e., more creatinine is being produced than eliminated), the plasma creatinine will be rising throughout the day. If you are going to use this equation in non–steady-state conditions, you must make the collection of the urine during a very short period of time (e.g., minutes rather than a day) to ensure that the plasma creatinine accurately reflects the concentration at the time of the urine collection.

?

THOUGHT QUESTION 4-3 We have assumed that creatinine and urea can be used as markers of the GFR because they are freely filtered across the glomerulus, and are not modulated by the more distal tubules. In reality, however, this is a slight over-simplification. It turns out that some filtered urea gets reclaimed by the tubules and some creatinine actually gets secreted by the tubules. How will this tubular handling of these substances influence the accuracy of creatinine and urea in estimating the GFR?

With respect to carbon dioxide, a byproduct of aerobic metabolism, the lungs act as an excretory organ. Venous blood returning to the heart carries carbon dioxide produced in the tissue. When the blood reaches the lung, carbon dioxide is cleared from the blood by alveoli that are being ventilated (the alveoli serve a role that is similar to the glomerulus with regard to this waste product). The equation for carbon dioxide elimination from the lung is analogous to the clearance equation for creatinine in the kidney.

$$\text{Lung:} \quad \text{Alveolar Ventilation} \propto \frac{CO_2 \text{ production}}{PaCO_2}$$

Alveolar ventilation (the number of L/min of air that enter and exit alveoli that are also receiving blood flow via the pulmonary capillaries) is analogous to creatinine clearance. Carbon dioxide production is analogous to the 24-hr urine creatinine collection (urine creatinine concentration multiplied by the volume of urine collected), and the partial pressure of CO_2 in the arterial blood is analogous to the plasma creatinine concentration.

As with creatinine clearance, this relationship assumes steady-state conditions. If disease processes reduce alveolar ventilation, the $PaCO_2$ rises until a new steady-state condition is established and CO_2 elimination is again equal to the amount of CO_2 produced.

ADEQUACY OF CLEARANCE

It is important to realize that ultimately we are more concerned about our ability to remove waste products in the context of how much we make every day—is the clearance of a particle effective in light of the amount of that particle produced? For instance, imagine two individuals each of whom has a GFR of 180 L/day, thus completely clearing 180 L of fluid daily of urea. The first individual is a 135-kg man who eats 160 g of protein per day, whereas the second is a 68-kg grandmother who does not eat much protein at all. Urea is a byproduct of protein metabolism; the large man is producing far more urea each day than the grandmother. A clearance of 180 L, therefore, is much less in the big man, *relative to what he needs to clear* with a huge daily production of urea and a large total body volume, than in the frail grandmother, *relative to what she needs* given her much smaller body and reduced production of urea.

To account for these differences, clearance is sometimes discussed in the context of the volume of distribution of the particle being removed. In human physiology, we often discuss clearances of urea. Since urea is a non-charged particle and freely crosses all membranes, its volume of distribution is equal to total body fluid. In the example above, the 135 kg man has a volume of distribution of urea of 81 L. The grandmother's volume of distribution is 41 L. Thus, if both have a clearance of 180 L/day, the man clears a volume of fluid equal to his whole volume of distribution of urea approximately twice each day, whereas the woman does so nearly four times. Her system is much more effective than his, relative to total body volume, despite the same total clearance.

 Use Animated Figure 4-5 (Adequacy of Clearance) to compare clearance relative to total body water (the volume of distribution of urea) between the 68-kg grandmother and the 135-kg man. As you run the clearance animation, notice how, despite the same volume of fluid cleared per time, the smaller woman clears her total body water more quickly than the man clears his. If each person is thought of as a tank, as depicted here, the woman in this particular example is more effective at clearing her tank, as measured by the number of times per day she is able to do this.

On an average, healthy individuals clear their volume of distribution of urea four times daily. In other words, the volume of distribution of urea, which is basically total body water, passes through the kidney, is filtered, and then reclaimed, four times daily. It is constantly recirculating, and is effectively cleaned four times a day. This constant cycling is necessary since the cells are continuously making waste products (like the fish in chapter one), and to keep the concentration of waste low, the kidneys must constantly filter out waste.

This principle of "relative effectiveness" of a given clearance is embodied in the concept of the overall **adequacy of clearance**, which is defined as the clearance divided by the volume of distribution. This is calculated by the simple formula,

$$\text{Adequacy} = \frac{\text{Clearance}}{\text{Volume of distribution}}$$

This term is often used to describe how much clearance is being delivered to patients on dialysis. In that setting, the native kidneys no longer work, and the patient is relying on an artificial dialyzer membrane. Therefore, in this case, the clearance is not the GFR; instead, it is a descriptive term used to describe the intrinsic filtering capacity of the dialysis process. However, the Kt/v (where K equals the dialyzer's intrinsic filtering capacity, t is the time during which the person is connected to the dialyzer, and v is the volume of distribution) still describes the adequacy of the amount of cleared fluid relative to the patient's volume of fluid that can be cleared.

USING THE SERUM CREATININE CONCENTRATION AS A MARKER OF GFR

We have described the process of defining the GFR based on the collection of waste products. The total amount of waste cleared per time (Urine concentration of waste multiplied by Volume of urine per unit time), divided by the fluid waste concentration (P), is a measure of clearance. Since urea and creatinine are freely filtered across the glomerulus, and not overly modified by the tubules, clearance of these particles provides a good marker of GFR. Collecting urine over 24 hours to make this measurement, however, is not an easy process, and clinically not useful given its burdensome nature.

Instead of collecting 24 hours of urine to estimate the GFR, it is possible to take a shortcut—one looks at the concentration of creatinine in the serum. This is not a true method for quantitatively measuring the GFR, but it does provide us with an estimate of the GFR without directly measuring it. Large population studies have evaluated how serum creatinine concentration relates to the GFR, and have provided mathematical population-based formulas to describe how to estimate the GFR from a serum creatinine concentration. Since this alleviates the need to perform a 24-hr urine collection, these formulas have become clinically useful in determining a patient's GFR.

The serum concentration of a waste product depends on the balance between the rate of production and the rate of removal. If you add and remove the same number of particles to a beaker per day, the concentration will not be affected, regardless of the rate of particle addition/subtraction. If, however, the rate of addition remains constant, but the rate of removal decreases, then the fluid concentration will increase.

Let us explore this a bit further. We begin with a large tank that has fluid with a concentration of 1 particle/L (see *Figure 4-9A*). You make a small hole in the tank to allow fluid to flow out at a rate of 2 L/day, discarding the filtered particles, and returning the "cleared" fluid. If the concentration of the fluid is 1 particle/L, then in one day, two particles will be

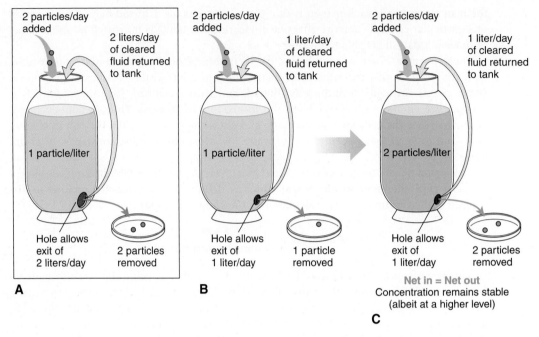

FIGURE 4-9 Equilibrium—the balance between net in and net out determines particle concentration. In Figure 4-9A, the amount of particles put into the beaker per day equals the amount removed, and thus the concentration does not change. In Figure 4-9B, the hole in the bottom of the tank has been reduced by half, so that the rate of flow is half as much. Consequently, the amount removed (1 particle/L × 1 L/day = 1 particle/day) is half as much as is being added to the tank, and the concentration rises. At some point, however, the concentration will reach 2 particles/L (Figure 4-9C). Now, since the concentration of fluid is 2 particles/L, the net particle removal will be 2 particles/day, even though the flow through the hole is still only 1 L/day; a new equilibrium has been reached and the tank's concentration will rise no further. During the time that the concentration of particles in the fluid is rising, we say that the system is *not* in steady-state conditions; when the new equilibrium is achieved, steady-state conditions have been restored.

removed. Rate multiplied by concentration gives the net amount of particles cleared. You add 2 particles/day into the beaker, so that two particles are being removed and added; steady-state conditions are present. The concentration will not change.

Next (Figure 4-9B) you narrow the hole so that only 1 L of fluid exits the tank per day. Now, only one particle will be removed. Since you have not changed how much you are putting into the tank (2 particles/day), the concentration will begin to rise in the tank (you are no longer in steady-state conditions). In fact, the concentration will continue to rise until the amount of particles you put into the tank equals the amount removed (Figure 4-9C). Since the amount removed is simply the flow of liquid multiplied by concentration of particles, and since the flow of liquid has been reduced by half (due to the smaller hole), the concentration of particles in the fluid will double. At the moment the tank's particle concentration doubles, two particles will now be removed even though flow through the hole remains at 50% of its original value. In other words, although the flow rate was cut in half, the same amount of particles is excreted because the concentration has doubled. A new steady-state condition has been established in which the amount added or produced equals the amount removed.

In a similar manner, the absolute serum concentration of urea or creatinine tells us little about the absolute GFR. A serum creatinine of 1 mg/dL in a muscular individual (who produces large quantities of urea) might reflect a GFR of 180 L/day, whereas a serum creatinine of 1 mg/dL in a small cachectic patient (who has little muscle mass and produces small amounts of urea) might reflect severe renal dysfunction. Nevertheless, the serum creatinine is very useful for following changes in the GFR in a particular individual over a time period during which muscle mass and protein intake are not expected to change; under these conditions, it is a clinically useful tool for assessing renal function over time.

This simple example highlights the elements that must be considered if serum creatinine (and blood urea nitrogen) is to be used as a marker of renal clearance. Muscle production of creatinine is usually constant over a time period during which an individual's weight is stable and she has not suffered any muscle damage; thus, the same amount is added to the body per day. The amount of creatinine removed is equal to the GFR times the serum creatinine concentration (rate × concentration). If the GFR falls by half, the serum creatinine concentration must double in order to re-establish a new steady state.

Given the fact that the production of creatinine is typically constant over short periods of time, we can use changes in the serum creatinine concentration as a reflection of the GFR. This relationship, however, does not hold true if the production of creatinine increases, such as in muscle breakdown syndromes, or decreases, such as in cachexia. Similarly, if the production of blood urea nitrogen increases unexpectedly, such as after a large protein meal, the level of urea in the blood will not accurately reflect an individual's GFR.

Figure 4-10 illustrates how the serum creatinine relates to the GFR. Individuals who have larger muscle mass, and thus produce more creatinine, have higher serum creatinine for the same degree of renal function as those with smaller muscle mass.

In both circumstances, however, the serum creatinine rises in proportion to the loss of function. A "normal" serum creatinine is typically considered less than 1.2 mg/dL in most laboratories. However, a level of 1.2 mg/dL might be normal for a very muscular individual, but reflects a huge loss (greater than 50% in some cases) of GFR in a smaller individual. Given the large fluctuation in "normal" serum creatinine, levels should always be interpreted against the individual's baseline normal state.

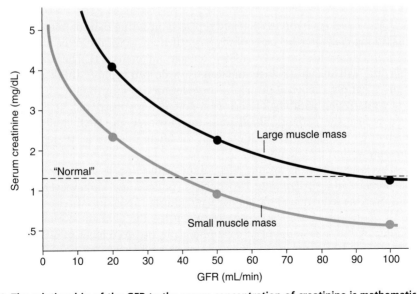

FIGURE 4-10 The relationship of the GFR to the serum concentration of creatinine is mathematically driven. If the amount of creatinine production in the body remains the same, the serum creatinine doubles when the GFR is cut in half. However, the "normal" creatinine depends on the amount of creatinine that a person makes, and can be quite different for different people.

THOUGHT QUESTION 4-4 A muscular individual undergoes a 24-hr urine collection, and is found to excrete 2 g of creatinine per day. Since his serum creatinine remains the same each day, the input of creatinine from muscle breakdown must equal his renal excretion.

A month later, he experiences an episode of renal failure, and loses exactly half of his renal function. At that moment, he is excreting less creatinine than he is making, and his serum creatinine will increase. At what point will his serum creatinine stop rising? If, once his creatinine reaches its new level, and thereafter remains constant, the 24-hr urine collection is reassessed; how much creatinine is he excreting on a daily basis at this time?

THOUGHT QUESTION 4-5 Imagine an experimental model in which you can control the GFR. A young muscular male and an elderly frail lady volunteer for the experiment. Both have a normal starting GFR of about 120 cc/min, or 180 L/day. The muscular male produces about 1.8 g of creatinine daily, and has a starting serum creatinine of 1 mg/dL. The frail woman makes only about 0.9 g of creatinine daily, with a baseline creatinine of 0.5 mg/dL. The experiment begins.

   On week 1, the GFR is reduced by half to 60 cc/min.
   On week 2, the GFR is reduced to 30 cc/min.
   On week 3, the GFR is reduced to 15 cc/min.

What will happen to each subject's creatinine during the subsequent weeks, assuming steady-state conditions are reached in each period?

PUTTING IT TOGETHER

A patient develops hypertension and is placed on a drug that inhibits the angiotensin converting enzyme (this class of drug is called an "ACE inhibitor"). These medications interfere with the body's ability to make angiotensin II. The patient asks you if this drug will alter his kidney function. How do you begin to think about this question? What physiological principles are relevant to this question?

   By interfering with angiotensin II, a potent vasoconstrictor, ACE inhibitors will help reduce the patient's blood pressure. However, the ACE inhibitor affects the efferent glomerular arteriole more than the afferent arteriole, thereby reducing the pressure within the glomerulus.

   This is actually a therapeutic effect of the medication, as the reduction of glomerular pressure in a patient with hypertension protects the kidney over the long term. However, the reduction of the glomerular hydrostatic pressure also leads to a reduction in the glomerular filtration. Since the patient has the same muscle mass, and thus is producing the same amount of creatinine daily, the decrement in GFR, and the corresponding decrement in creatinine excretion, will lead to an increase in the serum creatinine concentration. With time, however, since creatinine excretion is determined by the GFR multiplied by the serum creatinine concentration, the higher serum concentration will eventually compensate for the reduction of GFR, so that excretion once again equals production. At that point, the patient will reach a new steady state, albeit at a higher serum creatinine concentration before starting the medication.

Summary Points

- Our cells are constantly making waste, primarily in the form of urea. This waste distributes across our total body fluid.
- To prevent the accumulation of waste products within our body, our kidneys filter waste from the fluid traversing the capillary loop; this filtrate enters the urinary space. Thereafter, waste-free filtrate is reclaimed, leaving the waste to be eliminated in the urine. The net result is excretion of metabolic byproducts and preservation of the body's vital electrolytes and water.
- The GFR equals the flow (mL/min) of filtrate that exits from the capillary loop into the urinary space.
- The GFR is determined by the balance within the glomerular capillary of outward hydrostatic pressure and the inward oncotic force.
- Unlike other capillaries within the body, the glomerular capillary loop is a high-pressure low-resistance system, allowing the maintenance of a strong outward driving force along its length; this results in net loss of fluid from the capillary.
- Due to the fact that the filtrate does not contain protein (which cannot pass through the glomerular capillary) and the high *filtration fraction*, the inward oncotic force increases along the length of the capillary, so that a *filtration equilibrium* is eventually reached.
- The myogenic reflex allows the kidney to autoregulate its blood flow; this serves as a protective mechanism to maintain the GFR at a relatively constant level despite changes in systemic blood pressure.
- The rennin–angiotensin system is an important modulator of the GFR; activation of this system primarily leads to vasoconstriction of the efferent arteriole, which sustains appropriate glomerular capillary pressure in the setting of hypotension.
- Clearance refers to the amount of fluid that is totally cleared of a particular substance.
- Clearance is calculated by comparing the amount of substance filtered in relation to its starting concentration. The basic formula for clinical measurement of clearance is: clearance = UV/P.
- The amount of clearance relative to the volume of distribution of waste is termed the "adequacy" of clearance, and describes the relative effectiveness of the process by which the kidney removes toxic byproducts of metabolism.
- If a particle is freely filtered across the glomerulus, and is neither absorbed nor secreted by the tubule, then the clearance of that particle per unit time equals the GFR.
- Serum creatinine is a useful clinical marker of GFR.

Answers TO THOUGHT QUESTIONS

4-1. Although the afferent and the efferent arterioles do indeed act as resistors in series, there is one major reason why the efferent arteriole constriction does not lead to a significant decrease in flow through the afferent arteriole: the circuit is open, not closed. In other words, the effect of efferent arteriole constriction is felt within the capillary loop, stimulating filtration, thus dispersing any hydrostatic pressure changes. The glomerulus has low resistance to filtration and is, therefore, almost like a pressure valve; changes in pressure in the capillary are "blown off" by generating a filtrate.

4-2. The loss of some glomerular tufts will reduce the overall number of capillaries in parallel, thereby reducing the capacity of the circuit and increasing the resistance across the capillary plexus. This will be associated with an increase of pressure within the remaining tufts.

There are two possible outcomes to this event. On the one hand, the increase in capillary resistance might lead to decreased renal blood flow. On the other hand, the increased capillary pressure might increase the GFR.

Typically, in many human diseases, the latter occurs. Despite the loss of units available for filtration, the remaining capillary loops experience increasing hydrostatic pressure, which leads to increased filtration. Hyperfiltration often occurs early in renal disease processes. Although the GFR may be sustained by this mechanism, this compensatory mechanism occurs at the expense of increased intraglomerular pressure. Prolonged elevations of intraglomerular pressure can lead to further damage to the glomeruli, perpetuating renal damage. Thus, in early renal disease processes, glomerular pressure may increase, sustaining the overall GFR, despite loss of functioning renal units. Renal blood flow probably does not change. With continued damage; however, the GFR eventually falls.

4-3. In calculating the GFR, we are simply dividing the amount of filtered substance by the serum concentration in order to calculate the rate of filtration. We use the urine concentration multiplied by the urine volume to assess total filtered substance. This holds true only if the tubules do not alter the amount of substance, i.e., do not secrete the substance into the tubule or absorb the substance from the tubule.

In some scenarios, urea gets reclaimed along the tubule. In this setting, the disappearance of urea from the tubular fluid due to tubular reclamation will falsely underestimate the GFR, as it "seems" as less urea has been filtered. Conversely, in some scenarios, creatinine gets secreted along the tubule, so that it "seems" as if more creatinine is being filtered than actually occurs. Therefore, urea-based formulas have a tendency to underestimate the GFR, whereas creatinine-based formulas have the tendency to overestimate GFR. Typically, these inaccuracies are worse in the settings of severe renal failure. In that case, the average of a urea- and a creatinine-based GFR estimation is used; the overestimation and underestimation of the GFR from the two techniques, when combined, balance each other out.

4-4. The man loses half of his renal function. Initially, his excretion of creatinine, which is simply GFR multiplied by plasma concentration of creatinine, falls by half. At that point in time, therefore, he is putting more creatinine into the blood (from muscle breakdown) than he is excreting from the blood (from renal excretion).

Consequently, his serum creatinine will rise. As the concentration rises, however, renal excretion (GFR multiplied by plasma concentration of creatinine) increases too, so that, at some point, the amount of creatinine excreted will once again equal the amount produced.

In this individual, since his GFR was reduced by half, his serum creatinine concentration will eventually double. At that point, however, creatinine production equals creatinine excretion. So, unless he has an unexpected loss of muscle mass, his second 24-hr urine collection will still measure 2 g of creatinine.

4-5. The creatinine of both individuals will double with each decrement of GFR (*Table 4-1*).

TABLE 4-1					
		BASELINE	WEEK 1	WEEK 2	WEEK 3
Creatinine (mg/dL)	Man	1	2	4	8
	Woman	0.5	1	2	4

The importance of this question illustrates the difficulty of using serum creatinine as an estimation of GFR. Since muscle mass is not often known in clinical medicine, the relationship of a single measurement of serum creatinine concentration to underlying renal filtration is not clear. In this example, a serum creatinine of 1 mg/dL is normal for the muscular male, yet the same level underscores a huge loss of function in the frail woman. Most clinical laboratories define "normal" creatinine based on large population-based studies, and an increase of creatinine from 0.5 mg/dL to 1.0 mg/dL, might still be interpreted and reported as "normal" function when, in fact, she has lost half of her kidney function. Thus, interpreting the serum creatinine concentration is not always straightforward and requires careful correlation without clinical information available to you.

Review Questions

DIRECTIONS: Each of the numbered items or incomplete statements in this section is followed by answers or by completions of the statement. Select the ONE lettered answer or completion that is BEST in each case.

1. The widely available class of medications termed NSAIDs (non-steroidal anti-inflammatory drugs) cause vasoconstriction of the afferent arteriole. What would you expect a patient's creatinine to do after taking several doses of NSAIDs for a week?

    A. Increase
    B. Decrease
    C. No change

2. The class of anti-hypertensive medications called angiotension converting enzyme (ACE) Inhibitors lead to dilation of the efferent arteriole. How will the serum creatinine change for patients on these medications?

    A. Increase
    B. Decrease
    C. No change

3. A patient taking NSAIDs and using an ACE Inhibitor develops diarrhea after travelling abroad. The combination of these medications alters the risk of renal failure in which way?

    A. Higher
    B. Lower
    C. No change

4. Since creatinine is freely filtered by the glomerulus and not secreted or reabsorbed by the tubule, it can be used to estimate the GFR. Some commonly used medications can cause tubular secretion of creatinine. If a patient is taking one of these medications, will the use of excreted creatinine as a marker of GFR still be accurate?

    A. Yes
    B. No, excreted creatinine will underestimate the true GFR
    C. No, excreted creatinine will overestimate the true GFR

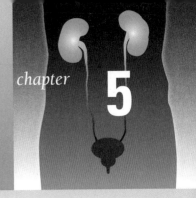

chapter

5

Reclaiming the Filtrate
Tubular Function

LEARNING OBJECTIVES

By the end of this chapter, you should be able to:

- characterize the basic architecture of the renal tubule.
- describe how water moves across tubular epithelial cells.
- describe the distribution of tight junction proteins and aquaporins throughout the renal tubule.
- describe how solute particles move across tubular epithelial cells.
- communicate the importance of the Na/K ATPases in generating a vector of electrochemical force.
- describe the individual proteins responsible for sodium, bicarbonate, chloride, phosphate, and glucose reclamation.
- outline the different segments of the renal tubule and detail which transport proteins are found within each segment.

Introduction

In Chapter 2, you learned that most cell membranes in the body as well as the endothelial layer lining the body's blood vessels form semipermeable barriers, which permit passage of water and select particles. Yet as discussed in Chapter 3, the epithelial barrier of the renal tubule is notably different. It has the potential to be a fully impermeable membrane. Under certain conditions, neither small particles nor water can pass across the renal tubule.

To achieve this impermeable state, the tubule has several important structural traits. First, the plasma membranes of the individual cells lining the tubule have unique architectural modifications that "waterproof" the cell. Specialized lipids within the membrane bilayer prevent the movement of even the smallest molecules across the cell membrane. In addition, to prevent fluid from moving between neighboring cells, interlocking proteins create "watertight" junctions that connect the epithelial cells. The combination of these lipids within the cell membrane, and the tight junction proteins between cells, creates a unique impermeable barrier.

There are other sites of impermeable epithelial layers in the body, most notably the bladder and the skin. The bladder is predominantly a urine holding receptacle while the skin functions to prevent the loss of body fluid to the surrounding elements. Both create a barrier to the movement of fluid. The renal tubule, however, has the incredible responsibility of moving almost 180 L of fluid across its membrane daily. To eliminate excess water and electrolytes, as well as toxic products of metabolism, the glomeruli within the kidneys filter huge amounts of fluid. For the body to survive, however, it must then reabsorb most of that filtrate along the tubules, leaving only the toxins and excess water and solutes to be removed in the urine. Almost all of the glomerular filtrate must be transported from the tubular lumen, across the tubular epithelial cells, and into the interstitial fluid of the body. Thus, despite its intrinsic impermeability, the tubules must possess mechanisms to transport both water and particles efficiently. In addition, these mechanisms need to be regulated in order to respond to the needs of the body, which vary depending on what is ingested from and lost to the environment.

Several important modifications within the renal tubular epithelium facilitate these processes. Transporter proteins within the membranes of epithelial cells allow the transcellular movement of molecules across cell membranes. In addition, specialized proteins between cells control the paracellular movement of molecules; the presence and conformational nature of tight junction proteins control the movement of molecules between neighboring cells. As filtrate flows along the renal tubule, these proteins act in a coordinated manner to move particles across cell membranes or between cells, from the tubular lumen back into the body. There are several different families of transporter proteins, about which you will learn in this chapter, each of which has its own carrier molecule and specific function within the tubule. Their presence and activity within different segments of the tubule ultimately determine the function of that segment.

We are about to take a conceptual journey along the path of a single tubule, focusing on the important protein transporters of each segment. Because each segment expresses a unique complement of transporter proteins, each segment transports particles and water differently; the final goal is to ensure that the body's balance of sodium, glucose, potassium, and other particles, along with water, is optimal. By the end of this journey, we hope you will understand the basic molecular machinery of the renal tubule and the processes by which the majority of the glomerular filtrate is reclaimed. To appreciate the effects of many disease processes and the drugs that are used to treat them, you must have a strong foundation in these concepts. In future chapters, with the knowledge of how the individual tubule segments function together to create the final urine, we will focus on how these transporter proteins are regulated and how this regulation permits the kidney to alter the composition of the urine and of the body fluids.

Water Movement Across the Tubule

The kidney can create urine that is more concentrated (up to 1,200 mOsm/kg) or more dilute (down to 50 mOsm/kg) than the plasma (285 mOsm/kg). To do this, individual tubule segments must be able to transport sodium without water and water without sodium. In other epithelia, sodium and water are transported so that the osmolality of the fluid on both sides of the epithelium is the same. To separate the movements of sodium and water, the renal tubule must have some segments that have extremely low water permeabilities and other segments with extremely high water permeabilities; the former permit sodium reclamation without water, whereas the latter allows water movement to follow sodium movement.

How do renal epithelia block the movement of water? Since net movement of water across the tubule is determined by passage via paracellular and transcellular pathways, we must focus on each possible route. Transcellular movement of water is prevented by unique modifications of the apical membranes of specialized epithelial cells. These cell membranes are tightly packed with lipids, in essence, "repelling" or blocking water movement through the lipid bilayer. Paracellular movement is determined by the presence or the absence of tight junctions between cells, which retard water movement. For example, in the thin descending limb, there is a relative paucity of tight junction proteins, and consequently, paracellular water movement occurs freely. However, in the thick ascending limb and the collecting duct, the presence of abundant tight junction proteins prohibits paracellular water movement.

Since tubular epithelial cells are intrinsically impermeable to water, moving water across the transcellular route requires specific water transporters. These water transporters, termed **aquaporins**, are specific for water movement and do not allow particles to pass. Aquaporins are a large class of proteins, with several different types described. They are embedded into cell membranes and specifically conduct water molecules while preventing the passage of other molecules. Although water movement across a cell membrane was thought historically to occur passively via small membrane "pores," we have learned that water movement is much more complex. The presence of aquaporins greatly enhances the speed and the efficiency with which water molecules may pass and greatly enhances the water permeability of any membrane. Aquaporin I, the first to be discovered, is found in the membranes of red blood cells. It is also expressed in the membranes of the cells lining the proximal tubule and thin descending segment. Aquaporin II is found within the apical membrane of the collecting duct cells, whereas aquaporins III and IV are found on the basolateral membrane of the collecting duct.

In summary, as shown in *Figure 5-1*, the net water permeability of the renal tubule is determined by two factors: the presence or absence of tight junctions (controlling paracellular movement), and the presence of aquaporin channels, which modify the intrinsic impermeability of tubular membranes (controlling transcellular movement). When the distribution of water channels is combined with the distribution of tight junctions, a full understanding of the tubule's total water permeability emerges. Although the proximal tubule has many tight junctions, it also has extensive aquaporin I channels, which make it permeable to water. However, the ascending limb of the tubule has the greatest concentration of tight junctions and no aquaporins and thus is completely impermeable.

Use Animated Figure 5-1 (Water Permeability) to inspect the distribution of aquaporin channels and tight junctions, as well as to get an overview of water permeability along the length of the renal tubule. Note how the water permeability of the collecting duct can vary, as described below.

The collecting duct permeability is unique, primarily because of the presence of aquaporin II. Unlike other aquaporins, aquaporin II is subject to regulation, i.e., permeability of this segment of the tubule is subject to control mechanisms responding to the needs of the body for water. Aquaporin II is regulated by the hormone **antidiuretic hormone**, or **ADH** (sometimes called vasopressin because of its secondary role in regulating vascular tone).

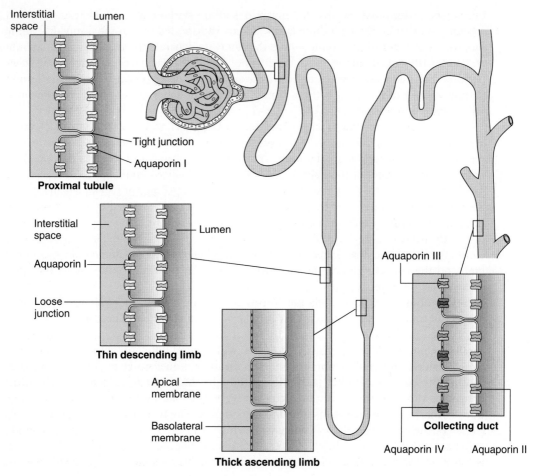

FIGURE 5-1 Water permeability of the renal tubule. Given that the apical membrane of the renal tubule has important modifications that make it water impermeable, water cannot flow across the cell membrane unless there are specific water channels, called aquaporins, inserted into the membrane. Water movement between neighboring cells can only occur if the cells do not have tight junctions. Thus, the water permeability of the tubule is determined by the presence or absence of both aquaporins and tight junctions. The presence of aquaporins makes the proximal tubule water permeable. The absence of aquaporins and the presence of tight junctions make the thick ascending limb impermeable. Aquaporin II is unique in that it can be regulated (whereas other aquaporins are constitutively expressed). The presence or absence of aquaporin II in the collecting duct determines its water permeability.

Under certain stimuli (to be discussed in detail in Chapter 7), ADH is released by the brain and, upon reaching the kidney, stimulates the expression of aquaporin II in the apical membrane of the collecting duct. Moving the aquaporin channel along its production chain, from cell nucleus to endoplasmic reticulum, and finally to the Golgi complex where it is packed for transport to the cell membrane, is a complex multistep process.

Since the expression of the tight junctions and aquaporins I, III, and IV is fixed, the water permeability characteristics of most of the tubule's segments are predictable. The proximal tubule, thin descending limb, and distal convoluted tubule are water permeable; the thick ascending limb is not. However, the permeability of the collecting duct, as noted above, depends on the presence of aquaporin II, which is regulated by ADH. The importance of this ability to control the water permeability of the collecting tubule will become clear in the coming chapters.

Although aquaporins provide a pathway for water movement across the membrane, they do not provide the force to move the water. In the kidney, this force is provided by an osmotic gradient. In order for water to be reclaimed, a solute gradient must generate the osmotic force to pull water through the open aquaporin channels. Along parts of the tubules, reclamation of solutes creates concentration microgradients, so that water will follow. In the collecting duct, a different type of concentration gradient is established. This process of moving solutes across the tubule will be explored next. The mechanisms underlying the creation of a concentration gradient along the collecting duct will be detailed in Chapter 7.

Solute Movement Across the Tubule

Having examined how the intrinsic architecture of the renal tubule determines water permeability, we will now investigate the kidneys regulation of reabsorption of solutes. Since small charged particles flow freely across the glomerulus, the concentration of small particles within the first part of the tubules mirrors that of serum. Thus, if 180 L is delivered to the tubules daily, with a concentration of sodium that is the same as serum (say 140 meq/L), approximately 25,000 meq of sodium reaches the tubule daily. There are also about 18,000 mmol of chloride, 4,500 mmol of bicarbonate, 900 mmol of glucose, and 720 mmol of potassium. Reclaiming all this solute is indeed a challenge! Moreover, as discussed in Chapter 2, filtrate passes from the high-pressure (hydrostatic pressure) system within the glomerular capillaries into the low-pressure system of the tubules. There is no hydrostatic gradient to drive solute reclamation, i.e., movement of molecules from tubule to the renal interstitium.

The tubules are charged with the process of reclaiming thousands of sodium, chloride, potassium, calcium, and other small electrolytes on a daily basis. This must occur across an intrinsically impermeable barrier and without the benefit of a pressure gradient. How this process occurs is discussed in this section. We will begin with the power workhorse of the tubules, the Na/K ATPase, which generates the driving force for this process. We will then proceed with a description of the unique transport proteins in each segment of the tubules and outline how these proteins determine that segment's function. Based on the presence of the cell Na/K ATPases, and the unique membrane proteins, each segment creates a distinct electrical and chemical gradient that facilitates the process of tubular solute reclamation.

THE Na/K ATPase WORKHORSE

The Na/K ATPase is made up of two subunits (α and β) and is expressed in virtually all mammalian cells. It plays a crucial role in maintaining the ionic concentration within cells by creating an electrical and chemical gradient that not only determines the cell's resting membrane potential but also controls key cellular mechanisms and functions. The alpha subunit is composed of 10 segments spanning the cell membrane. It functions as a sodium pump. By binding to ATP, three intracellular sodium ions are captured. Subsequent hydrolysis of the ATP molecule phosphorylates the cytoplasmic loop, inducing a conformational change and extruding the three sodium ions from within the cell to the extracellular space. In exchange, two extracellular potassium ions are moved into the cell. The inward flux of the potassium leads to dephosphorylation of the cytoplasmic loop, shutting off the pump's activity. The beta unit functions as a molecular chaperone, interacting with external stimuli and regulating how the alpha unit is folded into the cell membrane. In summary, the Na/K ATPase exchanges three positive sodium ions for two positive potassium ions. The movement of three Na^+ ions out of the cell in exchange for two K^+ ions leads to a negative voltage inside of the cell relative to the outside and causes the cell to have a potassium concentration in the range of 150 meq/L and a sodium concentration in the range of 10

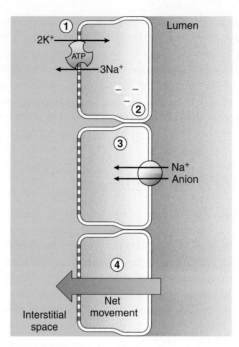

FIGURE 5-2 The Na/K ATPase "workhorse." The Na/K ATPase is situated on the basolateral side of renal tubule epithelial cells. Because it exchanges three Na^+ ions for two K^+ ions, it creates a low intracellular sodium concentration and a negative charge. This creates a vector of electrochemical force that spans the epithelial cell from tubular lumen to interstitium. The placement of transporters within the apical membrane allows Na^+ to flow from the tubule into the cell, down its electrochemical gradient. The movement of many anions is coupled to the movement of sodium.

to 30 meq/L. By contrast, the extracellular fluid has a potassium concentration of 4 meq/L and a sodium concentration of 140 meq/L.

ELECTROCHEMICAL GRADIENT ALONG THE TUBULE

In most cells, Na/K ATPase appears on the cell membrane surface and moves ions between the intracellular and the extracellular space; the cell functions with a uniform cell surface, i.e., the Na/K ATPase is distributed throughout the cell surface. By contrast, epithelial cells are polarized; the cell surface facing the "outside world" has different characteristics than the one in contact with the body's internal environment. In the renal tubule, Na/K ATPase appears only on the basolateral or blood side of the cell and never on the apical or urinary side of the cell. By creating a low intracellular sodium and negative voltage, the Na/K ATPase provides an electrochemical gradient that drives the movement of sodium from the urinary space across the apical membrane into the cell. By coupling transport of other solutes to the entry of sodium, the cell uses the energy of the electrochemical gradient created by Na/K ATPase to drive the transport of other solutes. As seen in *Figure 5-2*, this force eventually is translated across the whole epithelial cell, creating a net vector of electrochemical force from lumen to interstitium.

The ATP needed to power the Na/K ATPase is generated by mitochondria, which lie immediately adjacent to the pump molecules, along the basolateral membrane. The highest density of Na/K ATPase activity is found in the proximal tubule, thick ascending limb, and distal convoluted tubule. It is therefore not surprising that the kidney consumes an enormous amount of oxygen per gram of tissue. Although the total mass of the kidneys is only 0.5% of the total body weight, they consume approximately 7% of the oxygen uptake of the entire body. Approximately 20% of the cardiac output perfuses the kidney, thereby maintaining a relatively high renal tissue oxygen concentration, which facilitates the oxidative metabolism needed to provide energy for the process of reclaiming all these particles. Any interruption of the flow of blood and oxygen to the kidney leads to prompt damage to proximal tubules and thick ascending limbs, resulting in acute renal failure.

The Proximal Tubule

The proximal tubule must reclaim 60% to 80% of the constant deluge of solute-laden filtrate it receives. Of the approximately 180 L that is filtered across the glomerulus daily, only about 50 L reaches more distal segments of the renal tubule. Thus, the proximal tubule reclaims about 130 L/day. It has several unique architectural features that support this function, as illustrated in *Figure 5-3*.

It is the most abundant of the tubule system; it ranges in length from 12 to 24 mm, has a typical diameter of 50 to 65 microns, and is characterized by extensive twisting and coiling upon itself. In total, the proximal tubules comprise the majority of the renal cortex. Furthermore, the epithelial cells lining the tubule have highly redundant microvilli, which greatly expand the surface area for reabsorption. The basolateral membrane also has many infoldings, which add surface area for Na/K ATPase and volume within the cell for the mitochondria needed to power the pump.

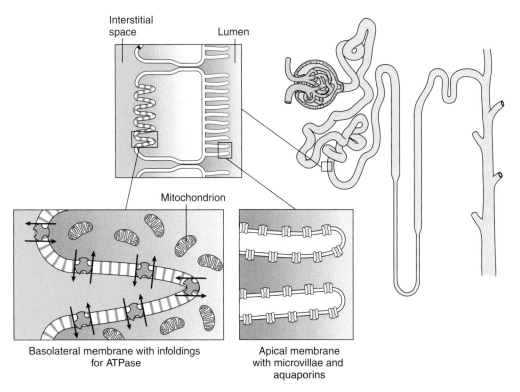

Interstitial space | Lumen

Mitochondrion

Basolateral membrane with infoldings for ATPase

Apical membrane with microvillae and aquaporins

FIGURE 5-3 The proximal tubule. The proximal tubule is the longest segment of the renal tubule, with many infoldings. Along the basolateral membrane, there are many Na/K ATPases to provide energy for particle reclamation. Mitochondria are abundant in these proximal epithelial cells to support the Na/K ATPases. In addition, the proximal epithelia cells have microvilli along their apical surface, further increasing their surface area. These structural modifications are important to enable most of the filtered load to be reclaimed in the proximal tubule.

Absorptive processes in the proximal tubule focus primarily on sodium, chloride, bicarbonate, phosphate, and glucose, whereas retrieval of potassium is relegated to more distal parts of the tubule. Almost 80% of the filtered $NaHCO_3$ and 50% of the filtered NaCl is absorbed within the proximal tubule. The electrochemical gradient created by the Na/K ATPase provides the energy for tubular reclamation. As we will learn next, specific apical proteins provide the pathway for individual solute movement. Although each transport protein has unique conformational specificity for a particular solute, they all share a common dependence on the electrochemical gradient derived from sodium and potassium exchange to effect movement of particles from the lumen to the interstitial fluid. Some of the transporters piggyback movement of a particular solute onto the movement of sodium. **Cotransporters** are proteins that move a molecule in conjunction with a sodium ion. There are also **exchangers** that move a molecule in the opposite direction of sodium. Cotransporters and exchangers differ from channels; channels allow movement of a particle down its gradient, without depending on sodium movement. Nevertheless, all these proteins capitalize on the electrochemical gradient initially established by the Na/K ATPases. In all figures in this book, ATPases, channels, cotransporters, and countertransporters are each represented with a unique symbol, as seen in *Legend 5-1*.

THE Na/H EXCHANGERS

The Na/H exchangers (NHEs) are proteins found along the apical membrane of the proximal tubule, and they reclaim one sodium ion from the lumen in exchange for one hydrogen ion. The exchange of sodium ion for a hydrogen ion has two important consequences: sodium reabsorption and bicarbonate reclamation, as illustrated in *Figure 5-4*. Since this exchange process must occur repetitively to reclaim sodium, two issues arise. First, how does the body provide sufficient amounts of intracellular hydrogen to feed the exchange,

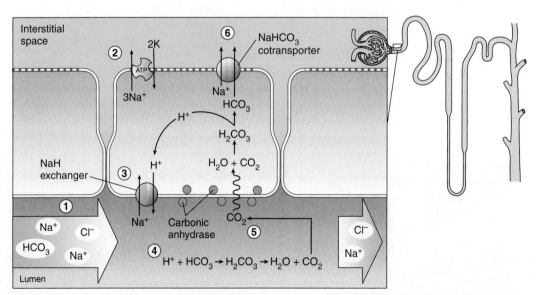

FIGURE 5-4 The sodium–hydrogen exchanger (NHE). (1) The initial filtrate that passes across the glomerulus and enters the proximal tubule has a concentration of sodium, chloride, and bicarbonate similar to serum. (2) The Na/K ATPases on the basolateral membrane create the electrostatic force for particle reclamation. (3) The NHE on the apical membrane exchanges a sodium ion for a hydrogen ion. (4) The extruded hydrogen ion instantly combines with bicarbonate, a reaction catalyzed by the enzyme carbonic anhydrase. (5) This leads to the formation of carbon dioxide, which passes down its concentration gradient from tubule into the cell. There, again in the presence of carbonic anhydrase, it splits into hydrogen and bicarbonate. The hydrogen ion recirculates into the tubule via the NHE. (6) The bicarbonate is extruded across the basolateral wall by a $NaHCO_3$ cotransporter. The net effect is reclamation of sodium and bicarbonate from the tubular lumen.

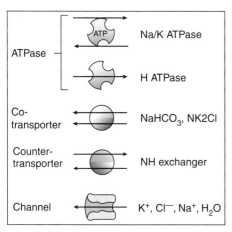

LEGEND 5-1

ATPase: Examples include the NaK ATPase

Cotransporter: Ions are moved in the same direction. Examples include the NK2CL, NaCl, and NaHCO₃ cotransporters

Countertransporter: Ions move in the opposite direction. Examples include the NHE

Channel: Examples include water channels, sodium channels, and potassium channels

and secondly, what happens to all the hydrogen ions that enter the lumen of the tubule? Since hydrogen ions lead to an acidic environment, they must be transformed into, or buffered with, another molecule.

The presence of **carbonic anhydrase**, both within the proximal tubule and along its brush border, resolves these two important challenges. Carbonic anhydrase catalyzes the conversion of carbon dioxide and water to bicarbonate and a hydrogen ion, as seen in the reaction below.

$$CO_2 + H_2O \leftrightarrow H_2CO_3 \leftrightarrow HCO_3^- + H^+$$

The catalytic rate is incredibly fast, usually in the range of 10^5 reactions per second. Thus, the hydrogen ion extruded into the lumen combines with filtered bicarbonate and is transformed into CO_2 and water. This CO_2, as a volatile gas, readily diffuses across the apical membrane into the cell lumen, combines with water to form carbonic acid, and once again, in the presence of carbonic anhydrase, it forms bicarbonate and hydrogen ion. The hydrogen ion recycles through the NHE, and the bicarbonate exits the cell into the interstitial space via a NaHCO₃ cotransporter.

The net effect of this process is to allow hydrogen recycling around the NHE while moving bicarbonate from the lumen back into the interstitial fluid. Thus, as illustrated in *Figure 5-4*, the combination of the NHE and carbonic anhydrase in the apical membrane, along with the basolateral membrane NaHCO₃ cotransporter, leads to net reclamation of sodium and bicarbonate.

Use Animated Figure 5-2 (Proximal Tubule Bicarbonate Reclamation) to review the reactions described above. You can see how the recycling of hydrogen ions is linked to the reclamation of bicarbonate, with carbonic anhydrase and the NHE playing crucial roles in the process.

 THOUGHT QUESTION 5-1 Carbonated drinks fizz slowly upon opening, as the CO₂ comes out of solution. However, as soon as one takes a sip, the fizziness of the liquid in your mouth seems to decrease. Why? How might the presence of carbonic anhydrase in saliva play a role?

THOUGHT QUESTION 5-2 How would the lack of carbonic anhydrase in tubular cells affect sodium and bicarbonate reclamation?

PARACELLULAR CHLORIDE MOVEMENT AND THE CHLORIDE EXCHANGERS

Because of the presence of the NHEs along the proximal tubule, $NaHCO_3$ is avidly absorbed. In the early part of the proximal tubule, there are no chloride transporters. Thus, as the filtrate moves along the proximal tubule, the concentration of chloride increases. Since chloride is freely filtered across the glomerulus, its concentration initially in the tubule is the same as serum, typically about 100 mmol/L. By the time the filtrate has reached the later segment of the proximal tubule, and sodium and water have been reabsorbed from the filtrate, the concentration has risen by about 20% to 120 mmol/L.

The increasing intraluminal chloride concentration provides a chemical gradient that drives chloride movement "passively," i.e., without the need for additional energy expenditure, along the paracellular pathway, down its concentration gradient. Paracellular chloride movement is a major mechanism for chloride reclamation. Specific chloride transport proteins exist, however, within the later parts of the proximal tubule to enable transcellular reclamation of chloride, thereby supplementing this passive process. There are many types of chloride transport proteins, typically in the form of an anion exchanger. One chloride exchanger, termed Pat-1 (from the gene Slc26a6), exchanges one chloride for one of several anions, including formate and/or oxalate.

THE GLUCOSE TRANSPORTERS

Since glucose plays such a critical role in metabolism, its reclamation is a high priority. Glucose, the source of energy for aerobic metabolism, must be transported into all cells within the body. Most commonly, a specific form of glucose transporter, termed **glucose transporter facilitator (GLUT)**, allows the movement of glucose down its concentration gradient. In the presence of insulin, glucose can move across cell membranes. Since glucose is freely filtered across the glomerulus, the concentration of glucose within the tubule is the same as in the interstitium and the blood; consequently, glucose reclamation cannot rely on differences of concentration. Instead, active reclamation is needed to prevent loss of glucose in the urine.

The renal tubule has specific glucose transporter proteins that piggyback glucose transport onto active sodium transport. The negative intracellular voltage and low intracellular sodium powered by the Na/K ATPase provide a strong gradient for sodium flux from the lumen into the cell. To reclaim filtered glucose, **Na^+-coupled glucose transporters (SGLT)** link the movement of Na^+ down its electrochemical gradient to the "uphill" reabsorption of glucose, even when the concentration of glucose inside the cell is higher than that in the tubule's lumen. The glucose absorbed is either used by the cell to supply energy for active transport or transported from inside the cell to the basolateral side via GLUT transporters. Similar pathways function for the reabsorption of amino acids and other organic molecules from the glomerular filtrate.

Several different isoforms within the SGLT family have been identified. In the early proximal tubule, SGLT2 predominates. It is a low-affinity but high-capacity cotransporter. In other words, although it does not tightly bind to glucose molecules, it has the ability to transport large numbers of them. Conversely, in the later part of the proximal tubule, another SGLT cotransporter (termed SGLT1) is present. It is a highly selective transporter, with an affinity for glucose 10 times higher than the SGLT2 of the early proximal tubule, yet it has a lower capacity. Its high-affinity low-capacity nature allows it to scavenge the few residual glucose molecules that were not absorbed earlier. The combination of these transporters makes glucose reabsorption efficient and quite complete. Beyond the proximal tubule, there are no glucose transporters within the apical membrane of the cells lining the renal tubules.

For normal individuals, who filter about 95 mg of glucose per minute across the glomerulus, almost all filtered glucose is reabsorbed within the proximal tubule. If any glucose escapes reclamation in the proximal tubule, it will find its way into the urine, a condition called **glucosuria**. Given the efficiency of proximal tubule reabsorption, normal individuals almost never have glucosuria. Because glucose spills into the urine only when the rate of its filtration exceeds the capacity of the proximal tubule to absorb it, glucosuria usually occurs only when the serum glucose in high, as occurs in diabetes mellitus. Because proximal tubule glucose reabsorption is so complete, testing the urine for glucose can be used to screen for diabetes.

> **?**
>
> **THOUGHT QUESTION 5-3** **A diabetic patient forgets to take his insulin, and his serum glucose levels rise to 400 mg/dL. Will this make him initially urinate more or less than usual? Why?**

As part of the routine evaluation of a patient's urine, the presence of glucosuria is assessed. Typically, a dipstick (a piece of specially treated paper) is placed into the urine, and depending on the amount of glucose detected, it changes color. Since almost no glucose should be in normal urine, any color change suggests an abnormality. As noted above, the most common cause of glucosuria is diabetes. The high serum glucose leads to an increased amount of filtered glucose, overwhelming the absorptive capacity of the proximal tubule. Glucosuria can be seen in pregnancy, often as a consequence of the development of insulin resistance during pregnancy, a condition termed gestational diabetes.

There are several important clinical scenarios, however, in which glucosuria is due to a decrease in the reabsorptive capacity of the proximal tubule. In some patients, the proximal tubule's capacity for glucose reabsorption diminishes, (it can decline by up to 50%) and glucosuria develops despite normal serum glucose. Several disease processes can affect the absorptive capacity of the proximal tubule more broadly, inducing a proximal tubule wasting syndrome in which glucose, phosphate, and other solutes are lost inappropriately. Finally, mutations in the renal glucose transporters, leading to a change in the affinity for glucose or a decrease in the total number of transporters along the proximal tubule, can also lead to glucosuria.

> **?**
>
> **THOUGHT QUESTION 5-4** **In an attempt to discover new treatments for diabetes mellitus, a pharmaceutical company is trying to develop a drug that blocks proximal tubule glucose reclamation. The resulting increase in glucosuria might lead to improvement of serum glucose. They ask your advice as to whether they should attempt to block the SGLT cotransporter or the GLUT transporter? Which would you choose? Why? What might be the side effects of each drug?**

THE PHOSPHATE TRANSPORTERS

Phosphate, which plays a critical role in many metabolic pathways, is freely filtered in the glomerulus and predominantly reabsorbed in the proximal tubule. As with glucose, proximal tubule cells couple the flux of phosphate across the apical membrane to the transport of Na^+ down its electrochemical gradient. The cell deploys a specific **sodium phosphate cotransporter**, called **NaPi IIa** on its apical membrane. As you will learn when you study the hormonal regulation of bone metabolism, the parathyroid gland monitors serum-free calcium levels. When phosphate levels rise, phosphate binds to calcium and lowers the free calcium level. Reduced serum-free calcium triggers the release of parathyroid hormone (PTH) from the parathyroid glands. As one action to restore free calcium toward normal, PTH reduces the numbers of NaPi IIa cotransporters in the proximal tubule apical membrane. This reduction diminishes proximal tubule phosphate reabsorption, leading to phosphate wasting in the urine and a drop in the serum phosphate levels.

EDITOR'S INTEGRATION

The kidney plays an important role in bone metabolism via its contributions to the body's regulation of calcium and phosphate. In addition to being a target organ for PTH action in the proximal tubule, the kidney is essential for the production of the active form of vitamin D, which is critical for the absorption of calcium from the intestine.

?

THOUGHT QUESTION 5-5 The gene that encodes the NaPi IIa protein is called SLC34A1. Certain mutations in this gene lead to a protein that is not as efficient in phosphate reclamation as the normal gene. What type of problems might such a person with such a mutant gene have?

SUMMARY OF FILTRATE COMPOSITION ALONG THE PROXIMAL TUBULE

The actions of the apical transporters described above ultimately determine the composition of the filtrate along the proximal tubule as well as the tubular charge within the lumen. The abundance of NHEs, Na phosphate, and Na glucose cotransporters in this segment of the tubule drives the reabsorption of sodium, bicarbonate, glucose, phosphate, and other molecules, such as citrate, amino acids, and other organic acids.

In the early proximal tubule, chloride is not absorbed, and its concentration increases along the proximal tubule as water and other solutes, such as bicarbonate, are reclaimed. Once the filtrate reaches the later segments of the proximal tubule, however, the presence of chloride anion exchangers allows chloride to move down its concentration gradient from tubular lumen to the interstitial compartment. As these negatively charged chloride ions leave the lumen for the peritubular fluid, the lumen acquires a slight positive charge (estimated at +4 mV), which provides an important force for the paracellular movement of cations. Approximately 50% of filtered potassium, 60% of filtered calcium, and 15% of filtered magnesium are reclaimed in the late proximal tubule due to this electrostatic force.

By the end of the proximal tubule, approximately 67% of the glomerular filtrate has been reclaimed. This process is primarily driven by the movement of sodium bicarbonate and then sodium chloride. Almost 17,000 meq of sodium, 13,300 meq of chloride, and 3,000 meq of bicarbonate are reclaimed within the proximal tubule daily. Because of the presence of aquaporin channels along the proximal tubule, water follows particles. No osmotic gradient develops between the lumen and the surrounding interstitium of the proximal tubule; the osmolality of the fluid in the proximal tubule remains around 300 mOsm/kg. Thus, since 67% of the filtrate particles have been reclaimed, 67% of the filtered water is reclaimed as well—almost 121 L/day. The remaining filtrate then moves into the deeper aspects of the renal tissue, flowing down the descending limb of the Loop of Henle into the medulla, around a hairpin loop, and back up the ascending limb.

Use Animated Figure 5-3 (Proximal Tubule Filtrate Composition) to explore the changes in the composition of the filtrate. The overall size of the stream in the figure and the proportions and sizes of the individual elements of the stream give an idea of the proximal tubule's role in the reclamation of water, ions (other than potassium), and substances such as glucose.

Our journey will continue as the kidney enters a more discriminating region of the tubule in which solute and water can be handled independently.

Descending Limb of the Loop of Henle

Since the nephron reabsorbs over 99% of the glomerular filtrate, and the proximal tubule reabsorbs two-thirds, the nephron distal to the proximal tubule must reabsorb the remaining third (or 60 L/day) of filtrate. The segment immediately following the proximal tubule, the descending limb of the Loop of Henle, has few mitochondria and little Na/K ATPase. Because these cells lack the machinery for active reabsorption, they must use a different mechanism to reabsorb filtrate. The descending limb penetrates deep into the renal medulla. Mechanisms that we will discuss later cause the accumulation of high concentrations of sodium and urea in the interstitium of the medulla; consequently, the interstitial osmolality reaches levels of 600 mOsm/kg or higher. The descending limb is very porous with respect to water and urea. The junctions between the cells are leaky and the cells express abundant water channels (aquaporin I) on their membranes. As the tubular fluid progresses into the descending limb, water moves rapidly across the epithelium until the osmotic gradient between tubular lumen and interstitium dissipates. As a result, of the 60 L of isotonic filtrate that begins the journey down the thin descending limb, approximately 30 L of water exit into the interstitium, leaving about 30 L of hypertonic filtrate to begin the climb up the ascending limb of the Loop of Henle.

 Use Animated Figure 5-4 (Descending Limb Fluid Movement) to explore the changes in the tubular fluid as it moves down the descending limb. Similar to Animated Figure 5-3, the overall size of the stream and the proportions and sizes of the individual elements of the stream give an idea of the role of the descending limb; you can see that water has exited the tubule, leaving a more concentrated (hypertonic) tubular fluid as mentioned above.

Ascending Limb of the Loop of Henle

In contrast to the descending limb, where water is reabsorbed without particles, the ascending limb reabsorbs particles without water. On a daily basis, 30 L of filtrate enter the ascending limb with an osmolality of 600 mOsm/kg (total of approximately 18,000 mOsms). Since 67% of sodium, chloride, and bicarbonate are absorbed in the proximal tubule and there is no particle reclamation in the thin descending limb, approximately 8,250 meq of sodium, 6,500 meq of chloride, and 1,500 meq of bicarbonate arrive in the ascending limb daily (total of 16,250 meq). The remaining particles include potassium, calcium, magnesium, and urea.

The thick ascending limb extracts tremendous amounts of particles from the lumen into the surrounding interstitium. By effectively removing particles while remaining impermeable to water, the thick ascending limb "dilutes" the filtrate, earning it the nickname, "diluting segment." Almost 75% of the particles that enter the ascending limb are reabsorbed along its route. Consequently, by the time the filtrate moves beyond the ascending limb into more distal segments, its concentration has fallen dramatically, typically reaching levels as low as 50 mOsm/L; this is less than 10% of the concentration of the filtrate that entered this segment of the tubule. On a given day, almost 13,500 mOsms must be reclaimed. To accomplish this task of intense particle reclamation, the ascending limb has a very high density of Na/K ATPase along its basolateral membrane. Not surprisingly, per gram of tissue, the thick ascending limb uses more energy than any other section of the kidney. This energy requirement partly explains why the thick ascending limb is particularly at risk for injury in states of renal hypoperfusion or hypoxia; without the oxygen and substrates to support cellular function, tubular damage results.

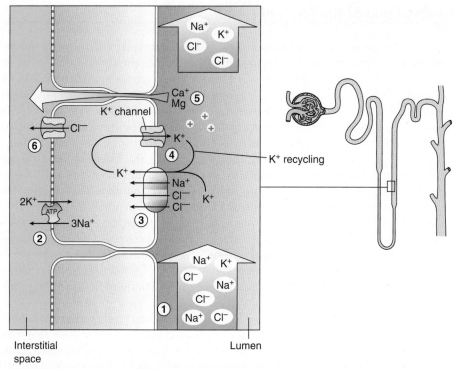

FIGURE 5-5 The thick ascending limb. The NK2Cl cotransporter is located in the apical membrane of the thick ascending limb of the Loop of Henle. (1) Filtrate in the ascending limb has a very high concentration of sodium and chloride, with relatively less potassium. (2) The Na/K ATPase provides the electrostatic gradient (the cell becomes negatively charged relative to the interstitium). (3) The NK2Cl cotransporter couples movement of one sodium and one potassium with two chloride ions. Since this is an equal movement of charged particles, there is electrical neutrality. (4) Potassium recycles back into the tubule via a potassium channel. Given the relatively lower concentration of potassium than sodium in the tubular filtrate, having this potassium recycling is important to provide sufficient potassium ions for the NK2Cl cotransporter to continue functioning. (5) The recycled potassium creates a positive charge in the lumen relative to the cell and the interstitium, which drives the paracellular reclamation of other important cations such as calcium, magnesium, and potassium. (6) The reclaimed chloride ions exits the epithelial cells via basolateral chloride channels.

 Use Animated Figure 5-5 (Thick Ascending Limb Diluting Ability) to view the changes in the tubular fluid as it moves along the thick ascending limb. Similar to earlier figures, the overall size of the stream and the proportions and sizes of the individual elements of the stream give an idea of the role of the thick ascending limb; in contrast to the thin descending limb, you can see that water stays in the tubule while particles exit, leaving a significantly diluted tubular fluid as mentioned above.

THE NK2Cl COTRANSPORTER

The cells lining the thick limb couple reabsorption of Na^+ down its electrochemical gradient to the reclamation of two Cl^- and one K^+ by placing the NK2Cl cotransporter protein on their apical membrane (*Figure 5-5*).

This protein is a member of a large family of transporters that couple a cation to the movement of a chloride ion. By moving two cations along with two anions, this cotransporter moves particles in an electrostatically neutral manner. Basolateral Na/K ATPase generates a negative intracellular voltage and a low intracellular sodium level. NK2Cl allows one Na^+, one K^+, and two Cl^- ions to cross the apical membrane. K^+ subsequently exits the cell via an apical channel ("recycling" into the tubular fluid), while the Cl⁻ exits the basolateral side of the cell via a chloride channel, and the Na⁺ exits via Na/K ATPase. The net effect of these processes is that one positive charge and two negatively charged particles have been reabsorbed from the lumen; this leads to a transepithelial positive voltage (+3 to +10 mV)—the lumen is positively charged relative to the renal interstitium. This positive voltage drives the movement of cations such as Na^+, Ca^{2+}, and Mg^{2+} from the lumen to the basolateral side via specialized tight junctional proteins called claudins. Some potassium exits the cell via potassium channels on the basolateral membrane, contributing to potassium reabsorption.

This ability of the thick ascending limb to reabsorb Ca^{2+} and Mg^{2+} helps regulate serum levels and body stores of these two critical divalent cations. In addition, the unique method used by the thick limb to reabsorb Na^+ can be highly efficient, because two Na^+ ions cross from apical to basolateral side for every one Na^+ ion actually pumped by the Na/K ATPase, i.e., the establishment of the positive charge in the tubular lumen enables Na to be reabsorbed passively as well as via active transport.

For the NK2Cl to function, it must honor the 1:1:2 stoichiometry of the Na^+–K^+–$2Cl^-$ transport. As discussed above, approximately 8,250 meq of sodium and 6,500 meq of chloride are delivered to the ascending limb daily, but only about 240 meq of potassium. The constant recycling of potassium across the apical membrane keeps the cotransporter going.

Animated Figure 5-6 (NK2Cl Cotransporter) shows the mechanisms outlined above. As the animation plays, note how the recycling of K^+ via the apical channel leads to the lumen positivity that drives the movement of other cations.

Because the generation of a lumen-positive voltage drives the paracellular reabsorption of Ca^{2+} and Mg^{2+}, disruption of either the NK2Cl transporter, K^+ recycling, or the basolateral Cl⁻ channel will block reabsorption of these divalent cations.

NK2Cl has several unique features. It can remain active with very low luminal concentrations of sodium and potassium, yet it requires relatively robust chloride concentrations. Thus, the concentration of chloride, rather than sodium or potassium, is rate limiting in the cotransporter's activity. A group of diuretic medications (termed loop diuretics for their site of action on the Loop of Henle) blocks the NK2Cl cotransporter, interfering with the thick ascending limb's ability to reclaim sodium, chloride, and potassium.

The Distal Convoluted Tubule

The distal convoluted tubule begins just after the macula densa and connects the ascending limb to the collecting duct. It is mostly impermeable to water and reclaims about 5% of the filtered sodium. As in the thick ascending limb of the Loop of Henle, this ability to reabsorb solute independently of water contributes to the dilution of urine. Sodium reclamation is accomplished by an electroneutral NaCl cotransporter on the apical membrane of the distal convoluted tubular cells. Energy is supplied by basolateral Na/K ATPases, and chloride egress occurs via a basolateral chloride channel. A class of commonly prescribed diuretics, called thiazides, inhibits sodium chloride reclamation by competing for the chloride site on the apical NaCl cotransporter. By blocking Na reabsorption, the diuretic prevents the tubular fluid from being diluted, which reduces osmotically driven water reclamation in the collecting duct (which will be discussed in the section, The Collecting Duct, later in this chapter).

The distal tubule is also a major site of calcium reabsorption. The exact mechanisms of calcium reclamation are still being worked out. Most likely, a sodium–calcium exchanger on the basolateral membrane moves calcium into the interstitium, allowing calcium to flow from the tubule lumen into the cell via a calcium channel.

In Animated Figure 5-7, you can see how the fluid changes as it moves through the distal convoluted tubule; like the thick ascending limb, the distal convoluted tubule primarily reabsorbs particles without water, thereby further diluting the tubular fluid.

The Collecting Duct

The collecting tubule is the "fine tuner" of the filtrate. It has the unique capacity to respond to a wide variety of external signals and stimuli, including a range of hormones. In many ways the collecting duct is the interface between the tubules and the rest of the body, i.e., its function varies based on the needs of the body. Responding to a variety of stimuli, the collecting duct determines the final composition of the urine and, in doing so, makes the final decision about what is retained or excreted. Consequently, it plays a tremendous role in determining the composition of the body.

There are several different segments of the duct. The collecting tubule, which has a cortical and medullary component, leads into the collecting duct. Although there are some differences in the function of each one of these sections, there are more similarities than differences. For the sake of simplicity, we will call this whole section of the tubule the collecting duct.

There are two distinct types of epithelial cells within the collecting duct: the principal and the intercalated cell. The principal cells play a critical role in sodium reclamation, whereas the intercalated cell is more involved in acid secretion. The intercalated cell will be discussed in Chapter 9.

The principal cell has several important structural modifications that allow it to reclaim sodium in a regulated manner, so that it can respond to the overall sodium needs of the body. We will learn more about this integrated response system in Chapter 6, but for now, let us review the proteins within this cell, as seen in *Figure 5-6*. Like the earlier parts of the tubule, the activity of basolateral Na/K ATPase generates the negative internal voltage and low sodium to drive active sodium reabsorption. Sodium crosses the apical membrane, down its electrochemical gradient, via the Epithelial Na^+ Channel, **ENaC**. ENaC is a unique protein that sits within the apical membrane of the principal cell and has an affinity for sodium. Unlike transporter proteins, for which the entry of Na^+ is coupled directly to the entry of other ions or solutes, Na^+ moves through ENaC alone. The entry of Na^+ from the lumen creates a lumen-negative voltage (as high as –50 mV), which stimulates the secretion of K^+ into the lumen via an apical channel. In addition, the lumen-negative voltage enhances the secretion of H^+ by the adjacent intercalated cells. As we will learn in Chapter 6, volume regulatory hormones such as aldosterone stimulate ENaC activity, enhancing sodium reabsorption, as well as potassium and acid secretion.

    Animated Figure 5-8 (Principal and Intercalated Cells) shows the formation of the large negative voltage in the lumen of the collecting duct as a result of the movement of sodium. You can see how this lumen-negative voltage stimulates potassium secretion by the principal cells and hydrogen ion secretion by the intercalated cells.

Like the thick ascending limb (but unlike the proximal tubule), the collecting duct is inherently impermeable to water; when sodium moves from lumen to cell to the surrounding interstitium, water does not necessarily follow. Unlike the thick ascending limb, however, the collecting duct can become permeable to water when the body is in a water conservation state. As we will continue to learn about in Chapter 7, water will follow in this region of the tubule if aquaporin channels are inserted into the apical membrane of the tubular cells, thereby making the collecting duct water permeable. If they are not present, water does not follow solute in the collecting duct.

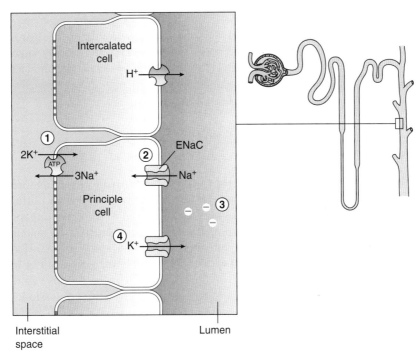

FIGURE 5-6 **The collecting duct.** The epithelial Na channel, or ENaC, is in the apical membrane of the principal cells in the collecting duct. (1) The Na/K ATPase generates the electrochemical gradient (inside of cell has a negative charge relative to interstitium). (2) Sodium passes through the ENaC from lumen into cell. (3) Because sodium is not coupled with another ion, the charge within the lumen becomes negative. (4) This lumen negativity drives secretion of potassium ions from the tubular cell into the lumen. The intercalated cell will be covered more fully in Chapter 9.

The collecting duct differs from the more proximal parts of the tubule in the manner in which electrochemical gradients are established. In the proximal tubule, the electrochemical gradient established by the Na/K ATPase stimulates an electrically neutral movement of ions from the lumen to the renal interstitium. For example, sodium is absorbed with bicarbonate or chloride. The net charge within the lumen does not change dramatically. Similarly, in the thick ascending limb, a Na^+ and a K^+ ion are reabsorbed with two Cl^- ions; although potassium recycling leads to mild lumen positivity, the overall change in the charge of the lumen is small. In contrast, sodium reclamation in the collecting tubule occurs across the apical lumen through an ion channel, not a cotransporter. Thus, sodium flows by itself, without an accompanying anion. As positively charged cations flow from lumen to cell, the lumen becomes negatively charged. This charge may be as much as −50 mV. This negative charge in the lumen has important effects on the handling of other solutes, particularly potassium.

? **THOUGHT QUESTION 5-6** Mutations in the proteins along the tubule lead to disease states that have been well described. The disorders called Bartter and Gitelman disease are characterized by underactivity of the NK2Cl protein and NaCl protein respectively. Liddle syndrome refers to overactivity of the ENaC ion cotransporter.

Describe the clinical consequences you would expect of each disorder based on your knowledge of the physiology of the tubule; specifically, comment on the blood pressure and potassium level that you might find in these patients.

THOUGHT QUESTION 5-7 The Na/K ATPases along the basolateral membrane of all tubular cells generate the electrochemical gradient that facilitates tubular reclamation of the filtered solute. How do the variations in apical membrane biology, specifically types of transporters or channels, affect the apical membrane permeability and thus, ultimately affect the remaining luminal charge and concentration of ions? Trace the tubule from proximal tubule to collecting duct.

Potassium Homeostasis

This chapter has been primarily devoted to describing the molecular machinery that facilitates tubular reclamation of the glomerular filtrate. In this final section of the chapter, we shift focus to describe how the tubule secretes potassium in the collecting duct.

Potassium is a critical ion in human metabolism. Its concentration is maintained within a very narrow margin in the serum, ranging between 3.5 and 5 meq/L. Higher concentrations can be lethal; by interfering with cardiac membrane polarization, hyperkalemia can induce life-threatening cardiac arrhythmias. Lower concentrations can result in profound muscle weakness. Thus, the body must regulate the serum potassium very closely. Although the average American diet contains approximately 100 to 200 meq of potassium daily, the serum concentration remains low since most of the body's potassium is contained within the cell. For any given intake of potassium, the ultimate concentration of the molecule in the serum depends upon the propensity for the ion to move into or out of cells (internal balance) and the elimination of potassium via the urine and gastrointestinal tract (external balance).

The movement of potassium from the serum into the cell is affected by insulin levels, the body's pH, and activity of the sympathetic nervous system. Abnormalities of the mechanisms by which potassium shifts into the cell can have a profound effect on the serum concentration. A patient with diabetes mellitus, for example, who is dependent upon daily injections of insulin, may become hyperkalemic if she misses one or more doses of his/her medication.

The storage of potassium within the cell creates a challenge for renal excretion of the ion. Of course, only ions dissolved within the serum are filtered across the glomerulus, whereas intracellular ions are not. While we filter 25,000 meq of sodium per day, only about 600 meq (180 L/day of filtrate multiplied by 3.5 meq/L serum K) of potassium is filtered daily. In individuals whose total amount of filtration is decreased due to kidney disease, the amount of filtered potassium can easily be outweighed by ingested potassium. Thus, to protect against hyperkalemia, the kidneys must have a means other than filtration across the glomerulus to excrete potassium; this other mechanism is secretion by the tubular epithelial cells into the collecting duct.

The key components facilitating potassium secretion are outlined in *Figure 5-7*. On the basolateral side of the principal cells, Na/K ATPases are present, which create an intracellular negative charge. These Na/K ATPases are unique in that they are responsive to the hormone aldosterone. Aldosterone, which is secreted when the renin–angiotensin–aldosterone system is activated, increases both the number and the functionality of Na/K ATPases on the basolateral membrane. In addition, there are both Na^+ and K^+ channels on the apical membrane. Thus, in settings in which aldosterone is released, Na/K ATPase activity is upregulated, driving sodium movement from the lumen into the cell via Na^+ channels, thereby creating a negative charge within the tubular lumen. The lumen negativity facilitates passive potassium secretion down the electrochemical gradient via potassium channels.

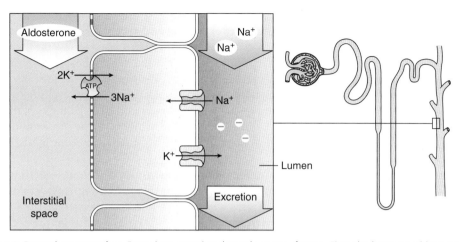

FIGURE 5-7 Potassium excretion. Potassium excretion depends on two factors. First, the hormone aldosterone must be present. It increases the activity of the basolateral Na/K ATPase, thus generating the gradient for sodium movement from the tubule into the cell. In addition, there must be an adequate distal delivery of sodium ions to supply the ENaC and generate a negative charge within the tubular lumen. This lumen's negative charge is the driving force for potassium excretion via an apical potassium channel.

Thus, in summary, there are two key components necessary to allow potassium secretion. First, aldosterone must be present to generate the movement of sodium out of the tubule lumen, thereby generating a negative charge to drive potassium secretion. In addition, there must be an adequate amount of sodium within the lumen. In other words, if there is no sodium in the lumen to begin with, no charge gradient can even be established. This scenario occurs when the total amount of filtered sodium decreases (due to a decreased GFR).

 Revisit Animated Figure 5-8 (Principal and Intercalated Cells) to view the effect of aldosterone on the principal cells. Notice how the increased activity of the Na/K ATPases leads to increased lumen negativity and hence enhanced potassium secretion.

? **THOUGHT QUESTION 5-8** After going for a jog on a hot summer, your body's normal response is to produce the hormone aldosterone to stimulate sodium reclamation. As discussed, aldosterone also drives potassium secretion. Can you explain why you do not become hypokalemic after a jog?

PUTTING IT TOGETHER

A patient ingests a toxin that interferes with tubule function. Over the next week, he notices that his urine output has increased and that he is quite dizzy upon standing up. In addition, he feels very weak and has trouble walking up stairs due to muscle weakness in his legs. On presentation to his doctor, he is noted to have low blood pressure. Blood tests show a very low serum phosphorus level and low serum bicarbonate, and he is noted to have glucose in his urine. How do we explain these findings? Which portion of the renal tubule is likely affected by the toxin? What compensatory factors might be triggered in other portions of the tubule? Predict what might happen to the serum potassium?

The proximal tubule is responsible for sodium and water reclamation, along with phosphate, glucose, and bicarbonate reclamation. Thus, damage to the proximal tubule can cause wasting of these particles in the urine. Since phosphorus is important for muscle function, low levels can lead to muscle weakness. The loss of sodium and water leads to low blood pressure, which often worsens upon standing (termed orthostatic hypotension) because of pooling of blood in the veins of the legs, thereby reducing preload of the right and left ventricles. Disorders of the proximal tubule, some of which are genetic and some of which are acquired, can occur in a range of disease states.

With the low blood pressure, the renin–angiotensin–aldosterone system will be stimulated and the ENaC transporters will be activated. Sodium reabsorption will be enhanced in the distal tubule; this will not be sufficient to overcome the sodium losses in the proximal tubule (remember, most Na is reabsorbed from the proximal tubule), but it will lead to excess loss of potassium in the collecting duct. The serum potassium will likely be very low.

Summary Points

- Approximately 180 L of glomerular filtrate enter the tubules per day. Almost all of it must be reclaimed.
- The presence of tight junctions between tubular cells, along with lipid bilayer modifications of cell membranes, makes the renal tubule inherently impermeable to both water and solute.
- Important proteins embedded within the apical membrane of cells along the tubule can greatly alter the epithelial barrier, thereby allowing solutes and water to pass from the lumen of the tubule to the interstitial fluid.
- Na/K ATPases, located along the basolateral membrane, generate an electrochemical gradient across the tubule (from lumen to cell). This gradient provides the driving force for filtrate reclamation.
- Aquaporins are specific water channels that can make the tubule water permeable. Several isoforms exist.
- NHEs are located along the early proximal tubule and help reclaim sodium and bicarbonate ions.
- Chloride ions are predominantly reclaimed in the later parts of the proximal tubule.
- Specialized glucose cotransporters link glucose reclamation to sodium reclamation in an active manner.
- Phosphate reclamation occurs via the NaPi IIa cotransporter, which is regulated by PTH.
- Little solute reclamation occurs in the descending limb of the Loop of Henle. However, about 30 L of water are reclaimed in this segment.
- Effective sodium and potassium reclamation occurs in the thick ascending limb.
- Fine-tuning of the filtrate occurs in the collecting duct. Most of the apical proteins in the collecting duct are highly regulated, so that the degree of reclamation of their respective molecules can also be controlled.
- The collecting duct plays an important role in fine-tuning water and solute balance for the body.

Answers TO THOUGHT QUESTIONS

5-1. The "fizz" of carbonated beverages is due to the slow release of CO_2 from carbonic acid, as evidenced by the gradual bubbling of an opened can of soda. However, saliva has the enzyme carbonic anhydrase, which catalyzes the release of CO_2, making the reaction much faster. Thus, as soon as the drink enters the mouth, CO_2 disappears.

5-2. Carbonic anhydrase allows the constant regeneration of intracellular hydrogen, fueling the NHEs, thereby allowing sodium and bicarbonate reclamation. A deficiency of this important enzyme would interfere with the proximal tubule's ability to reclaim these important solutes. Carbonic anhydrase inhibitors have been developed as a class of medications, used as diuretics, specifically to prevent the reabsorption of sodium (and bicarbonate). They are helpful for those patients whose kidneys are predisposed to salt retention.

5-3. As severe hyperglycemia develops, the filtered load of glucose (which is simply the GFR times the serum concentration) will overwhelm the absorptive capacity of the proximal tubule. Since there are no glucose cotransporters in any part of the tubule beyond the proximal segment, this glucose essentially becomes a nonreabsorbable molecule, which increases the osmolarity of urine and, therefore, works against passive reabsorption of water. The result is that hyperglycemia increases the daily production of urine. Since the increased volume of urine distends the bladder, which leads to an urge to urinate, these patients typically complain of urinating frequently. Since other conditions can cause urinary frequency (an irritated bladder from a urinary tract infection, for example), the total volume of urine per day, rather than the frequency of urination, should be assessed. Polyuria is the term used to describe an increased volume of urine per day and is defined as greater than 3 L of urine per day.

5-4. Glucose is a critical fuel in cell metabolism, and a constant supply must be delivered to all cells. GLUT transporters, found in almost all cell membranes, facilitate glucose uptake into all cells. Thus, one could imagine that although a drug that blocks GLUT will interrupt glucose reabsorption in the proximal tubule, it might also block glucose uptake by other cells.

For instance, the isoform GLUT1 is found within the capillary endothelium of the brain and is important in facilitating glucose movement across the blood–brain barrier, from serum into the cerebrospinal fluid. Mutations in GLUT1 interfere with this process, leading to low cerebrospinal glucose levels; patients with this problem develop seizures in the first few months of life, and their condition progresses over time resulting in severe neurologic defects. This remains a very rare condition, with less than 100 cases described. Nevertheless, it illustrates the importance of the GLUT transporters.

Unlike the ubiquitous GLUT transporters, the SGLT cotransporters are predominantly found in the apical membrane of the intestine and the proximal tubule, and their primary function is to absorb glucose from the respective lumens. Thus, their blockade would presumably affect net absorption of glucose, without affecting cell delivery to other tissues; this would likely lead to low serum glucose levels that would impair aerobic metabolism. Furthermore, a potential side affect of such a drug might be severe diarrhea due to glucose malabsorption (the increased osmotic load associated with high levels of glucose in the intestinal lumen would trap water and cause diarrhea, much as excess glucose in the renal tubule traps water and leads to increased urine volume). The blockade of proximal tubule SGLT could also prevent glucose reclamation and might lead to glucose wasting in the urine. The increased ambient glucose in the urine might lead to an increased risk of urinary tract infections and, in women, vaginal yeast infections.

5-5. If someone has a poorly functioning NaPi IIa cotransporter, phosphate will not be reclaimed, and phosphate wasting will occur. Such patients will excrete more phosphate in their urine than they eat and, consequently, will develop a net negative phosphate balance. Low levels of phosphate in the blood will result. Since phosphate is an important component of bone health, such individuals may develop thinning and weakening of the skeletal system, leading to fractures. Lastly, since phosphate is a mineral, the continued presence of large amounts of phosphate in the urine might lead to such high concentrations of the molecule that it will come out of solution, mineralize, and lead to the development of kidney stones.

5-6. Bartter and Gitelman syndromes are due to an underactivity of their respective proteins, leading to sodium, chloride, and potassium wasting. Since the presence of these solutes in the lumen of the tubule leads to an osmotic pressure that keeps water in the lumen, urine output increases and the patient becomes mildly volume depleted. Thus, these patients have low blood pressure due to sodium and chloride loss and also develop low levels of serum potassium (hypokalemia).

Liddle syndrome is due to overactivity of ENaC, leading to sodium retention and increased reabsorption of water when aquaporins are present; this often results in hypertension. However, since ENaC is a sodium-specific channel, its overactivity does not lead to potassium reclamation. In contrast, the lumen negativity generated by isolated sodium reclamation will facilitate both potassium and hydrogen excretion. Thus, patients with Liddle syndrome will have high blood pressure, as well as hypokalemia and metabolic alkalosis, the latter due to loss of hydrogen ions.

5-7. These Na/K ATPases along the basolateral membranes create a negative transepithelial potential of approximately −70 mV in the tubular cells and a very low concentration of sodium within the cell. By altering the permeability of the tubule to water and various ions, both the charge and the particle concentration change within the tubule, further facilitating the absorptive process. Detailed analyses of each tubular segment will follow.

As filtrate enters the proximal tubule, its solute concentration mirrors that of serum (140 mmol/L sodium, bicarbonate 25 mmol/L, chloride 100 mmol/L). The earliest section of the proximal tubule is permeable to sodium, bicarbonate, water, but not chloride. Thus, as sodium bicarbonate and water are reclaimed, the concentration of chloride within the lumen increases, reaching approximately 120 mmol/L. Consequently, toward the later segments of the proximal tubule, chloride begins to flow down its concentration gradient into the cells lining the proximal tubule and eventually into the peritubular fluid. The movement of the anion into the peritubular fluid is further facilitated by the intracellular negative charge. Thus, although the primary driving force remains the energy-dependent Na/K ATPase, by altering the sequential permeability to bicarbonate and chloride, the proximal tubule capitalizes on the resulting electrochemical gradient to facilitate the passive absorption of chloride down its concentration gradient, which increases the efficiency of the tubules and ultimately decreases its overall energy requirements.

In addition, the exit of chloride from the lumen leaves a slightly positive charge within the lumen. This lumen positivity repels positively charged ions out of the lumen via paracellular pathways, thereby facilitating the reclamation of potassium, calcium, and magnesium.

In the thick ascending limb, because an apical channel allows potassium to recycle back into the lumen, a lumen-positive charge develops as sodium and chloride is reclaimed by the NK2Cl. This lumen positivity facilitates the reabsorption of positively charged cations.

Finally, in the cortical collecting duct, in response to the basolateral Na/K ATPase, sodium is reclaimed from the lumen through a sodium channel, generating a lumen charge of close to -50 mV. This lumen negativity can facilitate the passive reclamation of chloride down its electrical gradient, as well the secretion of potassium into the lumen.

In summary, by altering the permeability to various particles along the tubule, the initial gradient generated by the Na/K ATPase is utilized to facilitate passive reclamation of particles down their respective electrochemical gradients. Understanding the process by which tubular permeability to various ions is varied along the tubule requires knowledge of the different transport mechanisms of each segment.

5-8. To secrete potassium, the principal cell requires two criteria: the presence of aldosterone and adequate tubular sodium. After a jog, aldosterone levels do in fact go up, facilitating conservation of whatever sodium makes it to the collecting duct. However, because the person is also volume depleted, his/her GFR is likely decreased, which diminishes the total amount of filtered sodium. In addition, because he is volume depleted, the majority of filtered sodium is reclaimed along more proximal portions of the tubule. Thus, although the aldosterone levels may be high, potassium wasting does not occur because little sodium is presented to the principal cell.

chapter 5

Review Questions

DIRECTIONS: Each of the numbered items or incomplete statements in this section is followed by answers or by completions of the statement. Select the ONE lettered answer or completion that is BEST in each case.

1. Along the length of the early proximal tubule, the concentration of sodium _____.

    A. increases
    B. decreases
    C. stays the same

2. Along the length of the early proximal tubule, the concentration of chloride _____.

    A. increases
    B. decreases
    C. stays the same

3. A patient is given an experimental drug for treatment of his cancer. One of the drug's side effects is destruction of the K channels on the apical membrane of the thick ascending limb. If you were monitoring laboratory tests of the patient's serum electrolytes, which value would you expect to become abnormal?

    A. Phosphate
    B. Chloride
    C. Magnesium
    D. Bicarbonate

4. Which of the following is an ion channel rather than a cotransporter?

    A. Sodium bicarbonate exchanger in the proximal tubule
    B. NK2Cl in the thick ascending limb
    C. Sodium chloride transporter in the distal convoluted tubule
    D. ENaC

5. A patient is diagnosed with hypertension and placed on a medication that blocks the hormone aldosterone. What will happen to his/her serum potassium?

    A. no change
    B. increase
    C. decrease

Maintaining the Volume of Body Fluid
Sodium Balance

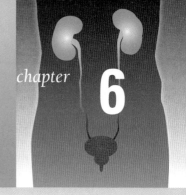

chapter **6**

CHAPTER OUTLINE

INTRODUCTION
INTERNAL SENSORS OF BODY VOLUME
- Baroreceptors
- Flow receptors
HOW THE BODY RESPONDS TO CHANGES
  IN SENSED VOLUME
- The renin–angiotensin–aldosterone system
- The natriuretic peptides
- Sodium handling

MAINTAINING BODY VOLUME—SODIUM
  HOMEOSTASIS
LIMITATIONS OF THE BODY'S SYSTEM
  OF SODIUM HOMEOSTASIS
CLINICAL MANIFESTATIONS OF SODIUM
  EXCESS VERSUS SODIUM DEFICIT
PUTTING IT TOGETHER
SUMMARY POINTS

LEARNING OBJECTIVES

By the end of this chapter, you should be able to:

- describe how our body regulates its volume of fluid.
- describe the complexities associated with the creation of an internal sensing mechanism of fluid volume.
- list the internal sensors of body volume and describe how they function.
- describe how sensors of body volume use changes of pressure or flow as surrogate markers of volume.
- describe how baroreceptors and flow receptors modulate sodium handling in the kidney.
- describe how the tubuloglomerular feedback system protects the body from sodium wasting in the setting of blood pressure changes.
- delineate the importance of natriuretic peptides and the renin–angiotensin–aldosterone (RAA) system in maintaining body volume.
- detail how changes in sodium balance lead to changes of total body fluid volume, without changes of fluid concentration.
- understand that regulation of sodium determines total body fluid volume.
- describe the role of the kidney, particularly with respect to sodium reabsorption in the tubule, in maintaining sodium homeostasis.
- delineate the limitations of the flow and baroreceptor system and the importance of sensed volume in maintaining hemodynamic stability.
- identify the factors that determine body volume and those that affect concentration.

Introduction

How much do you weigh today? How much did you weigh yesterday? How about last week? Most likely, your weight has not changed very much at all, and if you were to measure it in a week's time, it would remain unchanged. Admittedly, an individual's weight may change with fluctuations in body fat and muscle, but more acute variations likely reflect changes in total body fluid. Unless you have underlying illnesses, your body's total body fluid remains relatively constant, despite a large variation in dietary intake. By simply standing on your home scale, it is easy to measure your body's weight, and thus your body's fluid volume. But how can your body achieve a constant fluid status given the vagaries of our diet, our activity level, and our environment (hot and cold)? A scale is an external measure of your fluid volume. Your body needs an internal mechanism for monitoring total fluid. How is this accomplished?

The truth is that our body has no direct way of measuring total fluid volume. We do not have an internal scale. Fortunately, however, we do have alternative sensing mechanisms that ultimately lead to processes that regulate our body volume. These sensors, however, do not directly measure volume. Instead, they use other endpoints as surrogates of volume.

In this chapter, we will learn how our body internally senses and regulates our volume of body fluid. In addition, we will learn that changes in this sensed volume activate several hormonal axes, all of which culminate in altering the body's handling of sodium. The body's volume is adjusted, ultimately, by regulating its avidity for sodium ions. And although sodium retention might instinctively seem to affect serum sodium concentration, this is not the case. Indeed, as we will learn, regulation of sodium concentration in the body and total body fluid volume are related but distinctly different mechanisms.

Internal Sensors of Body Volume

BARORECEPTORS

As we have learned, the body has three major compartments, which are shown in *Figure 6-1*. To survive, the body must protect the volume within the vasculature to maintain tissue perfusion. Even brief hypoperfusion of critical organs can have serious consequences. Some of us have experienced vasovagal syncope, more simply known as fainting, when our blood pressure drops transiently because of a sudden dilation or expansion of the arteries and veins, which creates an effect similar to a sudden loss of intravascular volume; we are all acutely dependent on careful regulation of vascular volume.

Let us begin our exploration of body volume by imagining a sealed 5-L balloon that is placed into a second, larger balloon of fluid (*Figure 6-2*). Since the inner balloon is sealed, the volume of fluid within the balloon will remain 5 L. Now you take scissors and poke holes into the side of the inner balloon so that fluid flows freely across the surface of the balloon. How much fluid is now in the inner balloon?

Of course, the answer to this question is not immediately apparent. Since fluid is freely flowing in and out of the balloon, it does not really have a fixed volume. This scenario parallels the intravascular space. Water and sodium are freely permeable across the endothelial barrier; consequently, there is no separation of fluid between the intravascular and the interstitial space, and the volumes are intermixed. Hence, it is not possible for our bodies to directly measure intravascular volume.

Instead, our bodies rely on other mechanisms. Whereas intravascular volume cannot be measured, pressure within the vasculature can be easily assessed. And since blood pressure is determined in large part by the amount of fluid within our body, this gives us an

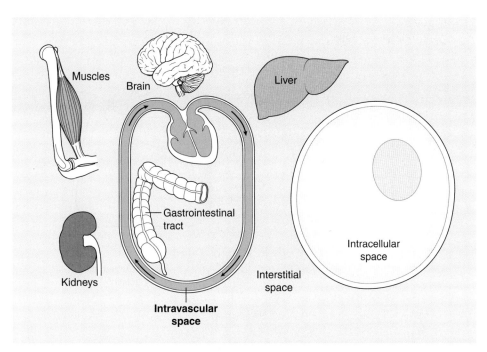

FIGURE 6-1 The intravascular compartment—link to vital organs. This is a very conceptual figure, emphasizing the importance of the intravascular compartment. The energy provided by the pumping motion of the heart generates movement of fluid through the blood vessels, allowing perfusion of the essential organs in the body. Obviously, the intracellular compartment extends to the cells within organs, not shown here.

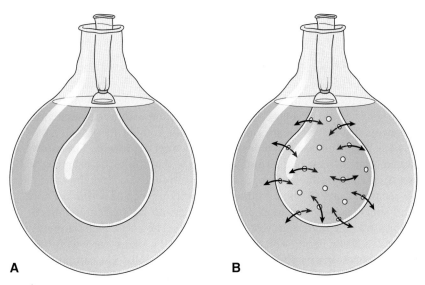

FIGURE 6-2 A balloon within a balloon. Panel 2**A** shows two impermeable balloons, one inside the other. Because the submerged balloon is tightly sealed with an impermeable barrier, no fluid either enters or exits the balloon, and the volume within it remains the same despite any differences that might exist in the osmolarity of the fluid between the balloons. One can determine the volumes of each balloon. However, once holes are cut into the balloon, as in Panel 2**B**, fluid freely exchanges between the inner balloon and the outer balloon. Thus, measuring a fixed volume within the inner balloon is not possible; it will be a dynamic variable that will depend on a number of characteristics of the balloons and the fluid within them.

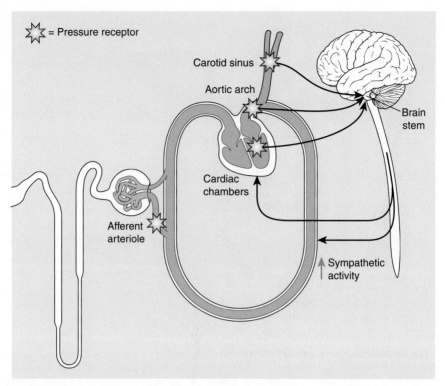

FIGURE 6-3 Baroreceptors. Receptors within the heart chambers, the aorta, and the carotid sinus detect changes in pressure. Travelling via nerve fibers to the brain, signals from the receptors can stimulate the sympathetic nervous system. In response to a decrease in pressure, these receptors can stimulate the heart rate, cardiac contractility and vascular tone, all of which act to restore intravascular pressure. Natriuretic peptides, released when the heart chambers are stretched, can affect sodium reabsorption in the kidney. Another pressure receptor sits within the renal afferent arteriole, which acts independently of the central nervous system, and directly stimulates renin release. Renin has important secondary effects, that act to increase sodium reclamation from the tubule.

approximation of vascular volume. **Baroreceptors,** which are situated in critical arteries, sense intra-arterial pressure. This pressure is dependent on a wide range of factors, including cardiac contractility, the intrinsic elasticity and permeability of the vessel wall, resistance, heart rate, and of course, total amount of fluid within the vasculature. The multiple components that determine pressure underlie the complexity of the system, and a change in any one factor can lead to alterations in intra-arterial pressure. The baroreceptors may be activated by an increase in the volume of fluid in the arteries, for example, while changes in vessel contractility without changes in volume of fluid can have the same effect.

As seen in *Figure 6-3*, important baroreceptors are located within the aortic arch and the carotid sinus (at the bifurcation of the external and internal carotid arteries). Signals are transmitted to the brainstem vasomotor region. The aortic arch baroreceptors are innervated by the aortic nerve, which combines with the vagus nerve as it travels back to the nucleus tractus solitarius (NTS) of the brainstem medulla. The carotid sinus baroreceptors communicate to the brain via a branch of the glossopharyngeal nerve.

Having processed the input from the baroreceptors, the brain generates efferent neural output via the sympathetic nervous system to try to correct disturbances that alter blood pressure. Immediately, occurring within one to two seconds, outgoing stimuli can change heart rate, peripheral vascular tone, and cardiac output, each of which can alter blood pressure and return it to normal. However, if the arterial baroreceptor stimuli persist, i.e., the initial response was inadequate to normalize pressure, signals mediated via the sympathetic nervous system also interact with the kidney. Specialized cells within the kidney, to be described later, can be stimulated to release **renin**. Renin is one of the most important hormones in salt homeostasis and regulation of blood pressure.

In addition to the aortic and the carotid baroreceptor, a unique baroreceptor is located within the afferent arteriole of the kidney; this receptor detects changes in pressure within this arteriole. Unlike the carotid and aortic baroreceptors, however, the afferent arteriole baroreceptors do not act via the brainstem. Instead, they directly stimulate granular cell release of renin. The regulation of renin release, therefore, does not require an intact sympathetic nervous system.

A type of baroreceptor is also located within the cardiac chambers. In the setting of increased pressure within the heart, these receptors are activated and, as we shall learn, can produce a range of downstream effects. Like the other baroreceptors, pressure within the heart may be altered by a variety of factors, including intrinsic myocardial function, the state of the intracardiac valves, and myocardial distensibility; changes in pressure may develop without changes in the volume of fluid within the vasculature.

In summary, in response to a drop in blood pressure, baroreceptors stimulate an increase in cardiac output and peripheral vascular resistance to restore tissue perfusion to vital organs. This occurs on an immediate basis, but may not be a long-term solution for the problem; the kidney helps to provide a more durable answer to the problem. By stimulating renin release, which eventually leads to the production of the hormone **aldosterone**, the baroreceptors stimulate the kidneys to retain sodium thereby increasing body volume and pressure in a manner that does not require ongoing stimulation of the sympathetic nervous system. The renin–angiontensin–aldosterone (RAA) axis will be explored in later parts of this chapter.

FLOW RECEPTORS

In addition to the baroreceptors described above, there is another type of receptor that helps monitor body fluid volume. It is located within the kidney, and monitors flow within the tubule. The macula densa is a modified epithelial cell of the thick ascending limb, and is part of the juxtaglomerular apparatus (JGA). As discussed in Chapter 3, the JGA is composed of the macula densa, the associated afferent arteriole that perfuses the glomerulus at the origin of that particular tubule, and granular interstitial cells, which are able to make the important peptide, renin. Thus, the macula densa, upon stimulation, can affect the afferent arteriole via two important pathways, thereby altering tubular flow and the production of renin. This is illustrated in *Figure 6-4*.

The exact mechanism by which the macula densa senses tubular flow remains an area of active research. Presumably, an NK2Cl cotransporter within the apical membrane is activated by tubular chloride, which induces changes in cell composition and membrane polarity, intracellular Na and Cl concentrations, and pH; exactly how these changes result in the generation of a signal to the glomerular arterioles is not well understood. Simply stated, the macula densa can detect and respond to changes in tubular flow.

The macula densa has two types of responses upon stimulation. Taking advantage of its proximity to the afferent arteriole, which controls the glomerular filtration rate (GFR) of the glomerulus associated with the tubule, the macula densa has the ability to moderate blood flow, and thus the amount of filtrate entering the tubule. This control mechanism is called **tubuloglomerular feedback**. Upon sensing increasing tubular flow, the macula densa releases adenosine, which causes vasoconstriction of the afferent arteriole; this decreases the GFR and limits the amount of fluid filtered by the glomerulus and flowing through the tubule.

This mechanism has important protective effects. The ability to regulate the GFR protects the individual from potentially devastating fluid loss associated with increases in glomerular perfusion. Remembering that a normal GFR is 120 cc/min, or 180 L/day, you can understand that even subtle increases of GFR will have large ramifications on tubular flow. The macula densa acts as a braking mechanism, preventing loss of body fluid associated with fluctuations of blood pressure and GFR.

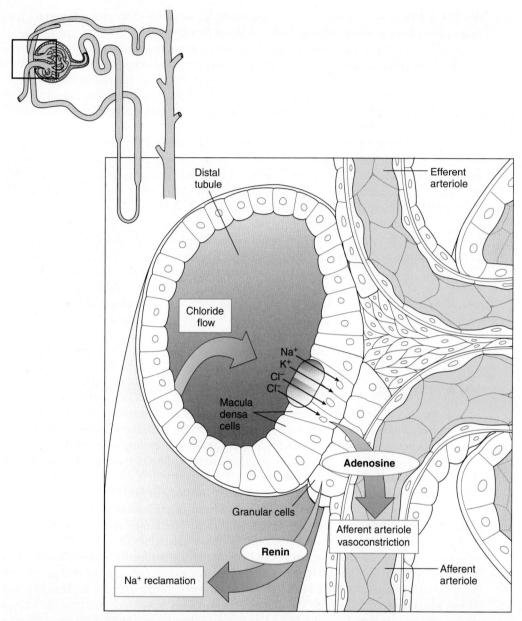

FIGURE 6-4 Flow receptor. The macula densa sits between the distal tubule and the corresponding afferent arteriole. It detects flow within the tubule (specifically chloride flow in the tubular fluid). In response to increases of tubular flow, the macula densa releases adenosine, which causes vasoconstriction of the afferent arteriole, further limiting filtration across the glomerulus, which leads to decreased tubular flow. More sustained changes in tubular flow can affect the release of renin from granular cells within the macula densa. Renin is a key regulator of renal sodium handling.

Tubuloglomerular feedback is a fast acting feedback system, designed primarily for dealing with the momentary fluctuations of GFR associated with blood pressure changes. More sustained changes of GFR, and thus tubular flow, lead to a different type of response. The fast response of the tubuloglomerular feedback system depends on the release of adenosine stored within the macula densa; more sustained mechanisms for regulating body volume include the stimulation of the RAA axis by the macula densa. We will discuss the RAA axis, which ultimately leads to tubular sodium avidity, in a few moments.

In summary, our body uses two types of receptors to detect intravascular volume. Neither one, however, directly measures volume; rather, they rely on surrogate indicators for volume. Baroreceptors sense pressure within the vascular compartment, whereas the macula densa senses flow within the tubular space.

How the Body Responds to Changes in Sensed Volume

THE RENIN–ANGIOTENSIN–ALDOSTERONE SYSTEM

As noted above, the macula densa, upon sensing sustained (more than several minutes) changes in tubular flow, responds by altering the release of renin, an important signal peptide in the control of body sodium. Decreases in tubular flow stimulate renin release; conversely, increased flow in the tubule inhibits further renin production of the protein. This process and the subsequent events triggered by it are illustrated in *Figure 6-5*.

Renin is produced as a pre-prorenin protein, which is eventually trafficked, modified, and readied for secretion. The packaged protein is stored in secretory granules, ready for immediate release upon stimulation. Renin circulates in the bloodstream, where it

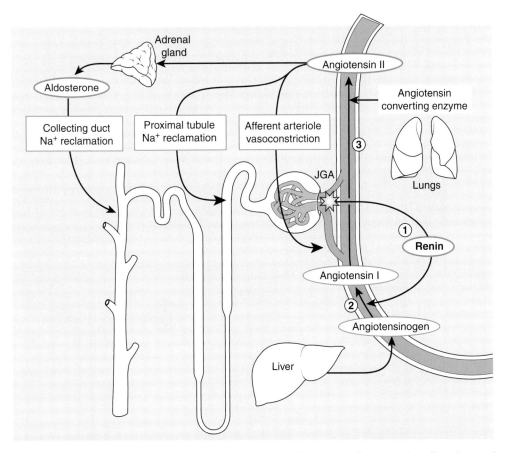

FIGURE 6-5 **The renin angiotensin aldosterone (RAA) system.** Upon release from granular cells in the macula densa, renin enters the systemic circulation (1). There, it catalyzes the conversion of angiotensinogen, produced by the liver, to angiotensin I (2). Angiotensin I travels to the lungs, where angiotensin converting enzyme (ACE) converts it into the biologically active angiotensin II (3). Angiotensin II has many subsequent effects, including systemic vasoconstriction, afferent arteriole vasoconstriction, and proximal tubule sodium reclamation. In addition, angiotensin II stimulates the adrenal gland to produce the hormone aldosterone, which is a key regulator of sodium handling in the kidney.

converts the protein angiotensinogen (produced in the liver), into its more active form, angiotensin I. Angiotensin I is further cleaved within the lungs by angiotensin converting enzyme (ACE), forming **angiotensin II**.

Angiotensin II has several important effects. As we learned in Chapter 4, it regulates the GFR by modulating afferent arteriole tone. In addition, it causes systemic vasoconstriction, and it leads to sodium reabsorption within the kidney. All of these actions share a similar goal—protecting systemic blood pressure. Angiotensin II release reduces GFR via constriction of the afferent arteriole, which leads to less filtration of sodium, although this effect is tempered by the relatively simultaneous constriction of the efferent arteriole to maintain filtration pressure. On balance, angiotensin II leads to increased salt and water in the body, which protects blood pressure while also maintaining filtration to eliminate potentially toxic metabolites.

The sodium retention effects of angiotensin II are mediated via at least two mechanisms. In the proximal tubule, angiotensin II leads to enhanced activation of the sodium hydrogen exchanger (NHE), thereby increasing sodium reclamation. In addition, angiotensin II acts upon the adrenal gland, which produces **aldosterone**, a hormone that also leads to sodium reabsorption by the kidney.

The primary targets of aldosterone are the principal cells of the collecting duct. Aldosterone binding has several effects, all of which facilitate tubular sodium reabsorption. As illustrated in *Figure 6-6*, aldosterone stimulates the trafficking of preformed epithelial sodium channel (ENaC) subunits to the apical cell.

As you will recall from Chapter 5, the ENaC protein is an important channel within the apical side of the collecting duct that allows sodium to be reclaimed from the lumen. In addition, in order to maximize the number of and time that such apical sodium channels are open, aldosterone helps stabilize the ENaC protein within the membrane, thereby limiting endocytotic return of the protein to the cytoplasm and preserving salt reclamation. This occurs by phosphorylation and subsequent inactivation of a cytoplasmic ubiquitin protein ligase (Nedd4-2), preventing it from degrading the ENaC protein.

In addition to its effects on ENaC, aldosterone also increases the activity of the basolateral Na/K ATPases. This results in an increase in the sodium electrostatic gradient across the cell, that facilitates sodium reabsorption from the tubular lumen.

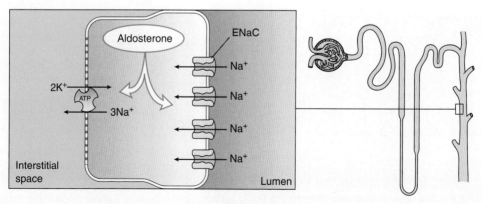

FIGURE 6-6 Aldosterone regulates tubular sodium handling. Aldosterone has important effects on the principal cell of the collecting duct. On the one hand, it increases the activity of the Na/K ATPases on the basolateral side, increasing the outward electrochemical gradient that facilitates sodium movement from lumen to interstitium. In addition, it increases the amount of ENaC proteins that are embedded in the apical membrane, thereby providing a route of sodium egress out of the tubule lumen.

In summary, when the macula densa senses changes in tubular flow, it responds by modulating the activity of the RAA system. In settings of decreased flow, the RAA system is activated, leading to sodium retention. In settings of increased flow, the RAA system is inhibited, facilitating sodium diuresis.

THE NATRIURETIC PEPTIDES

Whereas the macula densa within the kidney responds to changes of flow by modulating the RAA system, the baroreceptors stimulate a variety of mediators in response to changes in pressure.

A group of peptides plays an important role in natriuresis, or the excretion of sodium, in response to a perceived increase in body fluid volume. These natriuretic peptides include **atrial natriuretic peptide** (ANP) and **brain natriuretic peptide** (BNP). ANP is produced primarily in the cells of the right and left atria, whereas BNP, despite its name, is primarily produced in ventricular myocytes (it was originally discovered in the porcine brain, earning the name BNP). Both of these natriuretic peptides are produced in response to stretch of their respective compartments. Thus, increases in either volume or pressure within the heart, by causing wall stretch, induce release of the ANP and the BNP. The peptides circulate in the plasma and interact with their targets via high affinity receptors on the cell surface. These receptors are linked to a cGMP dependent signaling cascade; thus, activation of the receptors leads to an increase of intracellular cGMP, that mediates the action of the peptides. Natriuretic receptors have been found on a wide array of organs, including blood vessels, adrenal glands, and kidneys, reflecting the widespread effects of these peptides.

The natriuretic peptides can induce salt excretion by regulating both the GFR as well as tubular sodium reabsorption. They act to reduce the sympathetic tone of the peripheral vasculature, thereby reducing systemic vascular resistance. Consequently, cardiac output increases, allowing improved perfusion of the kidneys. In addition, the natriuretic peptides induce vasodilation of the glomerular afferent arteriole and simultaneous constriction of the efferent arteriole; this increases intra-glomerular pressure, which leads to increased GFR and sodium filtration.

The natriuretic peptides act directly on the tubules to decrease tubular sodium absorption. The peptides block the effects of the RAA system, noted previously to have potent salt retentive properties. In summary, by decreasing sodium tubular reabsorption and increasing sodium filtration, the natriuretic peptides facilitate renal salt excretion.

EDITOR'S INTEGRATION

A full understanding of blood pressure control requires the integration of renal and cardiovascular physiology. From a cardiovascular perspective, the blood pressure is a reflection of the cardiac output (the amount of blood pumped by the heart each minute) and the systemic vascular resistance (the resistance summed throughout the blood vessels of the body). By increasing intravascular volume via absorption of Na and water, the kidneys enhance cardiac output. By inducing vasoconstriction via the release of angiotensin, the kidneys increase the systemic vascular resistance. See *Cardiovascular Physiology: A Clinical Approach* for a further discussion of cardiovascular control of blood pressure.

SODIUM HANDLING

The hormonal regulation described above, which includes the natriuretic peptides as well as the RAA system, share a common end point—sodium handling. They affect the ability of the tubule to reclaim sodium, thereby increasing or decreasing the number of sodium particles returned to the body.

In the setting of sensed volume depletion, which is typically associated with decreased arterial pressure and decreased tubular flow and consequent down-regulation of the natriuretic peptides and up-regulation of the RAA system, the tubule becomes sodium avid; under these conditions, almost all the sodium filtered across the glomerulus is reclaimed. Does this reclaimed sodium, upon returning to the body, lead to hypernatremia? In other words, is serum sodium concentration (or osmolarity) changed?

The answer to this question is: "absolutely not!" This concept is one of the most fundamental issues in nephrology. Sodium reclamation in the distal tubule and collecting duct does not lead to changes in the body's concentration of sodium. This might not be instinctively obvious, so let us explore the explanation for this important observation.

One's initial response may be that as sodium particles are moved from lumen to the interstitium, water will follow, invoking the old adage "water follows salt." Is this true? Does water follow sodium in the collecting duct?

Although water and salt reabsorption are linked in the proximal tubule, water does not automatically follow salt in the distal tubule and collecting duct. Remember, as discussed in Chapter 5, the collecting duct has modifications within its lipid membrane and tight junctions between its cells, which together make the epithelial barrier impermeable to salt and water. Activation of the RAA system will increase sodium reclamation by increasing the number of pumps and transporter proteins within the tubule's wall, thereby making the tubule permeable to sodium. However, since water molecules cannot pass through the sodium transporter proteins, the tubule will remain impermeable to water. If water does not follow sodium in the distal tubule, we are left answering the question, why does sodium reclamation not lead to hypernatremia?

The answer is that the body's **osmoreceptor**, which senses concentration, is called into action. We will discuss the osmoreceptor in great detail in Chapter 8, but a few words are in order now. As the RAA system is activated and sodium reclamation occurs, the serum sodium will increase ever so slightly, perhaps by a single milliequivalent or so. This increase in concentration, albeit small, is sensed by the osmoreceptor cells within the brain. Osmoreceptors are specialized cells within the brain that detect small changes in concentration. As the concentration of sodium within the body increases, the osmoreceptors respond by stimulating the release of **antidiuretic hormone (ADH)** from the posterior pituitary. ADH, in turn, causes the synthesis of aquaporins, the important water channels we introduced in our discussion of the renal tubule in Chapter 5, which allow water to move freely across cell membranes. Aquaporins are inserted into the apical membrane of the cells lining the collecting duct, which increases the permeability of the tubule for water. Because of the high concentration of solutes within the medullary interstitium (600 to 1,200 mOsm), water moves from the lumen into the interstitium, and eventually, back to the vascular space.

In summary, in the setting of sensed volume depletion, the baroreceptors and the JGA respond by stimulating sodium reclamation via the RAA system. As this sodium is returned to the body, a slight increment in serum concentration occurs, activating the osmoreceptors, which lead to release of ADH, thereby resulting in water reclamation from the tubule. The net result is isotonic expansion of the body's fluid with no change in serum sodium concentration.

? **THOUGHT QUESTION 6-1** Assume you eat about 10 g of salt each day. How much sodium do you eat per day? How does the body deal with this sodium load?

Maintaining Body Volume—Sodium Homeostasis

As we have learned, sodium handling determines overall body volume. Net sodium retention will lead to isotonic expansion of the total body volume, and net sodium loss will lead to isotonic volume loss.

Maintaining sodium homeostasis is critical to protecting the body's volume of fluid. Sodium intake predominantly comes from one source—food. Sodium loss from the body occurs through several sources, including sweat, stool, and most importantly, the kidney. Typically, the total amount of salt lost through sweating is small, although varies widely depending on individual acclimatization and environmental factors. Given the relatively small amount of stool formed on a daily basis, normal bowel movements are not an important source of salt loss. However, this can change dramatically with gastrointestinal illnesses that lead to large quantities of diarrhea. Typical viral gastroenteritis, usually a mixture of secretion and malabsorption in the intestine, results in stool losses of approximately 35 to 45 meq of sodium per liter, whereas secretory diarrheas such as cholera can produce liquid stool with as much as 140 meq/L. Although salt losses may be impressive during these illnesses, salt loss through the stool is minimal in healthy individuals.

If an individual eats 250 meq of sodium daily, and if the typical amount of sweat and stool loss is small, the kidney must be able to eliminate the difference in order to maintain sodium balance. And, if that person decides to eat 500 meq of sodium the following day, the kidneys must excrete that extra sodium intake in order to maintain a steady body volume. Ultimately, it is the kidney's handling of sodium that determines the body's net sodium balance, and thus, the body's total body volume.

Net renal sodium excretion is determined by two factors: sodium filtration minus tubular sodium reclamation. The amount of filtered sodium is primarily determined by the GFR. For an average individual with a GFR of 180 L/day, and a serum concentration of 140 meq/L, about 25,000 meq of sodium are filtered daily. Clearly, the great majority of this sodium is reclaimed along the tubules; if this were not true, fatal volume depletion would occur within minutes. The tubule's ability to reclaim sodium is one of its most important functions, often preserved even in the setting of marked tubular dysfunction. Indeed, there are very few scenarios in which the tubules lose excessive amounts of sodium.

Nevertheless, the range of tubular sodium avidity is quite large. In settings of minimal dietary salt intake, tubular sodium reclamation can reach almost 100%, so that all that is filtered is reclaimed. On an average diet, in which 250 meq is ingested daily, tubule avidity decreases to approximately 99% of the filtered load. Remember, if a person eats 250 meq of sodium, she must excrete 250 meq of sodium to remain in steady state. If she has a normal GFR, and thus filters 25,000 meq of sodium daily, she must excrete 1% of her filtered sodium load.

This relationship between the amount of sodium filtered across the glomeruli and the amount of sodium reclaimed across the tubules is termed the **fractional excretion of sodium (FENA)**. On an average American diet, with normal renal function, a typical FENA is 1%. If a person increases her sodium dietary intake to 500 meq, in order to remain in steady state, her FENA must increase to 2%.

 THOUGHT QUESTION 6-2 What is the maximum amount of sodium one might consume before body fluid volume becomes excessive? Explain your reasoning.

In summary, the ability to alter tubular sodium avidity is fundamental to the maintenance of total body sodium, and thus, net volume, homeostasis. Healthy kidneys have an enormous capacity to respond to changes in dietary sodium, decreasing fractional reabsorption during sodium excess and increasing fractional reabsorption during sodium deficit. These physiological processes maintain sodium balance.

Limitations of the Body's System of Sodium Homeostasis

To this point, we have described the mechanisms that allow the body to regulate total body volume. Let us summarize this system, and in doing so, begin to understand its limitations and weaknesses.

The body monitors the volume of fluid in the vascular space (and since the interstitial space is in equilibrium with the vascular space, the sensing mechanisms assess extracellular fluid volume under most conditions) by two different types of sensors. Receptors within the carotid body and the cardiac chambers use changes in pressure and myocyte stretch as an estimation of total body volume. A receptor within the distal renal tubule uses filtrate flow as its indicator of body fluid volume. Each receptor, when stimulated, triggers responses that lead to changes in sodium retention. If the serum concentration increases, the osmoreceptors are activated, which leads to thirst and release of ADH. Since almost all individuals have access to water, sodium retention necessarily induces enough water ingestion and retention to keep the serum concentration unchanged. Thus, from a physiologic perspective, the net effect of pressure and flow receptor induced sodium retention is an isotonic expansion of total body volume.

 Animated Figure 6-1 (Volume Sensing) summarizes this process. As you initiate a change in the body's fluid volume, observe how the integrated activity of the receptors leads to a change in sodium reclamation. In the figure, the overall process is illustrated with intermediate steps to show how the resulting slight change in sodium concentration then affects ADH release and thirst, ultimately restoring sodium concentration and leading to an isotonic change in body volume.

Hemodynamics, which refers to the laws that govern blood flow, is the primary determinant of pressure and flow in the vasculature and directly controls these receptors. Described simply by Ohm's law, which states that flow is proportional to the change of pressure divided by resistance, the hemodynamics of the body's blood flow determines the signals that the receptors perceive.

For example, in the setting of sudden blood loss, the volume of intravascular fluid falls, as does blood pressure, renal blood flow, and glomerular filtration. Consequently, the baroreceptors and the macula densa will sense a decrease in pressure and flow respectively, and the body will compensate with sodium retaining forces. It should be noted that the kidney cannot make new sodium; i.e. it cannot restore the amount lost in the hemorrhage. However, it can reduce renal sodium loss to almost nothing, so that whatever sodium is eaten in the diet, or given intravenously, remains in the body. In this manner, by retaining all the filtered sodium, the sensors help return the total body volume to its previous level.

EDITOR'S INTEGRATION

The activation of the baroreceptors in the setting of hypotension leads to other compensatory changes in the cardiovascular system to restore blood pressure towards normal. Baroreceptor signals result in activation of the sympathetic nervous system, which leads to vasoconstriction (increasing vascular resistance throughout the body) and increased contractility (force of contraction) of the ventricles, which increases the amount of blood pumped with each contraction of the heart (increased flow).

Let us consider a different example. Say an individual suffers a heart attack, so that her cardiac function decreases dramatically. The heart loses its ability to fully empty with each beat, and the heart cavity begins to dilate to accommodate ongoing venous flow; this leads to increased intra-chamber (atrium and ventricle) pressure and volume, and the stretch receptors are activated. Although the woman's total body volume has not changed from before to after her heart attack, the cardiac pressure receptors now sense pressure overload and stimulate the release of natriuretic peptides to facilitate renal sodium excretion.

However, the situation becomes more complex as one tries to predict the body's response to this problem. Although the cardiac receptors detect pressure overload, the carotid baroreceptors and the macula densa detect underfilling due to the decreased ejection of blood from the heart. With decreased cardiac output, blood pressure may fall, and the baroreceptors sense "underfilling" of the vasculature. Furthermore, the falling cardiac output undermines renal perfusion, glomerular filtration falls, and the tubular flow lessens. Because the GFR falls due to a failing cardiac pump, without a change in total body volume, the sensor is "tricked" into thinking there is total body volume depletion when, in fact, there has not been a change. Consequently, both the carotid baroreceptor and the macula densa sense a decrease in pressure and flow respectively, and their response is to activate sodium retention.

In this example the cardiac receptors detect increased pressure, suggesting too much volume, and the carotid baroreceptor and macula densa detect decreased pressure and flow respectively, suggesting too little volume. What is the net effect when there are different signals to the body's compensatory regulating mechanisms? Generally, the sodium retentive forces of the RAA system are more potent than the sodium losing forces of the natriuretic peptides. Thus, over time, unless the woman's heart function improves, she will remain in a sodium retentive state, and will retain a proportion of the sodium that she eats. Consequently, she will begin to develop volume overload. If this extra volume of fluid, some of which will remain in the vasculature, is able to improve cardiac hemodynamics, then the GFR will improve, tubular flow will increase, and the signal for sodium retention will diminish; the individual will be at a new steady state with an increased total body volume. However, in situations in which cardiac function is severely compromised, the increase of volume actually worsens the cardiac hemodynamics, so that the GFR worsens, tubular fluid delivery falls, and a vicious cycle ensues as the sensors simulate even more salt avidity.

EDITOR'S INTEGRATION

In the example, above, the term "tricked" is used in describing how the body's sensors are activated such that sodium is retained despite a stable intravascular volume when the heart's pump function is compromised by the myocardial infarction. In fact, the reabsorption of sodium and water is an important compensatory mechanism for a sudden decrease in cardiac function. The heart's ability to eject blood is determined, in part, by the amount of blood in the ventricle just before contraction occurs, which we call the "preload." By retaining sodium and water, preload is increased. The relationship between preload and the stroke volume, which refers to the amount of blood ejected with each contraction, is regulated by the Starling relationship (see Chapter 7 in *Cardiovascular Physiology: A Clinical Approach* for more information on this principle).

Importantly, in this scenario, volume depletion was not the initial problem; rather, the *sensation* of decreased volume, as perceived by the receptors in the carotid body and the macula densa, was the primary change. Thus, the addition of body volume will not directly rectify the initial problem. Only a change in the receptor stimulation—with correction of cardiac hemodynamics, or medications that will reduce the pressure within the cardiac chambers and/or improve flow to the macula densa—will re-establish sodium equilibrium.

Let us try another example. A young man develops sudden onset of pneumococcal pneumonia, and presents to the emergency room with high fevers and low blood pressure. His presentation would be consistent with sepsis, a condition in which an infection induces an overwhelming inflammatory response and a sudden release of cytokines, chemicals that alter the permeability of the vasculature, decrease the hepatic production of albumin, and cause dilation of many of the peripheral/extremity arterioles. These changes lead to the leakage of fluid from blood vessels (increased endothelial permeability and decreased inward directed oncotic pressure) with a net movement of fluid from the intravascular space to the interstitial space. Thus, although there has been no change in total body volume, the distribution between compartments has changed, so that the interstitial space fills at the expense of the intravascular space. In combination with dilation of the blood vessels, these physiological changes cause blood pressure to fall.

As part of this man's treatment, in order to improve his hemodynamics, intravenous saline is administered. Depending on the degree of sepsis, much of this fluid will continue to leak into the interstitial space, and the intravascular volume will remain low. Consequently, despite total body volume overload, the cardiac and carotid receptors, as well as other baroreceptors, will sense under-filling, and respond by inducing sodium retention. At some point, if the patient is to get better, either the administered fluid will be sufficient to raise the blood pressure or the sepsis syndrome will resolve and allow reconstitution of vessel integrity; the baroreceptor and flow receptor will then be turned off.

We will now examine one final example. Imagine a patient had a ligature (suture) placed around his renal artery, and the ligature was tightened in order to starve the kidneys of blood flow. The decrement in renal perfusion would lead to a fall in GFR, decreasing tubular flow to the macula densa, stimulating the RAA system, and producing sodium retention. The net effect would be isotonic volume expansion. Because the patient's cardiac function is normal and the capillaries are healthy, one-third of this volume would remain within the vasculature, leading to increased pressure. This may stimulate baroreceptor release of natriuretic peptides, but as mentioned above, macula densa stimulation of the RAA system has greater sodium retaining tendencies than the sodium losing properties of the natriuretic peptides; the net result is sodium retention. This increased extracellular volume would cause an increase in blood pressure in a normal individual, i.e., the person would develop hypertension. In the other disorders described above (heart failure, sepsis), blood pressure is usually low, due to a failing cardiac pump or leaky capillaries, respectively. In the condition in which the renal artery is narrowed (otherwise known as renal artery stenosis), the retained sodium, a consequence of renal under-perfusion, leads to *high* blood pressure. This is a clinically important distinction.

To restate the basic concept underlying these examples, baroreceptors and flow receptors ultimately control the body volume, but they do not directly measure the body's volume. They *sense* either pressure or flow, using these *sensations* as a surrogate of total body volume. Thus, their collective signals define the term "sensed" volume, referring to the perceived volume as interpreted by the body's baroreceptors and flow receptors. The activity of these receptors, driven by their sensed volume, often has no relationship to the actual volume of the patient. This concept is very important in understanding sodium balance.

Animated Figure 6-2 (Examples—Sensor Activity) summarizes these four examples. In each case, you can see how the patient's condition has affected the state of the various sensors and how the net signal is a sensed decrease in body volume, resulting in sodium retention. As noted previously, the sensors are not always in alignment; you can see this by looking at the state of the various sensors in congestive heart failure (CHF) and in renal artery stenosis.

In summary, the body has no mechanism to assess directly its total volume of sodium and water. There is no internal scale. Instead, we rely on surrogate markers of volume that detect either pressure or flow. These receptors define the body's "sensed volume." In addition, these sensing mechanisms have another limitation. They only monitor two small compartments of the total body, namely, the arterial tree and the renal tubular system. Consequently, one can accumulate huge amounts of extra interstitial volume, e.g., edema, and neither the baroreceptors nor the flow receptors would know it.

Clinical Manifestations of Sodium Excess versus Sodium Deficit

Changes in total body fluid volume are most easily noted by a change in body weight; patients with sodium retention will often be able to describe just how many pounds they have gained. Other clinical manifestations of sodium retention relate to the body compartments into which sodium distributes. As we discussed in Chapter 1, sodium is primarily extracellular, and distributed throughout the interstitial and the intravascular volume. Thus, sodium retention often leads to edema formation in dependent areas (i.e., areas in which the hydrostatic pressure is high). Patients may complain that their legs are swollen, they have trouble getting their shoes to fit, or that their socks leave marks on their legs.

Learning to assess the amount of fluid in the subcutaneous tissue, i.e., the determination of the patient's skin turgor, is one of the most important skills of clinical medicine. Typically, skin is loosely connected to the underlying supportive structures, and can be pulled away from the body, and pinched between finger and thumb. However, as edema accumulates in the soft tissues of the body, the underlying tissue beneath the skin swells, and no longer can the skin be easily pinched. As edema progresses, swelling becomes grossly visible, and when you push down on such a patient's leg, an indentation remains. Edema formation is often graded on a scale, from 1+ to 3+ depending on how deep the indentation is when you compress the area of the body being examined, although this rating system is quite subjective. Alternatively, when the volume of fluid in the interstitial space is depleted, the skin "tents," which means that it does not quickly return to normal position when it is pinched.

In addition to expanding the interstitial space, sodium accumulates within the intravascular space. This manifests clinically as hypertension, as the relative increase of intravascular fluid within the contractile arteries causes an increase in blood pressure. Sodium retention is one of the most important causes of hypertension.

We have just described several physical signs of volume overload. There are also symptoms of sodium retention about which the patient may complain. One of the earliest symptoms is **nocturia**, or the need to urinate at night. Upon lying supine, the hydrostatic pressure in the veins of the legs diminishes. If edema is present, the hydrostatic pressure of the tissue may exceed that in the veins, which leads to reabsorption of fluid into the vascular space. This results in increased renal perfusion, a rise in GFR, and the formation of extra quantities of urine. Patients will typically complain of needing to urinate about three to four hours after going to sleep; this is the time required for the urine to be formed, to accumulate in the bladder, and to stimulate the urge to void.

THOUGHT QUESTION 6-3 You may have noticed that the first thing you want to do after getting out of a swimming pool is to urinate. Why?

To this point, we have focused on the effect of salt retention on the systemic circulation. Intravascular volume expansion may also affect the pulmonary vascular volume and pressure. When edema fluid accumulates in the pulmonary interstitium, we call it **pulmonary edema**. Like nocturia, this may occur at night in association with the patient moving into the recumbent position; in these situations, the patient awakens with shortness of breath three to four hours after going to bed. This is called **paroxysmal nocturnal dyspnea**. Typically, patients awaken with a sputtering cough and shortness of breath, and must sit on the side of the bed, legs dangling down, for relief as blood empties from the pulmonary vasculature and hydrostatic pressure diminishes. With progressive fluid accumulation, patients can no longer lie flat at all, and will often require several pillows underneath their back to be comfortable when they get into bed. This is called **orthopnea**, and can be quantified by the number of pillows needed, as in one-pillow or two-pillow orthopnea.

EDITOR'S INTEGATION

The accumulation of fluid in the interstitium of the lung may lead to dyspnea by several mechanisms. The increased hydrostatic pressure of the interstitium may alter the distribution of gas flow to small airways and alveoli, which can lead to low oxygen levels in the blood (hypoxemia) via a phenomenon called "ventilation–perfusion mismatch." In more severe cases, fluid spills into the alveoli, further compromising gas entry into the alveoli and worsening hypoxemia. In addition, there are pulmonary receptors, called juxtacapillary or "J receptors," adjacent to the capillaries; when stimulated by the accumulation of interstitial fluid, these receptors send signals to the brain which lead to the sensation of dyspnea. For more details, see Chapter 8 in *Respiratory Physiology: A Clinical Approach.*

We have explored the clinical manifestations of salt excess. Now, let us discuss what happens when a salt deficit occurs. One might construct the scenario in which one eats 100 meq of salt, but the kidney loses 150 meq of salt, leading to a net loss. Although conceptually interesting, there are almost no clinical scenarios in which the kidney loses salt alone. It is always in conjunction with water. Thus, the use of diuretics blocks salt reabsorption by the tubule, leading to salt excretion. However, the diuretics also interfere with water reclamation, leading to equal amounts of water loss. Diuretic induced loss of salt is accompanied by loss of water, leading to isotonic volume loss of body fluid. Other bodily fluids, such as those lost via vomiting or diarrhea, often consist of equal amounts of salt and water, thereby leading to isotonic volume loss. The sensation of thirst resulting from volume depletion, however, may lead the patient to drink water. If she is not also eating salt, the ingestion of water may dilute the concentration of sodium in the body.

Volume loss is most easily quantified by measuring weight on a scale (assuming that one is looking at changes over a matter of hours or days during which weight loss or gain due to dietary or metabolic factors is less likely to occur). Changes in skin turgor typically represents about a 5% decrease in body volume. Upon standing, with the gravity driven shift of vascular volume to the legs, many volume depleted patients experience a drop in blood pressure with a consequent increase in heart rate; this finding, called orthostatic hypotension, usually signifies at least a 10% decrease in total body volume. This is one of the more sensitive clinical signs of volume depletion, and occurs before sustained changes in blood pressure. If volume depletion worsens however, hypotension ensues, that can lead to tissue hypoperfusion and death. Remember that total body water represents approximately 60% of body weight; thus, for a person who weighs 70 kg (with a total body volume of 42 L) and who is orthostatic, we would estimate that he has a total body volume deficit of 10% of body volume or 4.2 L.

PUTTING IT TOGETHER

Four patients come into the emergency room, one with hemorrhage, one with septic shock, one with a new myocardial infarction and consequent CHF, and one with renal artery stenosis.

How would you describe the volume of each compartment and as well as the sensed volume, as detected by the baroreceptor and flow receptors. Please complete the table below. (*Table 6-1*)

You can also use Animated Figure 6-3 (Volume and Sensor Status Quiz) to complete the table by dragging the pieces to the correct boxes. You can choose to get feedback on your progress as you fill in the table or try to complete it without hints.

In hemorrhage, there is consistency among all sensors, which appropriately detect the decrease in total body volume. All compartments, except for the intraceullar space (which is unchanged), are low. However, in all the other situations, there are inconsistencies between compartments. In sepsis, because of the leaky capillaries, which cause fluid to move from the intravascular space into the interstitial space, the intravascular volume is low. The baroreceptors and flow receptors detect low volume too. The interstitial space is increased, and the intracellullar space is unchanged. Since almost all patients with sepsis are sick enough to be in hospital and receive many liters of intravenous saline fluid resuscitation, the body's salt avid mechanisms lead to an increase in total body volume. The administered saline will not be excreted but, instead, will lead to peripheral edema.

In heart failure, the primary problem is depressed left ventricular function. The heart is unable to generate adequate blood pressure and, thus, the baroreceptors in the arterial tree emanating from the left ventricle, including the carotids and aorta, sense low volume. However, since the heart is failing and unable to pump effectively, the cardiac chamber baroreceptors detect overfilling. Meanwhile, the flow receptor and renal artery baroreceptor detects low flow and pressure. Thus, there is inconsistency between the different sensors. Indeed, in patients with CHF, the expected physiologic response is activation of the natriuretic peptides, based on stimulation of the cardiac chamber baroreceptors, and activation of the RAA axis, based

TABLE 6-1 SELF ASSESSMENT OF YOUR UNDERSTANDING OF BODY VOLUME					
	INTRAVASCULAR SPACE	BARORECEPTOR SENSED VOLUME	FLOW RECEPTOR SENSED VOLUME	INTERSTITIAL SPACE	INTRACELLULAR SPACE
Hemorrhage					
Sepsis					
Congestive heart failure					
Renal artery stenosis					

TABLE 6-2 PUTTING IT TOGETHER—SUMMARY OF CHANGES IN BODY VOLUME

	INTRAVASCULAR SPACE	BARORECEPTOR SENSED VOLUME	FLOW RECEPTOR SENSED VOLUME	INTERSTITIAL SPACE	INTRACELLULAR SPACE
Hemorrhage	↓	↓	↓	↓	No change
Sepsis	↓	↓	↓	↑	No change
Congestive heart failure	↑	↓↑	↓	↑	No change
Renal artery stenosis	↑	↑	↓	↑	No change

on stimulation of the kidney's sensors. Ultimately, although these two responses have opposing sodium forces, the relatively stronger RAA system wins out, and such patients become sodium avid, and sodium and water overloaded. Thus, the intravascular and the interstitial space become increased (again, cell volume does not change).

Finally, in the condition in which there is narrowing of the main renal artery (stenosis), the afferent arteriole and the macula densa both sense a low intravascular volume, which stimulates avid sodium retention. This leads to body volume overload, as sensed by the cardiac baroreceptors. Since the heart and blood vessels are normal, this increased volume will lead to an increase in blood pressure, as sensed by the carotid baroreceptor.

The completed table is provided above. (*Table 6-2*)

Summary Points

- We have no internal way to measure directly the total volume of body fluid.
- Changes in pressure or flow are surrogate markers of body volume. The baroreceptors and flow receptors detect this "sensed volume."
- There are many baroreceptors throughout the arterial vasculature. Changes in arterial pressure are determined by a wide variety of factors, including blood volume.
- The macula densa is a specialized epithelial cell within the renal tubule that senses flow of filtered fluid through the tubule.
- Changes in sensed volume modulate a cascade of responses, including the release of natriuretic peptides and the stimulation of the RAA axis, both of which culminate in changes in the way the kidney handles sodium.
- Angiotensin II protects arterial blood pressure by causing systemic vasoconstriction, reducing the GFR, and inducing renal sodium retention.
- Aldosterone is one of the major sodium retaining forces in the body. It stimulates distal tubule sodium reclamation.
- Clinical states of volume overload are due to problems with sodium handling. Typically, these conditions are associated with reduced "sensed volume," i.e., the cardiac output or blood pressure is reduced despite normal or expanded total body volume.
- Sodium retention by the kidney does not lead to hypernatremia.
- The indirect detection of body volume via the baroreceptors and flow receptors is not a perfect system. The limitations of this system contribute to important findings in a number of disease states.

Answers TO THOUGHT QUESTIONS

6-1.   On average, Americans consume about 10 to 15 g of salt a day. Most health guidelines suggest much lower goals. They typically make recommendations based on the amount of sodium, rather than salt. In addition, the sodium content of most intravenous fluids and medications is given in milliequivalents of sodium, rather than milligrams. Thus, it is important to understand the differences in all these terms, as you are likely to encounter them.

Grams, or milligrams, are a weight-based measurement. A mole, or millimole, refers to the number of particles, whereas equivalent, or milliequivalent, refers to the number of charged particles. Since sodium and chloride both have a single charge, one mmol equals one meq, yet a mmol of calcium, which has two positive charges, is equal to two meq. In order to convert from mg to meq, the weight must be divided by the atomic weight of the particle.

Sodium, with a molecular weight of 23, is about two-thirds as heavy as chloride, with a molecular weight of 35.5. Thus, 1 g of salt consists of one-third of sodium and two-thirds of chloride by weight. In other words, 10 g of salt is about 3.5 g of sodium. To convert from a weight-based measurement to a particle (or charged particle measurement), the weight must be divided by the atomic weight. Thus, since the combined weight of sodium and chloride is 58, 10 g of salt is made of about 0.172 mol of sodium and 0.172 mol of chloride.

Now, let us put these numbers in context. An American diet at the low end of the average range for salt intake, i.e., 10 g of salt, contains about 3.5 g or 172 meq of sodium. The recommended daily allowances are between 2 to 3 g of sodium. A small packet of salt (like that obtained from a fast food restaurant) has about 180 mg of sodium. Most cans of food contain about 800 to 1,000 mg of sodium, which is used for taste and as a preservative. A typical fast food hamburger loaded with bacon has almost 2,000 mg of sodium! One teaspoon of salt weighs 2.3 g.

As we have been discussing in this chapter, the kidney has an elaborate system for regulating salt and water. Under most conditions, the amount of sodium we consume is in excess of what we need. In response, the RAA system will be shut down and the kidney will excrete excess sodium.

6-2.   The maximum amount that one can eat before developing volume overload is defined by the maximum amount that the kidneys can excrete. For normal individuals, this amount is very large, although not known with certainty. Experimental studies suggest that the tubules can reduce their reclamation down to 70%. Thus, of a normal filtered load of 25,000 meq, about 7,500 meq of sodium can be excreted! It should be noted that this concept of maximal salt excretion was based on whole animal studies. It is unlikely that humans could tolerate such a high salt intake, and would likely develop pulmonary edema due to volume overload before the kidneys could excrete the salt load. Remember, 7,500 meq of sodium is equivalent to about 48 L of normal saline.

6-3.   The increased hydrostatic pressure on your body, generated by the surrounding water, moves fluid from the interstitium to the intravascular space, leading to an increased GFR, and thus, an increase of urine formation.

Review Questions

DIRECTIONS: *Each of the numbered items or incomplete statements in this section is followed by answers or by completions of the statement. Select the ONE lettered answer or completion that is BEST in each case.*

1. A 70-year-old man suffered a heart attack 2 months ago, resulting in congestive heart failure. The left ventricular ejection fraction (the percentage of blood that is ejected from the filled ventricle at the end of diastole; normal is >55%) is noted to decrease from normal to <15%. Consequently, with the decreased pumping of blood by the heart, his blood pressure is much lower. In addition, he develops lower extremity edema and shortness of breath. His renal function worsens, and his serum creatinine increases from 1 mg/dL to 1.5 mg/dL. The flow receptor detects a low flow state. How would you treat the patient?

    A. Administer normal saline
    B. Administer a diuretic to reduce total body volume
    C. No change in his management

2. An elderly woman develops congestive heart failure (low cardiac output leading to reduced sensed intravascular volume and secondary fluid accumulation). Because of increasing volume in her left ventricle, and consequent increased ventricular pressure, natriuretic peptides are released. How would this affect sodium handling in this patient?

    A. The kidney would excrete more sodium than ingested leading to volume loss.
    B. The kidney would retain more sodium than ingested leading to volume gain.
    C. The kidney's handling of sodium would not be affected.

3. A young healthy college student enjoys salty pretzels, chips, and beef jerky. Given this ingestion of salt, would there be permanent changes to body volume and to Na concentration over the course of many days or weeks?

    A. Body volume will increase, fluid concentration will increase
    B. Body volume will increase, fluid concentration will not change
    C. Body volume will not change, fluid concentration will increase
    D. Neither body volume nor fluid concentration will change

4. A middle-aged man with a history of high blood pressure enjoys salty pretzels, chips, and beef jerky. Will this ingestion of salt lead to permanent changes in body volume or concentration?

    A. Body volume will increase, fluid concentration will increase
    B. Body volume will increase, fluid concentration will not change
    C. Body volume will not change, fluid concentration will increase
    D. Neither body volume nor fluid concentration will change

Concentrating the Urine

Adapting to Life on Land

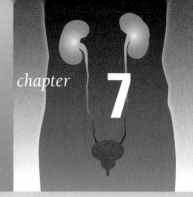

LEARNING OBJECTIVES

By the end of this chapter, you should be able to:

- describe the ongoing nature of water loss through the skin, gastrointestinal tract, and respiratory tract.
- categorize the ways in which the kidneys compensate for extrarenal water loss by making concentrated urine without affecting particle handling.
- identify the medullary interstitial concentration gradient and the permeability of the collecting tubule as the two fundamental criteria needed to retain water from the urine waste.
- explain the two key components needed to build a medullary interstitial gradient—countercurrent multiplication and urea handling.
- describe how the unique structure of the kidney's vascular supply prevents the dilution of the medullary gradient.
- delineate the structural differences in the renal tubule that result in countercurrent *multiplication* versus countercurrent *exchange.*
- describe the role of urea in the process that results in the concentration of urine.
- delineate how the water permeability of the tubule changes as it traverses the renal interstitium.

Reclaiming Water Without Affecting Particle Balance

Unlike animals that live in water, such as fish, we are surrounded by dry conditions, with consequent loss of water from the skin, as well as the respiratory and gastrointestinal tracts. This amount of water loss varies on a daily basis, depending on our activity level as well as the environmental conditions. To maintain normal concentrations of water and key molecules in our body despite these fluctuations in extrarenal water loss, we could either excrete more of the particles in our body, such as sodium, or retain relatively more water from our urine. Obviously, the first scenario could eventually lead to sodium depletion, which is not compatible with life if it were to continue for very long. Instead, our body retains water by making more concentrated urine. In doing so, it allows us to respond to wide ranges of insensible water loss without affecting our sodium stores. Ultimately, this response is dependent upon the fact that we can modulate water in the renal tubule independently of particles.

Maintaining the body's fluid concentration under these conditions is no easy task. Remember, since many cell membranes are permeable to water, water will flow passively toward areas of higher particulate concentration. Then how can we excrete concentrated urine full of particles, while at the same time moving water from the tubule back into the body?

The fascinating process used to accomplish this task will be the focus of this chapter. Specifically, we will explore how the kidneys are able to create urine full of particulate matter, including urea waste products and excess dietary solute intake, and at the same time, retain the ability to remove water from this concentrated waste. The unique structural design of the tubule is critical to this concentrating mechanism. As seen in *Figure 7-1*, the kidney is able to generate an area of high concentration in the tissue that surrounds the

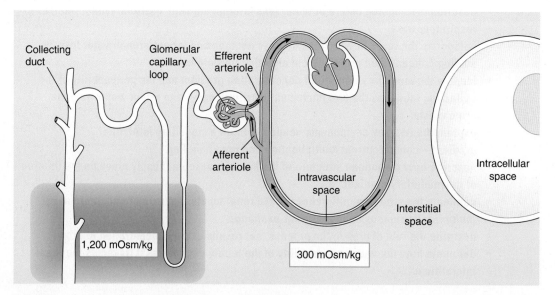

FIGURE 7-1 **A concentration "oasis" in the renal interstitium.** In order to move water out of the renal tubule, the concentration of the surrounding interstitium must be higher than within the tubule. The concentration of the interstitium in the medulla can reach 1,200 mOsm/kg. This is three to four times higher than elsewhere in the body. Despite the absence of physical barriers between the fluid surrounding the renal tubules and the remainder of the body's interstitial space, the unique architecture and vascular supply of the kidney prevents this concentration gradient from being dissipated, creating a "concentration oasis."

collecting duct. The concentration in this region of the kidney can exceed the concentration of fluid in the rest of the body by a factor of 4, a type of "concentration oasis." Although there is no barrier between this highly concentrated region and the rest of the kidney's interstitial space, the concentration gradient is not dissipated. As we will see, the unique structure of the tubules allows the maintenance of this concentration gradient.

We start our discussion with how our kidneys make a concentration gradient. Thereafter, we will discuss how this gradient is maintained, and not dissipated into the rest of the body. And finally, we will review how the antidiuretic hormone (ADH) alters the collecting tubule's permeability to water, thereby determining exactly how much water is reabsorbed from the urinary filtrate.

THOUGHT QUESTION 7-1 **A shark and a dolphin both have body osmolarities of approximately 300 mOsm/kg, yet both live in seawater whose concentration approaches 1,100 mOsm/kg. A dolphin is a mammal and extracts oxygen from air; a shark is a fish that must take in seawater to extract oxygen. Given the differences in the way that fish and mammals get oxygen, what hypotheses might you construct to explain how they deal with this challenge? Do they have ways of eliminating excess particles? How might that be accomplished?**

Building the Gradient

As seen in *Figure 7-1*, the concentrated area at the deepest part of the inner medulla is close to 1,200 mOsm/kg. As we shall discuss, preventing water from elsewhere in the body's interstitium from diluting this is important. However, **building** a concentration gradient between the tubular fluid and the interstitial fluid is an important first step in the process of concentrating the urine. Since the osmolarity in the interstitium can reach four times that within the tubule, much energy is needed to continue to move particles from the tubule into the interstitium against such a concentration gradient. Is there an efficient way to build this concentration gradient between the medullary interstitium and its surroundings?

Let us look again at a few simple diagrams, beginning with *Figure 7-2A*.

Imagine that you have a pipe embedded in a tank of fluid. Fluid within the pipe and within the tank is constantly flowing (not illustrated). In the pipe, the fluid has a concentration of 300 particles/L. The pipe is solid, impermeable to either particles or water. You purchase a special "particle pump" that extrudes particles from the pipeline. The pump has an intrinsic, limited power capacity. It can maintain a maximum concentration difference between inside and outside of the pipe of only 50 particles/L, at which point the pump goes into standby mode. The pump does not care what the starting concentration of the fluid is; it is only limited by the difference between the two areas. If it starts pumping fluid with a concentration of 200 particles/L, it will stop once it reduces the concentration in the tube's fluid to 150 particles/L; if it starts at 400 particles/L, it will stop when the concentration of the fluid is 350 particles/L. It is the difference between the two fluid concentrations (inside versus outside the pipe) that is important. In this example, since the fluid in the beginning of the pipe has a concentration of 300 particles/L, the pump will reduce the concentration in the fluid exiting the pipe to 250 particles/L.

Is there a way to improve the efficiency of the system? In other words, can we use the same pump to build a larger concentration gradient?

In *Figure 7-2B*, we place a bend in the pipeline, to form a hairpin loop with the particle pump in the ascending portion or limb of the loop. The simple change in shape allows

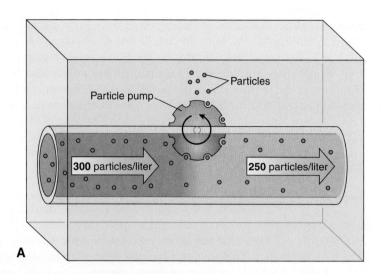

Particles

Particle pump

300 particles/liter

250 particles/liter

A

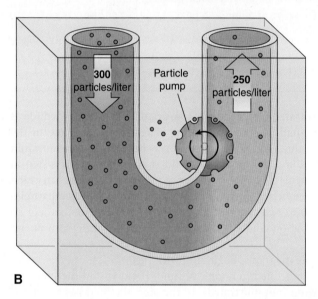

300 particles/liter

Particle pump

250 particles/liter

B

Holes allow water to leave pipe, thereby increasing concentration of remaining tubular fluid

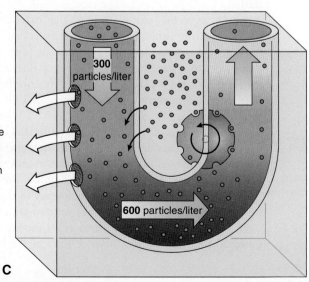

300 particles/liter

600 particles/liter

C

particles to accumulate around the tip of the loop, but does little to change the concentration within the pipe. Fluid with the same concentration (300 particles/L) will be delivered to the particle pump, generating the same gradient as before (50 particles/L).

Now, however, in addition to adding a hairpin loop, you place small little holes in the descending aspect of the loop, yet make no changes to the ascending aspect of the loop, as seen in *Figure 7-2C*. Initially, the pump will still extrude particles, generating the same gradient of 50 particles/L. Since the particles accumulate around the hairpin loop, the concentration of the fluid in the tank will increase. Since the descending limb is porous, however, particles will move down its concentration gradient into the descending limb, and at the same time, water will move out of the descending limb toward the more concentrated area. This movement of particles in and water out intensifies the concentration of fluid within the descending limb.

Remember, fluid is constantly flowing within the pipe. Thus, the "more concentrated" fluid within the descending limb is then pushed forward into the ascending limb. The pump will continue to generate its same gradient of 50 particles/L. It does not care, however, what the starting concentration is; the only thing that matters is the difference between the inside and outside of the tube. Thus, whereas the particle pump initially received fluid with a concentration of 300 particles/L, it is now the recipient of "more concentrated" fluid. Therefore, it can generate a higher concentration outside the pipe with the same amount of work. The key to this hairpin loop is the following concept: by allowing particles to move in and water to move out of the descending limb, increasingly more concentrated fluid is delivered to the pump, which can then continue to build a more concentrated gradient. This cycle continues and, over time, the concentration of the fluid approaching the ascending limb of the pipe substantially exceeds that of the fluid entering the descending limb.

By placing a loop into the system and by altering the permeability of certain sections of the tube, the net effect of the particle pump is multiplied. A much higher concentration can be generated along the pipe's length and in the surrounding fluid compared to the concentration of the original fluid that enters the pipe. This process occurs in the Loop of Henle, and is traditionally termed "countercurrent multiplication." Let us review the structure of the Loop of Henle, and see how its unique architectural design allows for the creation of the "countercurrent multiplier."

COUNTERCURRENT MULTIPLICATION WITHIN THE LOOP OF HENLE

As seen in *Figure 7-3*, the primary driving force, equivalent to the "pump" in the above example, remains the Na/K ATPase in the thick ascending limb. This ATPase extrudes sodium ions across the basolateral membrane into the interstitium, which results ultimately in the movement of sodium from within the lumen into the tubular epithelial cell

---

FIGURE 7-2 **The essentials of countercurrent multiplication.** In the following examples, an impermeable pipe is placed into a tank of moving fluid. In panel A, a single pump, with a fixed maximum pumping capacity, can generate a certain concentration gradient, in this case 50 particles/L. It should be noted that the fluid in the tank (outside of the pipe) is constantly been replaced (not shown) so that the particle concentration in the tank does not rise. A "hairpin loop", as seen in panel B, does little to change this gradient (still 50 particles/L difference between fluid in the pipe and in the tank), yet does allow the accumulation of a concentrated fluid in the region of the bend. The combination of a hairpin turn, combined with relative permeability in the descending limp (panel C), creates a unique scenario in which the effect of the pump's capacity can be greatly multiplied. By pumping particles from the ascending limp into the fluid surrounding the descending limb (thereby increasing the concentration of particles around the descending limb) water will leave the descending limb (and some particles may enter into the descending limb). Consequently, the concentration of the fluid being presented to the pump increases. Since the pump can generate a gradient above whatever concentration of fluid it is delivered, its ability to continue the cycle is multiplied. This is the basis of "countercurrent multiplication."

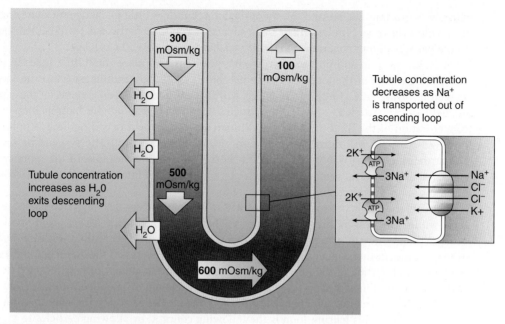

FIGURE 7-3 **Countercurrent multiplication in the Loop of Henle.** The combination of the hairpin loop, the Na/K ATPase pump in the ascending limb, and the permeability of the descending limb, allows the concentration gradient generated to be multiplied. The Na/K ATPase has a fixed amount of pumping capacity, and can only generate a fixed degree of concentration gradient. However, because the concentration of the fluid delivered to the pump is increasing, the Na/K ATPase can multiply the concentration gradient. In this figure, we have only illustrated water moving out of the descending limp in response to the increasing interstitial concentration; likely sodium flows from the interstitium into the thin descending limb as well, which further adds to the concentration of particles entering the ascending limb.

(it provides the environment that allows the NK2Cl transporter to work, as reviewed in Chapter 5) and then into the surrounding interstitium. The net effect is dilution of the tubular fluid and increased osmolarity of the interstitium.

Because of the hairpin configuration of the Loop of Henle, this extruded sodium surrounds the descending limb. There remains some controversy about the permeability of the thin descending limb to sodium, which raises the possibility that some of this extruded sodium from the ascending limb recycles back into the loop. However, more likely, the combination of aquaporin channels and an absence of tight junctions within the thin limb provides a pathway for water to move without sodium from the lumen of the descending limb to the interstitium of the renal medulla. Thus, in response to a growing interstitial gradient, water flows out of the descending limb, thereby concentrating the remaining tubular filtrate. In turn, this fluid progresses around the hairpin loop, and is presented to the ascending limb, where Na/K ATPases continue to extrude sodium ions and build the concentration gradient. In summary, the combination of a powerful Na/K ATPase pump, a hairpin loop, and structural features of the descending limb (the absence of tight junctions and the presence of plentiful aquaporin channels) all function to build a gradient between tubular fluid and the interstitium.

The maximal gradient that can be achieved is partly dependent on the length of the tubules. Short hairpin loops have less space to reabsorb water. Since quantitatively less water will be reclaimed from the tubule, a lower concentration of tubular sodium will be reached, and the Na/K ATPase will be presented with a less concentrated filtrate. Conversely, in longer loops, quantitatively more water will be removed; as a result, more concentrated fluid will reach the Na/K ATPase, which leads to a higher interstitial gradient. Animals that live in arid climates, such as the desert rats, have long Loops of Henle that can build interstitial gradients of almost 4,000 mOsm/kg.

The exact "maximum" concentration that can be attained by the Loop of Henle's **countercurrent multiplier** is uncertain. It is proposed to be approximately 600 to 800 mOsm/kg. Yet, the inner medullary regions of the interstitium reach concentrations of nearly 1,200 mOsm/kg. How is this additional concentration gradient built if not by the countercurrent multiplier? In fact, there is another important component to this process of building a gradient—the deposition of urea into the inner medulla. This second process is thought to contribute about one-third to half of the total concentration gradient. Urea handling will be discussed in the next section.

> **? THOUGHT QUESTION 7-2** Aquaporins, or water channels, provide a pathway for water to move across a cell membrane, and determine the water permeability of epithelial cells. Imagine that an individual was born with a lack of aquaporin channels in his Loop of Henle. How would that affect his ability to make concentrated urine?

THE IMPORTANCE OF UREA

Let us follow the filtrate as it passes beyond the Na/K ATPases in the thick ascending limb and into the distal tubule and the collecting duct. Since sodium, without water, has just been extruded actively from the lumen, the concentration of the filtrate as it reaches the distal tubules has fallen drastically, typically being diluted down to approximately 100 mOsm/kg. This region of the tubule is often termed the diluting segment, since the extrusion of particles without water obviously leads to a dilute filtrate remaining within the tubule. After the diluting segment, the fluid passes through the distal convoluted tubule. The tubule, which had been ascending from the medulla toward the cortex of the kidney, now reverses direction and moves back down toward the medulla. This redirection of the tubule brings the filtrate back to the same concentration gradient generated by the thick ascending limb's ATPases. In this final segment, termed the collecting duct, we find additional modifications in the tubular epithelium, which is regulated to refine further the body's water balance.

ADH has a particularly important role in the collecting duct. It orchestrates the movement of both water channels and urea transporters into the collecting tubule's membrane, thereby altering the tubule's permeability to these substances. In the presence of ADH, urea is able to contribute significantly to building the medullary interstitial gradient. This process is illustrated in *Figure 7-4*.

When ADH is present, aquaporin channels are inserted into the apical membrane of the outer and the inner collecting duct, which increases the epithelium's permeability to water. As water flows out of the tubule and into the interstitium, the filtrate remaining in the lumen becomes concentrated. The early section of the collecting tubule is impermeable to urea. Thus, as water exits, the concentration of urea remaining in the tubule increases dramatically.

By the time the filtrate has reached the inner medullary collecting duct, the lumen urea concentration can reach 600 to 800 mOsm/kg. In the presence of ADH, urea transporters are inserted into the inner medullary portion of the collecting duct. Whereas the outer sections of the collecting duct were urea impermeable, under ADH modulation, the inner medullary collecting duct is permeable and urea exits the lumen down its concentration gradient, into the interstitium. In this manner, when ADH is present, urea

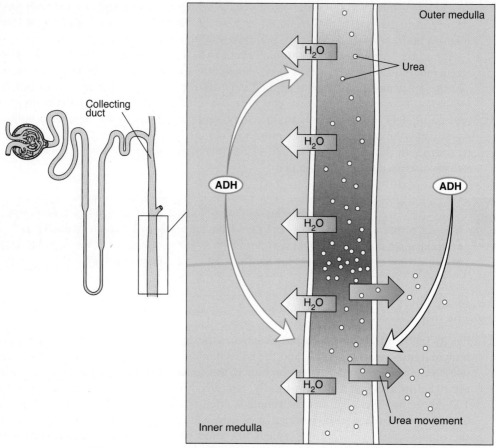

FIGURE 7-4 Urea contributes to the concentration gradient within the medulla. The concentration of the fluid in the interstitium can reach approximately 1,200 mOsm/kg. Approximately half of this is due to extrusion of sodium in the countercurrent multiplier. Urea accumulation accounts for the other half. ADH stimulates the expression of aquaporin in both the inner and outer medulla. ADH also stimulates expression of urea transporters in the inner medulla, but not the outer medulla. Thus, in the presence of ADH, the whole collecting duct is water permeable, whereas only the later section in the inner medulla is urea permeable. In this setting, the movement of water without urea in the outer medulla leads to increasing tubular urea concentration. Once the tubular fluid reaches the inner medulla, the now highly concentrated urea flows down its concentration gradient into the surrounding interstitium.

contributes to the generation of an interstitial gradient, i.e., to increasing the osmolarity of the interstitium.

In summary, in the presence of ADH, the collecting duct's permeability changes as it descends through the medulla. In the outer medulla, the tubule is permeable to water, but impermeable to urea. As water exits, the urea concentration increases. In the inner medulla, the tubule is permeable to both, and urea flows down its concentration gradient. Accumulation of urea in the interstitium adds to the medullary concentration gradient, which further enhances water movement from tubule to interstitium, thereby enhancing the concentrating ability of the kidney.

In the absence of ADH, neither water channels nor urea transporters are placed into the cells lining the collecting duct, and a urea concentration gradient is not built. Under these circumstances, the maximum inner medullary concentration falls to approximately 600 mOsm/kg, depending exclusively on the countercurrent multiplication of sodium (i.e., no additional gradient generated by urea movement).

Maintaining the Gradient

In the previous section, we have discussed the two methods of building a gradient within the interstitium. Maintenance of this gradient is critical to our ability to continue to concentrate urine. Given the large quantities of fluid that move through the kidney each day, there must be mechanisms that prevent the particles that have been placed in the inner portions of the medullary interstitium from being washed back into the blood stream. Why does the blood flow to the kidney not reabsorb the particles deposited in the interstitium? This will be the next topic of discussion—maintaining the gradient.

THE VASCULAR SUPPLY

As we learned in Chapter 3, there are three types of glomeruli within the renal cortex, as defined by their vascular supply. All glomeruli are supplied by penetrating interlobular arteries. However, after leaving the glomeruli to become the vasa recta plexus, the fate of the three different vasculatures is quite different. Vasa recta leaving glomeruli within the superficial cortex continue to head toward the kidney surface, directing blood away from the medulla. Vasa recta leaving midcortical glomeruli remain within the midcortex region and exit through the renal vein also without entering the medulla. Only the vasa recta leaving the deepest juxtamedullary glomeruli descend into the medulla.

Of the three pathways, only one vasa recta system enters the inner medulla and has the potential to dissipate the gradient established there. It is estimated that 90% of the renal blood perfuses the cortex alone, with only 10% entering the medulla and less than 2% reaching the deepest medullary regions. This vascular distribution helps to prevent washout of the medullary gradient. However, if we consider that 25% of the cardiac output perfuses the kidney per minute, then approximately 30 cc/min still reaches the deep inner medulla. On a daily basis, this is almost 45 L of blood per day! Then why does this large amount of blood not dissipate the concentration gradient within the inner medulla? This is the topic to be discussed in the next section.

COUNTERCURRENT EXCHANGE

There are unique structural modifications in the vasa recta, similar in design to the blood flow in penguins' webbed feet, that prevent the dilution of the medullary concentration gradient. Have you ever wondered how penguins can walk on the ice barefooted? Do they not get cold? What prevents them from losing all their body heat across their bare webbed feet? The design of the blood vessels in the penguin's legs prevents their body's heat from being lost via their cold feet; this basic design feature is also found in the organization of the medullary vasculature and prevents loss of the concentration gradient.

Let us take a closer look at the penguin. As illustrated in *Figure 7-5*, the blood supply within their webbed foot is in the shape of a hairpin loop. Unlike the hairpin loops we have discussed above, however, these thin endothelial cells have no active creation of gradients or differential permeabilities to water or particles. Instead, heat moves passively and freely from relatively warm areas (analogous to regions of high water concentration or low osmolarity) to relatively cold areas (analogous to regions of low water concentration or high osmolarity).

At the distal aspect of the web, exposed to the ice, cold meets the warm arterial blood as it is pumped from the systemic circulation, and heat is lost to the ice on which the penguin is standing. At the hairpin turn, the temperature of the animal's blood has dropped significantly. Yet, as the blood travels into the venous limb en route back to the body, it is

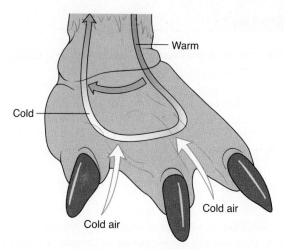

FIGURE 7-5 Countercurrent flow in a penguin's webbed foot. Warm arterial blood from the body flows toward the foot, where it is rapidly cooled. It passes through a hairpin loop into the venous limb, which runs in a countercurrent direction to the arterial limb. The venous limb is thus warmed by the arterial limb. The net effect of this anatomic arrangement of vessels is that there is a recycling of the warmth within the hairpin loop; this reduces the heat loss at the foot (and keeps the "cold" peripherally) and protects the animal. A similar mechanism in the kidney helps to maintain the high concentration of particles in the interstitium of the inner medulla.

once again exposed to warmer arterial blood by the countercurrent flow set up in the hairpin design. Warmth flows from the descending limb into the ascending limb, bypassing the most distal aspect of the loop, and cold is kept contained in a distal circuit; heat loss to the ice is minimized. A circular temperature flow loop arises proximal to the penguin's foot, thereby allowing the cold to remain within the distal aspect of the hairpin loop, and ultimately protecting the animal's body temperature. The unique countercurrent design of this hairpin blood supply maintains a temperature gradient in the web foot, with the cold kept distally and warmth proximally, while at the same time perfusing the animal's foot with blood.

In a similar manner, a countercurrent blood supply in the medulla maintains the concentration gradient while simultaneously perfusing important cells within the medullary interstitium.

As seen in *Figure 7-6*, the vasa recta arises from the efferent arteriole, descends alongside the tubules, continuing into the deepest parts of the inner medulla. The thin endothelial cells of the vasa recta are freely permeable to sodium and water, and thus the concentration of particles in the blood within the capillaries equilibrates with the surrounding interstitium.

Like the penguin's circulation, which constantly supplies the cold hairpin loop with warm blood, the descending loop of the vasa recta supplies the hairpin loop with relatively unconcentrated fluid, typically similar to plasma (290 mOsm/kg); fluid flows from regions of low osmolarity to high osmolarity. Analogous to the flow of heat in the penguin, in whom the arterial blood becomes colder as it approaches the loop's hairpin, water moves from the descending to the ascending limb of the vasa recta and the fluid becomes more concentrated as it descends into the inner medulla.

As the vasa recta descends into the concentrated medulla, water flows out of the blood vessel into the interstitium. After the hairpin bend, the opposite process occurs. Water enters from the interstitium into the vessel. This creates a circular loop of flow that maintains a high concentration of particles within the deepest parts of the medulla, preventing

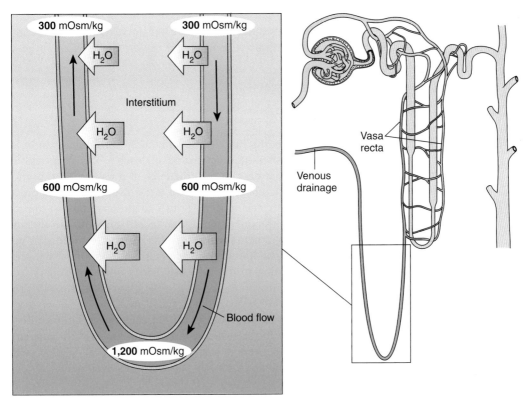

FIGURE 7-6 Countercurrent exchange in the vasa recta. Blood in the descending vessel begins with a relatively isotonic concentration. As the blood descends into the concentrated interstitium, water increasingly exits the vessel, and the blood increases in concentration. In the hairpin turn, the concentration reaches 1,200 mOsm/kg. In the ascending limb of the circuit, the opposite cycle occurs, with water entering the blood vessel, so that the concentration reapproximates serum as the vasa recta returns to the body. Water is moving out of the descending limb of the circuit and into the ascending limb, which limits the water that is available to dilute the interstitium of the inner medulla. In this manner, the concentration gradient of the interstitium is kept within the interstitium, and not dissipated into the systemic circulation. Note that movement of sodium, which likely occurs in the opposite direction of water, has not been illustrated in the figure.

them from being carried away into the venous circulation. In addition, since water exits the loop before reaching the hairpin, and then is reabsorbed, it bypasses the hairpin completely, preventing dilution of the inner medulla.

In this way, the **countercurrent exchange** of the vasa recta allows for perfusion of the deepest part of the medulla (bringing oxygen and nutrients to the tissue in the medulla), yet prevents the dissipation of the medulla's interstitial gradient. It should be noted that there are important differences between the countercurrent multiplier in the Loop of Henle and the countercurrent exchange of the vasa recta. Since the Loop of Henle is made of epithelial cells, depending on the presence of water channels and sodium transporters, there are significant permeability differences between the descending and ascending limbs. This allows the "multiplication" of the concentration gradient generated by the thick ascending limb. In contrast, the vasa recta is made up of thin endothelial cells, with equal permeability across all sections. Thus, no gradient is built; instead an "exchange" provides a circular flow of water in the upper limbs of the Loop, which prevents the water from washing out the particles that are in high concentration at the capillary loop tip.

? THOUGHT QUESTION 7-3 Would you expect the oxygen concentration of the innermost medulla to be—the same as arteries throughout the body? Lower? Higher? Explain your answer.

UREA RECYCLING

The Na/K ATPases in the thick ascending limb are continuously extruding sodium into the interstitium, yet the medullary interstitial osmolality plateaus at a concentration of around 1,200 mOsm/kg; it is clear that despite the efficiency of the vasa recta, particles eventually will be returned to the systemic circulation. In fact, this is a necessary process since the thick ascending limb must reclaim (i.e., return to the circulation) approximately 25% of the filtered sodium. Although sodium may "pool" transiently in the interstitium to provide the concentration gradient for reabsorption of water, it eventually must make its way back to the systemic circulation in order to maintain sodium homeostasis.

The other major particle contributing to the high osmolarity of the medullary interstitium is urea, the soluble form of nitrogenous waste. Unlike filtered sodium, which the tubules must reclaim, urea is destined to be excreted in the urine.

With this as a framework, the path of urea requires further elaboration. Unlike interstitial sodium, which eventually returns to the systemic circulation, much of the interstitial urea is channeled back into the tubular lumen, thereby entering a recycling process that keeps this waste product from returning to the body and allows its eventual excretion in the urine.

This process of urea recycling is facilitated by urea transporters, which have been identified in various segments of the kidney, as illustrated in *Figure 7-7*. By facilitating movement of urea, these transporters create a loop of urea flow. The inner medullary collecting tubule has urea transporters, which move urea into the interstitium. This urea is taken up by the vasa recta and, as discussed above, enters into the countercurrent flow within the distal aspect of the hairpin loop. Eventually, some urea escapes this cycle, and continues up the ascending limb of the vasa recta, potentially to return to the systemic circulation.

Yet, as the ascending vasa recta passes up toward the renal cortex, it passes next to the descending thin limb of nearby nephrons. These descending thin limbs also have urea transporters, which facilitate the movement of urea from the ascending vasa recta back into the tubule lumen. Consequently, urea is directed away from the systemic circulation into the tubule, and enters a loop of urea recycling. This process of urea recycling is important in two aspects. First, it continues to allow urea to participate in the inner medullary concentration gradient. Second, it prevents urea from returning to the body.

We have now discussed the major components of the medullary interstitial gradient. Let us put them all together.

Step 1. The driving force for the whole mechanism is provided the by Na/K ATPases in the thick ascending limb, which extrude sodium into the interstitium.

Step 2. The rising concentration of sodium in the interstitium provides a concentration gradient relative to the tubular fluid, which then pulls water out of the descending limb of the thin Loop of Henle. This further concentrates the luminal fluid, providing more concentrated substrate for the Na/K ATPases to work on, and thus "multiplies" the interstitial gradient further.

Step 3. The rising concentration of sodium in the interstitium also pulls water out of the urea impermeable cortical collecting tubule, thus increasing the concentration of urea within the tubular fluid. Once in the inner medulla, if ADH is present, urea transporters are inserted into the tubule, allowing highly concentrated urea to flow into the

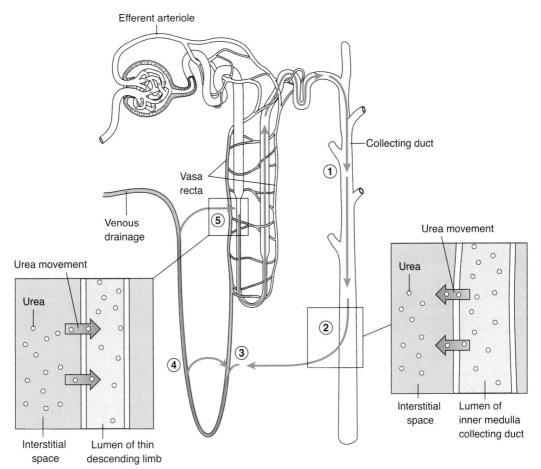

FIGURE 7-7 Urea recycling. Urea cycles in a loop-like fashion. This occurs via specific urea transporters placed in the inner medullary region of the collecting duct and in the descending limb of the Loop of Henle. (1) As water is drawn out of the collecting duct, the lumen urea concentration increases. (2) Urea then passes through urea specific transporters and enters the interstitium, where it helps generate the interstitial gradient. (3) Urea then diffuses into the blood across the permeable barrier of the descending vasa recta, passing through the hairpin loop, and into the ascending limb of the vasa recta. (4) Most of the urea recycles back into the descending limb as part of the countercurrent exchange. Some urea continues through the ascending limb, diffusing into more superficial parts of the interstitium. (5) Because of urea transporters in the thin descending limb of the Loop of Henle, the interstitial urea is then shuttled back into the tubule lumen. In this manner, urea, a potential waste product, is prevented from returning to the systemic circulation. It is contained within a local circuit that helps to both generate and maintain the interstitial concentration gradient.

interstitium, adding a second component to the development of high osmolarity in the medullary tissue.

Step 4. Urea enters the vasa recta. Much of the urea remains at the tip of the hairpin loop of the vasa recta, but the urea that escapes into the ascending limb of the vasa recta is channeled back into the descending limb of the tubule, creating a urea recycling pathway, which ensures that urea is ultimately excreted in the urine rather than returning to the body.

Step 5. The medullary concentration gradient, built by the accumulation of sodium and urea, is maintained by the unique architectural design of the vasa recta. Its hairpin loop functions to keep a high osmolar concentration at the hairpin tip.

These steps are summarized in Animated Figure 7-1 (Interstitial Gradient).

Reclaiming Water

We have now described how a gradient of increasing tissue osmolarity is generated and maintained in the renal medulla. Although it provides a force for water movement out of the tubule, this can only occur if the tubules allow the passage of water molecules. As discussed in Chapters 2 and 5, the collecting duct is impermeable to water in its baseline state. It is only when aquaporin water channels are inserted into the apical membrane that water can leave the tubule for the more concentrated interstitium. This, the final step in reclaiming water, is the release and subsequent action of ADH.

ADH is the orchestrating hormone for water regulation. The medullary concentration is relatively constant; fine-tuning of water reclamation is due to the presence of ADH, and the subsequent insertion of aquaporins into the epithelial cells of the collecting duct. How the body knows just how much ADH to release, and how much water to reclaim, is the subject of the next chapter.

> **?**   **THOUGHT QUESTION 7-4   You decide to go for a jog one summer afternoon. On your return, you go to the bathroom and notice that your urine is quite dark. Has either your kidney's medullary concentration or your body's ADH levels changed during the jog? Explain your answer.**

In summary, the kidney's ability to generate and maintain progressively higher tissue osmolarity in the deeper regions of the renal medulla and to alter the collecting tubules' water permeability are the two primary functions required for you to concentrate your urine. Countercurrent multiplication within the renal tubule helps generate the interstitial gradient, and countercurrent exchange within the vasa recta helps maintain it. Although both these processes require a hairpin loop, there are important structural differences between the tubules and the vas recta that are important to remember. In countercurrent multiplication, the tubules have variable permeability along their length, leading to the generation of an increasingly concentrated interstitial gradient. In countercurrent exchange, the capillaries are fully permeable to particles and water alike, leading to a circular current of water proximal to the distal tip of the vasa recta.

PUTTING IT TOGETHER

A 78-year-old man with a long-standing history of hypertension is brought into the emergency room with profound hypotension from an anterior myocardial infarction. He is stabilized, taken emergently to the cardiac catheterization lab, where an arteriogram reveals acute occlusion of his left anterior descending artery. A stent is placed, and the patient is taken to the ICU.

The nurses note that his urine output drops off to 5 cc/hr. The next day, his serum creatinine has risen from 0.8 mg/dl to 1.6 mg/dL, and you hear the renal consultant diagnose him with acute tubular necrosis (ATN), a condition in which tubular function is dramatically altered.

Why has the quantity of urine diminished? What do you think the concentration of his urine will be? If you infuse ADH, how would the urine concentration change in this patient?

This patient has suffered acute tubular necrosis due to profound and prolonged hypotension, i.e., there has been hypoperfusion or inadequate blood and oxygen delivery to the renal tubules. Since the thick ascending loop has a high-energy requirement, given its concentration of active Na/K ATPases, it is particularly susceptible to ischemic damage.

In this setting, the Na/K ATPases cease to function, and the kidney loses the critical first step necessary to generate a medullary concentration gradient. Without these "pumps", the osmolarity of the interstitium cannot be increased and the urine cannot be concentrated. Even if ADH is infused, and many aquaporin channels are inserted into the collecting tubule, there will be no concentration gradient to facilitate the movement of water from the tubule to the interstitium. Given this injury to the tubules, the urine will be "isosthenuric", meaning it will be neither dilute nor concentrated, but rather will have the same concentration as serum. So, this patient's urine osmolarity will be around 300 mOsm/kg.

If ADH is infused, the water channels in the collecting duct will increase its water permeability, but without a medullary interstitial gradient, no water will be reclaimed. Thus, ADH will not change the isosthenuric concentration of ATN urine. The urine volume is decreased because the severe tubular damage also leads to dysfunction of the glomeruli and reduced filtration of blood.

Summary Points

- Because we live in an arid environment, we are constantly at risk for becoming dehydrated, as defined by a relative deficiency of water to particles in our body and indicated by an abnormally high sodium concentration in the blood.
- Because we are constantly eating particles, in the form of sodium and protein, the kidneys must be able to excrete a particle rich waste product, i.e., concentrated urine.
- The high osmolarity of the renal medulla is key to absorbing water from the tubule and the production of concentrated urine.
- Both sodium and urea contribute to the building of the progressively concentrated medullary interstitium as one goes from the renal cortex toward the collecting system.
- The Na/K ATPases in the thick ascending tubules provide the driving energy to produce the high osmolarity of the renal medulla.
- Countercurrent multiplier and countercurrent exchange are two different processes; both are necessary for the urine to produce concentrated urine.
- The countercurrent multiplier plays an important role in increasing the total medullary concentration.
- There are three important aspects to the countercurrent multiplier—the Na/K ATPases in the thick ascending limb, the hairpin-shaped turn in the Loop of Henle, and the thin descending limb's permeability to water.
- Urea plays an important role in generating the medullary interstitial gradient.
- The renal medulla's interstitial osmolar gradient is protected by the structural design of the kidney's overall vascular flow and by the countercurrent exchange.
- The vascular supply of the kidney channels the majority of blood flow away from the medulla, helping to prevent the dissipation of the interstitial gradient.
- Of the blood that does perfuse the inner medulla, countercurrent exchange prevents the concentrated interstitium from being diluted.
- Urea recycling helps maintain the medullary interstitial gradient.
- Because the tubule is composed of epithelial cells, it is impermeable to water in its baseline state.
- ADH provides a rapid on/off switch that determines just how much water our kidneys retain; when present, ADH stimulates the insertion of aquaporins into the epithelial lining of the collecting duct, thereby making them permeable to water.

Answers TO THOUGHT QUESTIONS

7-1. The shark absorbs both sodium and water across its intestines and is exposed to large amounts of hyperosmolar fluid daily. Because of this excess sodium load, they must extrude particles. In their gills, they have a secretory sodium pump (NK2Cl—see Chapter 5), which actively extrudes particles from the animals' body. Thus, sharks maintain their serum osmolarity by actively excreting particles. Dolphins breathe through lungs. Since they do not have gills (and do not swallow large quantities of sea water), their plasma is not exposed to such large amounts of sodium. Their skins are impermeable to seawater. Like humans, they rely primarily on the concentration of their urine to protect their serum osmolarity rather than extrusion of particles. Their urines typically range from 800 to 2,000 mOsm/kg.

7-2. The countercurrent exchanger helps generate the concentration gradient within the medullary interstitium. It is dependent on several unique features. First, Na/K ATPases in the thick ascending limb provide the initial force to extrude sodium ions from the tubule into the interstitium. Because of the hairpin turn of the Loop of Henle, these extruded sodium ions now surround relatively dilute fluid flowing along the descending thin limb. The thin limb must be water permeable in order to allow water to exit the lumen, thereby increasing the concentration of the fluid remaining in the tubule, which is subsequently presented to the pumping Na/K ATPases in the ascending limb of the Loop of Henle. Thus, in the setting of aquaporin deficiency, the thin descending tubule will be less permeable to water, interrupting the multiplication process, and thus will prevent the concentration of the urine.

7-3. The unique vascular supply of the kidneys delivers blood first to the glomerulus, and then forms a second capillary network in a "series" configuration. This second capillary structure is the vasa recta, which delivers blood to the energy-dependent thick ascending tubules, and then descends farther down into the deepest parts of the inner medulla. With respect to water movement, the anatomic configuration of the vasa recta protects the interstitial gradient of the inner medulla. However, when one considers the role of the vasa recta in supplying oxygen to the kidney, this vascular route places the inner medullary region at risk for hypoxia.

The amount of blood within the vasa recta is dependent on the amount of fluid that is filtered across the more proximal glomerulus (more fluid filtered from the blood passing through the glomerulus leaves a smaller volume of blood continuing to the vasa recta). In addition, the Na/K ATPases present in the thick ascending limb consume oxygen. Thus, the inner medulla receives quantitatively less blood and the blood it does receive is relatively hypoxic. Furthermore, the countercurrent exchange of the vasa recta, while setting up flows of water and sodium that keep the most distal tip highly concentrated, sets up a similar flow of oxygen, which ultimately keeps the distal tip hypoxic, i.e., oxygen flows from the descending limb to the ascending limb of the vasa recta leaving little to reach the tip of the capillary loop. Whereas the pO_2 of the outer cortex is close to 100 mm Hg, it falls to approximately 5 to 10 mm Hg in the inner medulla.

7-4.   In order to reclaim water from the urine, we need both a concentrated medullary inter-stitium and a water permeable collecting duct. The former is an energy-dependent and time-consuming process, and takes hours to days to build a highly concen-trated medullary interstitium. Conversely, in the presence of ADH, aquaporins move quickly from within the cell to the apical membrane (minutes to hours). Thus, the modulation of water channels is a much more efficient and timely way to control the water avidity of the kidneys. Therefore, ADH plays more of a role in the hour-to-hour modification of our urine concentration. Most likely, your med-ullary concentration has not changed dramatically (perhaps increasing due to the presence of ADH effect on urea handling), while the levels of ADH have increased dramatically from the resting state to the period following the exercise.

7

Review Questions

DIRECTIONS: Each of the numbered items or incomplete statements in this section is followed by answers or by completion of the statement. Select the ONE lettered answer or completion that is BEST in each case.

1. Imagine that two friends go out for a hiking trip into the hot desert of Arizona. They both are equally well conditioned, and seem to sweat the same amount. Mike, who is a vegan, eats mostly vegetables, supplemented by sodium tablets and water to prevent dehydration and to replace his sodium loss. Jeff tries to recreate his usual meat and potatoes diet and brings along protein bars, yet consumes similar amounts of sodium and water. After a long day of hiking during which they both run short of water, they return to base camp and provide a urine sample.
    Which of the following statements is true?

    A. Mike and Jeff's urines will have similar concentration.
    B. Mike's urine will be more concentrated.
    C. Jeff's urine will be more concentrated.
    D. Neither Mike nor Jeff will be able to make concentrated urine.

2. Two women visit their respective physicians and are found to have high blood pressure. The first physician prescribes 25 mg of hydrochlorothiazide, which blocks sodium reclamation at the distal convoluted tubule. The second prescribes 20 mg of furosemide, which blocks the sodium/potassium/chloride (NK2Cl) channel in the thick ascending limb. Both women are avid long distance joggers. Which one is more likely to get dehydrated (i.e., have difficulty concentrating her urine)?

    A. The woman placed on hydrochlorothiazide
    B. The woman placed on furosemide
    C. Since diuretics affect sodium handling, not water, neither woman is at risk for dehydration.

3. Following a new health craze suggesting that excessive water intake is healthy, a young man drinks about 15 L of water per day. Not surprisingly, he spends most of the day in the bathroom, urinating many liters of dilute urine. He then decides to stop drinking water, and wants to test how concentrated he can make his urine (he is a budding nephrologist). Relative to the concentration of his urine before the health craze, what would you expect his maximal urine concentration to be?

    A. His maximal urine concentration would be less.
    B. His maximal urine concentration would be more.
    C. His maximal urine concentration would not be affected by his water intake.

Maintaining the Serum Concentration

Water Balance

chapter **8**

CHAPTER OUTLINE

INTRODUCTION
THE CONCENTRATION OF OUR BODY'S FLUID
DETECTING THE BODY'S CONCENTRATION:
  THE OSMORECEPTOR
OSMORECEPTOR CONTROL OF ADH RELEASE
  AND THIRST
NON-OSMORECEPTOR CONTROL OF ADH
  RELEASE AND THIRST
SERUM OSMOLALITY

APPLICATION OF THE PRINCIPLES OF WATER
  REGULATION
  • Disorder of osmolality: a water problem
  • Disorders of decreased concentration
  • Disorders of increased concentration
  • Disorders of urine volume
PUTTING IT TOGETHER
SUMMARY POINTS

LEARNING OBJECTIVES

By the end of this chapter, you should be able to:

- **recognize that water flows freely across the major fluid compartments in our body.**
- **define the terms "osmolarity" and "osmolality," and how they are measured.**
- **define the major particles that determine osmolality.**
- **explain how changes in body water lead to changes in serum osmolality.**
- **describe how the body senses its own fluid concentration via the osmoreceptor.**
- **define the mechanisms that lead to the release of ADH.**
- **describe the difference between calculated and measured osmolality.**
- **explain the relationship of urine volume to solute and water homeostasis.**
- **describe an analytical approach to disorders of hyponatremia and hypernatremia.**

Introduction

As we described in Chapter 2, the body is composed of three major compartments or spaces: the intracellular, the interstitial, and the intravascular spaces. Although the barriers that separate each compartment differ with respect to their permeability to electrolytes, both the cell membrane and the endovascular lining of blood vessels are fully permeable to water. Thus, except for a few important exceptions that we will address later, there are no concentration gradients between the major body compartments. Water flows freely across all barriers, equalizing the concentration among the spaces. Of course, the type of particles may differ among these compartments. For example, cells have a relatively large amount of potassium, yet little sodium, whereas the serum has more sodium and little potassium. Because water flows freely across all the surfaces, however, the total concentration of all particles within each compartment is the same.

The ability of water to cross most cell membranes creates important challenges for our body. In the setting of water excess, for example, water will distribute into all compartments, including the cells of the brain, causing cell swelling. Since neuronal cells have excitable properties sensitive to small changes in the local environment, subtle changes of neuronal cell volume can induce a wide range of clinical symptoms, ranging from mild headaches to mental confusion and even seizures and death.

In order to preserve normal cellular function, mammals have evolved efficient homeostatic mechanisms to protect the body's osmolality. Small changes (<1%) in plasma osmolality trigger a wide range of neuroendocrine and behavioral responses that re-establish the equilibrium. Human plasma osmolality is vigorously protected to maintain a range somewhere between 280 and 300 mOsm/kg.

Given the arid environment in which we live, this is no easy task. On an average day, we lose approximately 1 L of water through evaporation from our skin and respiratory tract. This obviously increases in warmer climates, and is highly dependent on our daily activity. On an average diet, at least 0.5 L of water is required in urine in order to clear our body's toxic waste. Thus, each day, we must replace this loss with ingestion of adequate water (minus the small amount that is derived from cellular metabolism). Thanks to various health crazes, the preponderance of coffee shops, myriad types of bottled drinks, and a wide range of other social and cultural practices, most Americans have no problem ingesting adequate amounts of water. In fact, most of us are in a state of great water excess, and the body is more often challenged to rid itself of extra water rather than to conserve in the setting of water restriction. Both these processes are equally important, however. In order to maintain plasma concentration, the body must be able to excrete water in times of excess, and conserve water in times of deficit.

The Concentration of Our Body's Fluid

Our bodies are primarily composed of water. There are many particles dissolved into that water, including electrolytes such as sodium, potassium, chloride, and bicarbonate, along with molecules such as glucose and urea. Other particles, such as triglycerides and proteins, do not dissolve, but rather exist in a separate phase, in a manner similar to an oil slick floating upon the water. Within the aqueous phase, the relationship of the particles to dissolved water is expressed as a concentration.

How can we measure the concentration of particles within our own body? As we discussed in Chapter 2, the presence of particles within a solution alters the inherent kinetic potential between the water molecules. Adding salt to a pot of boiling water transiently stops the boil, for example, as the added particles change the relationship between the water molecules, increasing the boiling point of the solution. In a similar manner, the particles within our blood change the inherent boiling point, as well as the freezing point, of blood (for these purposes, we are referring to the serum or non-cellular component of blood). Boiling points of blood are infrequently measured in commercial labs; most rely on freezing point depression. On average, whereas water freezes at 0°C, blood typically freezes at a slightly lower temperature, around −0.52°C.

Capitalizing on the predictable effect of particles on a solution's freezing point, one can measure the freezing point of an individual's serum and, in comparison to freezing points of known solutions, determine exactly how many particles are present. This measurement

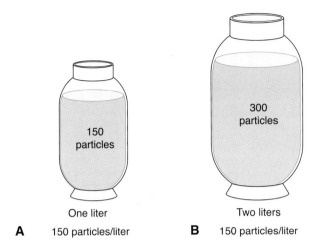

FIGURE 8-1 Fluid concentration vs. fluid volume. The concentration of a fluid describes the relationship between the number of particles and the volume of a fluid; it tells us nothing about the total amount of particles and water. Container **B,** with 300 particles in 2 L, contains more particles than does Container **A,** but the two containers have the same concentration, 150 particles/L.

cannot distinguish what types of particles are contributing to the overall concentration; it simply tells you the total number of all particles within a particular solution. **Osmolality** is the term used to describe the number of osmotically active particles within 1 kg of solution. **Osmolarity** refers to the number of osmotically active particles within 1 L of solution. Since 1 L of serum weighs 1 kg, we can use these terms interchangeably with respect to the body's fluids. In summary, the serum or plasma osmolarity simply describes the number of dissolved particles within the aqueous phase of blood.

Let us look at *Figure 8-1* for a moment. Two different sized tanks are present. In *Figure 8-1A*, there are 150 particles in 1 L of water. The concentration is 150 particles/L. In *Figure 8-1B*, there are 300 particles in 2 L of water. The concentration is 150 particles/L. Thus, despite the total amount of particles and the volume of water being much greater in *Figure 8-1B*, the concentrations of the two solutions are the exactly the same.

The simple scenario is an important (and often overlooked) reminder regarding the difference between concentration and volume. Concentration tells us only about the relationship between the amounts of particles and water, but tells us nothing about the absolute amounts. Thus, serum osmolality says absolutely nothing about the total amount of particles or the total volume of water, but simply describes the relative relationship of both.

In this chapter, we describe the mechanisms with which our body assesses and responds to changes in concentration. This stands in contrast to our previous discussions about the body's control of the volume of body fluid, in which case there was little regard for concentration. Importantly, as we will learn, the changes in body concentration are primarily due to either excess or deficit of water, rather than loss or gain of particles.

Detecting the Body's Concentration: The Osmoreceptor

The internal measurement of the body's osmolality belongs to a group of neurons called **osmoreceptors**. These cells are defined by their intrinsic capacity to both sense and respond to the changes in serum osmolality. Osmoreceptors are likely to be found in many areas within the brain, but recent studies have suggested that one area may be of particular importance: the organum vasculosum of the laminae terminalis (OVLT). The OVLT sits anterior and ventral to the third ventricle, and has a unique blood supply. Unlike the

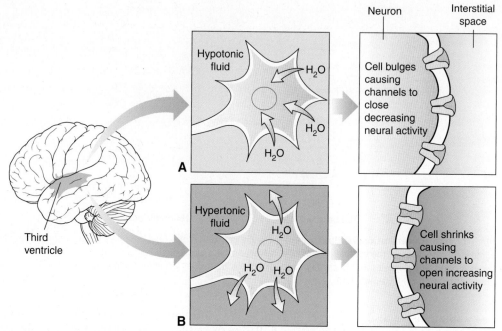

FIGURE 8-2 The osmoreceptor. The osmoreceptor is located within the brain, and senses serum osmolality. A stretch receptor within the cell membrane responds to changes in cell size. In Panel 2**A,** fluid outside the neuron has a lower concentration than within the neuron, causing water to flow into the cell. The resulting cell swelling closes the receptor, and neuronal activity is decreased. Conversely, in Panel 2**B,** the concentration of fluid outside the neuron is higher; fluid leaves the cell, the cell shrinks, and the stretch receptor is activated, increasing neuronal activity.

remainder of the blood-brain barrier, where tight junctions connect adjacent endothelial cells, the OVLT has a fenestrated, leaky endothelium. The cells here are not part of the cerebrospinal fluid sanctuary, but instead are exposed directly to the chemical environment of the systemic circulation. Thus, they are good sensors of the body's osmolality.

The cellular mechanisms of how the osmoreceptors detect serum osmolality have recently been described. The OVLT cells have membrane bound cation channels that are sensitive to mechanical stimuli. The activity of these channels is inhibited by membrane stretch and, conversely, activated by membrane shrinkage. Activation of the channels leads to an inward flux of cations, which increases the neuronal action potential firing frequency. As illustrated in *Figure 8-2*, upon being exposed to hypotonic fluid, the osmoreceptor cell swells as water flows into it. This results in stretch of its cell membrane, which decreases the activity of the mechanosensitive channels and causes hyperpolarization and inhibition of neuronal firing frequency. Conversely, water leaves the osmoreceptor when it is exposed to hypertonic fluid, and its cell membrane shrinks stimulating the mechanosensitive channels to open. The influx of cations depolarizes the membrane and increases neuronal action potential firing frequency.

The importance of cell size change, as water either enters or leaves, explains an early experimental observation. Injection of hypertonic sodium chloride into dogs precipitated drinking, but an equal amount of urea had little effect. Since the cell membrane of the osmoreceptor is impermeable to sodium chloride but permeable to urea, the former causes an efflux of water and cellular shrinkage, whereas the later induces no change in cell volume.

Having sensed serum osmolality, the osmoreceptors trigger secondary responses, which are mediated through two pathways that lead to two different clinical outcomes: concentration of the urine and thirst. OVLT axons connect to the supraoptic nucleus in the hypothalamus, the source of antidiuretic hormone (ADH) production. ADH, otherwise known as vasopressin, is the major hormone responsible for the process of concentrating the urine, a critical step in water conservation. In addition, OVLT neurons connect via unspecified pathways to the insula and anterior cingulate gyrus within the cortex, the regions of the brain thought to be involved in the perception of thirst. These two neuronal pathways allow the osmoreceptor to coordinate two very important physiological responses. When faced with hyperosmolality, the osmoreceptor activation causes release of ADH, which prevents the loss of water in the urine, and stimulates thirst, a powerful urge to drink water.

Osmoreceptor Control of ADH Release and Thirst

The osmoreceptors are sensitive to small changes in plasma osmolality; changes as little as 1% to 2% cause release of ADH and stimulation of thirst. However, these mechanistic responses do not occur simultaneously. Consider the often-quoted hikers warning: "The first sign of dehydration is darkening of the urine. If you wait until you are thirsty, you are already in a water deficit." This simple observation correlates with physiological principles.

Although there is variability among individuals, the osmoreceptor generally activates the ADH pathway before the thirst pathway (*Figure 8-3*). In other words, our first response to increasing plasma concentration is to concentrate the urine. Thirst develops somewhat later. This timing is important; it allows us to go about our daily activity, conserving water through concentrating the urine, rather than constantly searching for a water fountain. In healthy adults, the osmotic threshold for ADH secretion ranges from 275 to 290 mOsm/kg, averaging approximately 280 mOsm/kg. The osmotic threshold for thirst typically ranges from 285 to 305 mOsm/kg, averaging approximately 290 mOsm/kg. These are generalizations, however, and controversy exists within the literature about the exact numbers. But on average, the threshold for release of ADH occurs at an osmolality about 5 to 10 mOsm/kg lower than for the stimulation of thirst.

OVLT osmoreceptor stimulation of ADH occurs along a distinct pathway. Axons project from the OVLT to the supraoptic nucleus and paraventricular nucleus of the

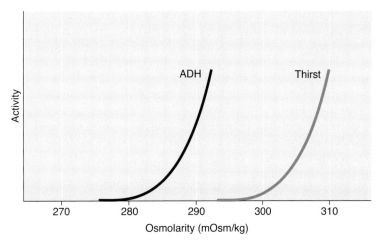

FIGURE 8-3 The body's response to increasing serum concentration. Changes in body osmolality induce release of ADH and stimulate thirst. ADH is stimulated at a lower osmolality than is thirst. ADH and thirst are the two mechanisms available to the body to correct serum hyperosmolarity; ADH leads to water reabsorption in the collecting duct and thirst increases water ingestion.

hypothalamus, continuing down the neurohypophyseal tract into the posterior lobe of the pituitary. Osmoreceptor depolarization results in the release of the excitatory neurotransmitter glutamate within the synapse, which in turn stimulates the synthesis of ADH. Its biosynthesis occurs from a precursor peptide that is produced in the supraoptic nuclei, packaged in secretory granules, and cleaved progressively as it moves down the axon into the posterior pituitary where it is released into the systemic circulation.

Osmoreceptor-stimulated ADH release is an exquisitely sensitive pathway, which allows precise fine-tuning of the serum osmolality. Changes in plasma osmolality of as little as 1% will change plasma ADH by an average of 1 pg/mL, an amount sufficient to greatly concentrate the urine and conserve water. In addition, vasopressin release has a set "break point" phenomenon. As illustrated in *Figure 8-3*, at plasma osmolality below a threshold level, plasma ADH is completely suppressed (levels are undetectable). Above that point, plasma ADH concentration rises steeply in direct proportion to plasma osmolality. In addition, the slope of the rise in ADH also differs among individuals. In some people, small changes (0.5 mOsm/kg) in osmolality will have the same effect on ADH release as large changes (5 mOsm/kg) in others. Many factors can affect this relationship between plasma osmolality and ADH release. Medications, including psychotropic drugs, along with volume depletion, hypercalcemia, angiotensin, and possibly sex hormones change the slope; age has been shown to alter the set point too.

Non-osmoreceptor Control of ADH Release and Thirst

In the previous section, we have described how the brain's osmoreceptors internally sense the plasma's concentration and respond to perturbations by modulating ADH release and thirst. These two mechanisms for responding to changes in osmolarity are critically important to the preservation of the body's chemical composition. However, there are also important mechanisms by which ADH release and thirst occur, which are independent of the osmoreceptor and plasma concentration. Even in the setting of severe hypo-osmolality, if these non-osmotic stimuli are present, the body will retain water and lower the plasma concentration even further.

Perhaps the most important non-osmotic stimulus of both ADH release and thirst is a decrease in sensed body volume, which is usually manifest as a decline in blood pressure. Although small decreases in blood pressure (on the order of 5% to 10%) have little effect, once the blood pressure falls by 20%, ADH rises to levels many times greater than what is necessary to maintain antidiuresis, i.e., water reclamation in the collecting duct. Conversely, an acute rise in blood pressure suppresses ADH secretion. Since perfusion of vital organs is critical for the survival of the organism, it makes sense that blood volume would be protected even if it will lead to a drop in serum osmolality.

Use Animated Figure 8-1 (Control of ADH Release) to explore the relationships between plasma osmolality, volume and blood pressure status, and ADH release. First change osmolality and observe the change in plasma ADH levels for a normal ADH release curve. Then experiment with changing blood pressure or volume status and notice how the ADH release curve shifts.

The processes by which this hemodynamic-driven release of ADH occurs are not fully known. Neurogenic afferent nerves from the left ventricle, pressure receptors in the aorta and carotid sinus, as well as humoral mechanisms have all been postulated to be potential pathways. Despite the absence of a definitive explanation for how this occurs, the biologic value of such a pathway is obvious. Although water retention is an inefficient way to improve intravascular volume (only 1/9 of the water stays in the vascular space—see Chapter 2), the body responds with every mechanism available to it, including water

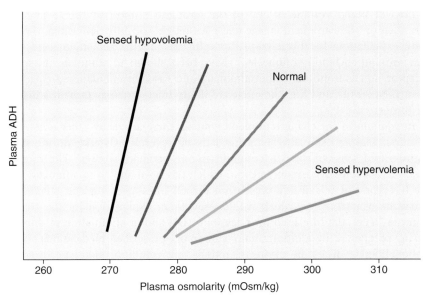

FIGURE 8-4 **The effect of sensed volume on the relationship of osmolality and ADH release.** Decreases of sensed volume "sensitize" the system, so that smaller changes of osmolality induce larger amounts of ADH release. Conversely, if the body senses volume expansion, there is a higher threshold for release of ADH and a less vigorous response to progressive hyperosmolarity.

retention, to restore the blood pressure when confronted with severe hypotension. In times of pending hemodynamic collapse, the body will sacrifice concentration for volume. Since reduced cerebral blood flow associated with hypotension causes death much more rapidly than a fall or rise in plasma osmolality, this prioritization makes sense.

The relative importance of the osmoreceptor versus hemodynamic stimulation of ADH release must be put into context. The osmoreceptor system is tenfold more sensitive than the hemodynamic system: a 1% to 2% change in osmolality stimulates the equivalent ADH release as a 20% to 30% change in blood pressure. The presence of hypotension does not disrupt the osmoreceptor regulation, but instead changes the sensitivity of the system (both the set point and the slope of the response), as illustrated in *Figure 8-4*. In the setting of sensed hypovolemia, the amount of ADH released increases for a given plasma osmolality.

In addition to sensed blood volume, various other stimuli affect the release of ADH. Nausea is a potent stimulus, and can increase ADH levels to 1,000 times basal level. Emetic drugs like morphine, nicotine, and alcohol, as well as conditions such as motion sickness, vasovagal syncope, acute hypoglycemia, and hypoxia all induce ADH release.

Like the non-osmotic stimuli of ADH release, a wide array of events can lead to an increase in thirst. As a conscious perception of the need to drink, thirst is a complex biologic process that involves many different parts of the brain and is influenced by a variety of biologic, psychological, and environmental factors. In many ways, drinking liquids has become a cultural phenomenon, rather than a physiologic one. From Starbucks coffee to Nalgene water bottles, we are constantly bombarded with stimuli to drink. How this affects the perception of thirst is not clear. Nevertheless, the perception of thirst is often divorced from any abnormality in plasma osmolality. As an illustration of this phenomenon, the infusion of physiologically excessive amounts of water into the stomach of a rat, bypassing its mouth, does not extinguish the need to drink. The animal continues to drink despite a low plasma osmolality. The passage of water across the lips and mouth in itself provides a sense of satisfaction, especially for those with the tendency toward dry mucus membranes (mouth breathers, disorders of the salivary glands).

Loss of blood volume is one of the strongest stimuli of thirst. Thirst among the wounded on the battlefield is legendary. Although not fully delineated, there are mechanistic explanations for this relationship. Infusions of renin and angiotensin, the hormones that respond to blood volume loss, have been shown to stimulate thirst. In addition, receptor signals from the cardiopulmonary and vascular circulation are carried along the Cranial Nerves IX and X to the nucleus solitary tract, and may provide a distinct pathway for this sensation.

In addition to the changes in blood volume, there are many other non-osmotic stimuli of thirst. Plasma osmolality typically falls by several mOsm/kg during pregnancy, yet an increased sense of thirst is common among pregnant women. The corpus luteum of the ovary secretes a hormone relaxin, which has been shown to stimulate thirst. In fact, the receptors for relaxin are present on the OVLT, suggesting that relaxin may directly affect the osmoreceptor, which would provide an explanation for the "resetting of the osmostat" (i.e., the threshold for release of ADH and/or stimulation of thirst is changed) during pregnancy. In addition, many commonly prescribed medications stimulate thirst. Anticholinergic drugs, by drying secretions, are common offenders. In addition, many psychiatric drugs as well as psychiatric illnesses have been associated with an increased perception of thirst. Cold water seems to satiate thirst more than an equal volume of room temperature water.

Serum Osmolality

You place 1,000 mg of glucose and 100 mmol of sodium chloride into 1 L of water. What is the osmolarity of the solution? There are several important concepts to be learned in this example. Osmolarity refers to the number of particles per solution. It does not care about the size of the particle, nor the charge; only the number is important. Thus, one particle of sodium chloride (NaCl) has the same osmolar contribution as one mmol of sodium. If the sodium chloride dissociates into separate sodium and chloride particles, there will be 2 mmol, 1 mmol of sodium and 1 mmol of chloride, and the osmolarity of the solution would be twice that of the solution with undissociated sodium chloride.

It turns out that 100 molecules of sodium chloride typically dissociate in a manner that leads to 175 particles (75 of sodium, 75 of chloride, and 25 of sodium chloride). Thus, in order to obtain the osmolarity of sodium chloride in solution, you multiply the sodium concentration by 1.75.

As for the glucose, again, we are not concerned with the size or weight of the particle. Thus, the 1,000 mg of glucose must be divided by its molecular weight (180) in order to determine the number of particles. The glucose in this example provides 5.6 mOsm and the sodium chloride 1.75 mOsm. The osmolality of the solution is 7.35 mOsm/kg.

Serum osmolality can be calculated from the following formula.

$$\text{Osmolality} = 2(Na) + BUN/2.8 + glucose/18$$

This formula, which divides the blood urea nitrogen (BUN) and serum glucose levels [which are measured in weights per unit volume (mg/dL)] by their respective molecular weight, calculates the number of particles per weight of fluid. We multiply the measured serum sodium by 2 to account for all the negatively charged anions, such as chloride. Since sodium chloride typically dissociates into 1.75 rather than 2 particles, as noted earlier, this calculation slightly overestimates osmolality. However, there are other cations and anions that we typically do not measure in our routine laboratory evaluation, but still contribute to osmolality, such as calcium, magnesium, and potassium. Multiplying the sodium by 2, instead of 1.75, is a "fudge factor" that allows correction for these unmeasured particles.

In our current practice of clinical medicine, the basic laboratory panel includes an assessment of sodium, chloride, potassium, bicarbonate, BUN, creatinine, and glucose, otherwise known as the "chem-7." Using the formula shown earlier, the calculated osmolality is obtained from these measured laboratory values. However, the most accurate method of assessing osmolality is by direct measurement of the freezing point depression of the blood sample. When ordering a measured, rather than a calculated, osmolality, the laboratory performs a direct measurement of the blood's freezing point. This is a true osmolality, always more accurate than the calculated value.

There are certain conditions in which the calculated osmolality (as determined from the measured chem-7 panel) and the directly measured osmolality differ. This implies that some other type of particle is present, which is not represented by the items in the routine chemistry panel. Most often, these "non-measurable" particles are associated with ingested alcohols, including standard recreational alcohols as well as highly toxic alcohols such as ethylene glycol (antifreeze) or methanol.

Application of the Principles of Water Regulation

To reinforce the principles we have been discussing, and to help you see how these principles are applied to common clinical scenarios, we provide several examples in which the application of what you have learned helps you understand how the body strives to maintain a constant serum osmolality.

DISORDERS OF OSMOLALITY: A WATER PROBLEM

The challenge for every case of hypo-osmolality or hyperosmolality is to determine why there is either a water excess or deficit, respectively. Conceptually, one might argue that the loss of particles, such as sodium without water, would lead to changes in body concentration. Although this is conceptually true, there are almost no clinical scenarios in which the body loses particles in excess of water. For example, sweat is usually hypotonic, so that relatively more water than particles is lost, tending toward hyperosmolality. Gastric loss (vomiting) is usually isotonic because the epithelial layer along the gastrointestinal mucosa does not have tight junctions and is permeable to water. Similarly, the fluid lost in illnesses associated with diarrhea tends to be isotonic or hypotonic. An understanding of these physiological principles illustrates why hypo-osmolality is due to water retention, not particle loss.

One might also want to argue that problems with water excess, in addition to causing changes in serum concentration, will also affect body volume, i.e., intravascular or interstitial volume. Well, this is somewhat true, although the impact is less than you might initially think. For example, if a patient drinks 10 L of water, and does not urinate at all (say he is a dialysis patient and makes no urine), then clearly, his serum sodium concentration will fall and the volume of his total body fluid will increase by 10 L. However, the great majority of that fluid (as discussed in Chapter 2) will distribute into the cells, including his brain cells. Because the brain is surrounded by a tight cranium, and because of its sensitive neurologic function, it is highly intolerant of changes in cell size. Thus, the patient would begin to develop neurological symptoms, including headache, seizures, and even death. The effect of the portion (one-ninth) of the 10-L water that remained in the intravascular compartment would pale in comparison to the devastating effect of the portion (two-thirds) of the 10-L water that expands cells. Thus, in clinical medicine, accumulation of water, as evidenced by a decreased serum osmolality, is defined as a "water disorder" rather than a "volume disorder" precisely because of where that water distributes.

DISORDERS OF DECREASED CONCENTRATION

We have now described the underlying mechanisms whereby the body protects against the changes in plasma osmolality. Clinically, when a patient is found with aberrations of serum osmolality, it is our job to find out why. As of this point, there is no way to measure the direct activity of the osmoreceptors within the OVLT. Thus, it is impossible to determine with any certainty whether clinical disorders of osmolality are due to abnormalities within the osmoreceptor or due to the presence of non-osmotic stimuli. We are left to sort out the possibilities based on our clinical physiologic assessment of the patient. A key element in our reasoning is an evaluation of the response mechanisms, namely, the activity of ADH and thirst. In this section, we discuss how to approach clinical disorders of osmolality.

As described earlier, the chem-7 panel is ordered as the first step in the evaluation. From this, the calculated osmolality is easily obtained. In clinical medicine, concentration disorders are usually encountered when someone notices either an abnormal serum sodium value on the chem-7 panel or an abnormal calculated osmolality (which is derived from the chem-7).

The first step in evaluating hypo- or hypernatremia, however, is to confirm that the hyponatremia correlates with the total serum osmolality. Remember, our osmoreceptors detect the changes in total plasma osmolality, not the changes in the plasma sodium level. Osmolality is not only determined by the presence of electrolytes such as sodium and chloride, but also other particles such as urea, glucose, and potentially alcohols. Thus, although we more commonly discuss sodium levels, they must always be interpreted in context of the total serum osmolality.

> **?** **THOUGHT QUESTION 8-1** **A young man with Type I diabetes stops taking his insulin. He visits his primary care physician and is found to have the following laboratory values (normal range in parentheses): Sodium 120 meq/L (136 to 144 meq/L), potassium 3 meq/L (3.6 to 5.0 meq/L), chloride 90 meq/L (96 to 105 meq/L), bicarbonate 20 meq/L (22 to 26 meq/L), BUN 20 mg/dL (5 to 15 mg/dL), creatinine 1 mg/dL (0.6 to 1.2 mg/dL), and glucose 800 mg/dL (70 to 110 mg/dL). Why is he hyponatremic? What is his total plasma osmolality?**

There are several important examples of measured hyponatremia but normal or elevated total plasma osmolality. The most common example is hyperglycemia in patients with diabetes. Since the glucose cannot cross into the cell membrane (because of the lack of insulin), it creates an osmolar gradient, which results in the movement of water from intracellular to the extracellular region thereby diluting the serum sodium. Mannitol, which also does not cross cell membranes, is often administered to the patients with cerebral edema in order to shift water out of the cell, reduce cell size and, hopefully, decrease intracranial pressure. With this shift of water out of cells, the serum sodium level decreases. However, in both these examples, the actual number of particles in the plasma is increased. Thus, although both hyperglycemia and mannitol may lead to "hyponatremia" as detected on the chem-7 panel, the patient is actually hyperosmolar, as detected by a directly measured osmolality.

In the example of hyperglycemia, detection of these additional particles is simple since the glucose is part of the routine chem-7 panel. However, detecting mannitol can be trickier because mannitol is not assessed in the chem-7 panel. Thus, the calculated osmolality in a case of mannitol exposure would be low. One would need to ask the lab to directly measure a plasma osmolality using freezing point depression. In this manner, since the addition of mannitol will lower the freezing point, one can detect the presence of particles not accounted for by the calculated osmolality. The patients given mannitol will have an "osmolar gap," or a difference in the calculated (from the chem-7) and the measured (from freezing point depression) osmolality (a difference or gap of more than 10 mOsm/L between calculated and measured osmolarity is considered the evidence of the presence of an unknown extra particle). They will have hyponatremia, calculated hypo-osmolality, but measured (and hence true) hyperosmolality.

Now that we have discussed examples in which the serum sodium does not reflect the total body osmolality, let us move on to the more common scenarios in which abnormalities in sodium do reflect abnormalities in the total amount of body water, rather than a shift from one compartment to the other.

When faced with hypo-osmolality, the predominant question is why the body cannot correct the concentration abnormality. As we have discussed, the sensing mechanism is the osmoreceptor. In hypo-osmolar states, the osmoreceptor should be deactivated, which leads to a cessation of release of ADH, formation of dilute urine, and decrease in thirst and associated water intake. In approaching problems of osmolality, one must try to determine why the osmoreceptor is unable to turn off these mechanisms, rid the body of excess water, and re-establish a normal plasma concentration.

> **?** **THOUGHT QUESTION 8-2** **A patient is placed on strong diuretics, which interfere with the kidney's ability to reclaim sodium. Will this sodium loss lead to hyponatremia? Explain your answer.**

Let us start off with a clinical example. A patient is found to have a serum sodium value of 120 meq/L, with a low measured osmolality of 250 mOsm/kg. Looking at *Figure 8-3*, we would expect that the patient's thirst and ADH axis would be totally extinguished at this level of osmolality. The patient confirms that he is not particularly thirsty, and does not drink more than his wife (estimated at 2 to 3 L/day). So, it does not seem like excessive water intake is the problem.

The next step in your evaluation is to assess whether ADH is being produced, despite the low osmolality, which would lead to water reclamation from the urine. Unfortunately, ADH levels cannot be measured clinically. Instead, we use the urine concentration as a marker of ADH activity. A dilute urine means ADH activity is off; the presence of concentrated urine means that ADH activity is on. Remember, there are exceptions to this rule. As we discussed in Chapter 7, ADH is just one component necessary to concentrate the urine to very high levels. Countercurrent multiplication, urea recycling, as well as tubular responsiveness to ADH are all required to generate highly concentrated urine. With that caveat, however, the urine osmolarity usually reflects the ADH axis and provides a measure of urine concentration.

Typically, dilute urine is defined as urine osmolarity in the range of 40 to 80 mOsm/L, whereas concentrated urine is generally considered anything above 350 mOsm/L. Isosthenuria, meaning that the urine is neither concentrated nor dilute, refers to a urine concentration that is similar to the concentration of serum. These are gross generalizations, and values must always be interpreted within the clinical context. As individuals age, they lose some ability to maximally dilute or concentrate their urine. Thus, maximally concentrated urine for an 18-year old may be close to 1,000 mOsm/L, whereas it may be approximately 600 mOsm/L for an 80-year old. Conversely, most young individuals can dilute their urine down to 40 mOsm/L, whereas older people cannot get down to such levels.

Let us return to the clinical example. We have established that the patient does not seem to have a problem with thirst. Since his serum osmolality is very low, we would expect that his ADH production would be nonexistent. Remember the step-off nature of the ADH curve; its production drops off dramatically as hypo-osmolality develops. You send off a urine osmolarity, and it returns at 400 mOsm/L. Thus, despite having a low plasma osmolality, the patient is still producing ADH and concentrating his urine. This is the mechanism for perpetuating his hypo-osmolality, i.e., he cannot eliminate the excess body water in the urine because of ADH-induced water retention.

Now that you have identified the mechanism explaining the water retention, your final step is to explain why ADH is being produced inappropriately (given the serum osmolality) in this patient. Either the osmoreceptor is faulty and producing ADH incorrectly, or there are non-osmotic stimuli for ADH production.

We do not have the ability to assess the osmoreceptor function directly; thus, it is not possible to resolve whether the problem lies with osmotic or non-osmotic stimuli. We are left to our clinical judgment. Yet, armed with the knowledge of the most common causes of non-osmotic stimuli, we can resolve this issue with a reasonable amount of certainty.

As we discussed previously, hemodynamic disturbances are a common cause of non-osmotic stimulation of ADH release. Our first thought, therefore, is to assess whether there is evidence of sensed volume deficiency. Remember, the body will sacrifice concentration for volume, i.e., retain water in the presence of low blood pressure even if it leads to low serum sodium. If the baroreceptors within the carotids sense a low pressure, they can stimulate ADH release independently of the osmoreceptor. Thus, we must determine whether hemodynamic factors are leading to the release of ADH.

In order to do this, we need a good history, physical examination, and assessment of the renin–angiotensin–aldosterone axis. Is there any evidence in the patient's history of volume depletion as a consequence of vomiting or diarrhea? Furthermore, is there the appearance of volume depletion on physical exam (skin tenting, orthostatic changes in heart rate and blood pressure)? And finally, is the renin–angiotensin–aldosterone axis turned on? The most clinically useful measure of this axis is the urine sodium concentration since aldosterone release leads to sodium reclamation in the distal tubule.

The clinical history, exam findings, and urine sodium concentration must be used in combination to accurately assess the activity of the baroreceptors. One test in isolation does not give us the full picture. For example, if a healthy person is placed on diuretics, she will become volume depleted and activate her baroreceptors. If this becomes severe enough, this may cause ADH release. However, her urine sodium concentration will remain elevated, despite the volume depletion, since the diuretics block sodium absorption from the tubule and cause persistent urinary sodium loss.

In returning to the example, the patient tells you that he has not had any vomiting or diarrhea. His physical examination is completely normal. And his urine sodium is 100 meq/L (in a volume-depleted individual, urine sodium is typically less than 20 meq/L). He does tell you that he was recently started on an antidepressant. What is your diagnosis?

Let us summarize. He is not particularly thirsty. Furthermore, his urine is inappropriately concentrated for someone with such a low serum osmolality, suggesting that the hyponatremia is ADH related. Next, we attempt to delineate whether this ADH release is driven by osmotic or nonosmotic stimuli. Since non-osmotic stimuli are so common, we should think about this pathway first. Within the category of non-osmotic stimuli of ADH, hemodynamic stimuli are the most common cause of ADH release. Given his normal history, exam, and high urine sodium, however, there is no evidence that his baroreceptors are activated. Thus, there is no reason to suspect that activation of the baroreceptors is driving ADH release.

We are left with considering other conditions that cause inappropriate release of ADH in the setting of hypo-osmolality. This is a condition called syndrome of inappropriate antidiuretic hormone (SIADH) in which the production of ADH becomes divorced from serum osmolality and sensed volume status. All of his findings can be explained by excessive production (or unregulated production) of ADH.

DISORDERS OF INCREASED CONCENTRATION

Conditions of increased serum concentration are less common than those of decreased concentration, but are equally important to understand. The physiological principles are the same.

Let us consider the following scenario. You are on duty at a local hospital, and the lab calls you with a critically abnormal value: the sodium is 152 meq/L. How do you begin to think about this problem?

In looking at *Figure 8-3*, at a concentration of 150 meq/L (or an osmolality of 300 mOsm/kg), the patient's thirst and ADH axis should be activated. You speak with the patient, and indeed, he notes being incredibly thirsty, suggesting that the thirst axis is functioning normally. The patient tells you his urine is very dark too, and when looking more carefully at the labs, you notice that urine osmolarity has been checked. It is very high, at 500 mOsm/L. Thus, both the thirst axis and the ADH axis seem to be responding normally. Why then is the patient hypernatremic?

On further questioning, it turns out that the patient is quite elderly, lives by himself, and is bed bound following injuries sustained in a fall. He is unable to get out of bed to reach the faucet, and depends on his neighbor to bring him food and water. A visiting nurse had drawn the blood sample for laboratory analysis. You contact the visiting nurse, and arrange for better home services for the elderly patient; his case of hypernatremia was simply due to lack of access to water.

Let us change the circumstances a bit in another example. The scenario begins in the same way—you are contacted by the hospital for a serum sodium value of 152 meq/L. Upon calling the patient, you discover that she is very thirsty, and spends most of the day drinking water. Her urine osmolarity is also available, and, unlike the scenario above, is actually quite low at 50 mOsm/kg. This is abnormal. As mentioned, normal osmoreceptors should sense the hyperosmolality, stimulate ADH release, and cause water extraction from the tubules, leading to very concentrated urine; her urine, however, is dilute.

There are two possible explanations for the finding that her urine is dilute in the face of a concentrated serum. Either ADH is not being made, or the tubules are resistant to ADH. These conditions are collectively known as diabetes insipidus, and are defined by dilute urine in the setting of concentrated serum. When this condition is due to the lack of ADH, it is called central diabetes insipidus, whereas renal tubular resistance to ADH is called nephrogenic diabetes insipidus. Since ADH cannot be measured in a clinical laboratory, distinguishing between these conditions requires one to administer exogenous ADH and assess the response.

In central diabetes insipidus, the problem is due to lack of ADH production, and the tubules work well. Thus, administration of exogenous ADH would result in increased urine concentration. In nephrogenic diabetes insipidus, however, the tubules are resistant to ADH, and administration of the hormone results in little change in the urine concentration. This patient has dilute urine in the setting of a concentrated serum, earning her a diagnosis of diabetes insipidus. ADH is administered, and her urine osmolarity increases from 50 to 400 mOsm/L, confirming the diagnosis of central diabetes insipidus.

? **THOUGHT QUESTION 8-3** A woman presents to your office with complaints of being thirsty all the time and having to urinate all the time. She has a history of bipolar disorder and has been on lithium for many years. Her blood sugar is normal. You check a urine osmolality and discover it to be quite low, at 50 mOsm/kg. What are the possible mechanisms that could explain these findings?

DISORDERS OF URINE VOLUME

What determines how much urine we make per day? In this chapter, we have discussed the body's mechanisms for maintaining water homeostasis, so that our net intake balances our net consumption and loss. Fluctuations in our ADH levels, by either diluting or concentrating our urine, determine exactly how much water we excrete. Thus, the urine volume is partly determined by the degree of water excretion.

However, water is just one component of urine. There are also many particles within urine. Metabolism of the food we eat produces breakdown products such as urea, which must be excreted. The excess salt from our diet must also be removed, and, as we discussed previously, there is a finely tuned mechanism to assure that sodium intake equals sodium excretion. These particles collectively constitute the second determinant of urine volume, namely, solute excretion. It is the combination of water and solute excretion that ultimately determines urine volume.

In normal physiology, the hormonal axis that controls water excretion (ADH) and the hormonal axis that controls sodium excretion (renin–angiotensin–aldosterone) function independently of each other. Remember, the osmoreceptor measures and responds to fluid concentration, and the baroreceptor and flow receptor act as surrogate markers of body volume. The stimulation of their respective axes of function occurs independently of each other. In addition, the amount of food that an individual eats varies on a daily basis, so that the excretion of urea varies accordingly. Consequently, the amount of water, salt, and urea that is excreted is determined largely by the amount of water, salt, and urea (as protein) that is ingested. Since the amounts of each one may vary on a daily basis, the body is able to modify the excretion of that substance without affecting any of the other substances.

It is not possible to predict how much urine an individual makes without making some assumptions. First, we know that on an average diet, most people consume 600 mOsm of solute (including sodium and urea), which means they must excrete 600 mOsm in their urine. This assumption at least allows us to estimate the number of particles excreted. In order to determine the volume of urine, we must also estimate the concentration of the urine in which those particles will be excreted.

Depending on how much water an average person drinks, her ADH axis may be completely extinguished, resulting in dilute urine, or completely activated, leading to concentrated urine. As we discussed, most individuals can dilute down to about 40 mOsm/L (the kidney cannot make completely particle-free urine), and can concentrate up to approximately 1,000 mOsm/L. If, for example, the individual is consuming 600 mOsm of foodstuffs, and thus excreting 600 mOsm of particles in the urine, and drinking lots of water so that her urine osmolarity is decreased to 40 mOsm/L, then she will make 15 L urine. If, on the other hand, she is excreting the same 600 mOsm, but instead drinking very little water so that her urine becomes fully concentrated, then she will make 600 mL urine per day.

Normal urine volume is considered anything above 25 mL/min (600 mL/day), and less than 3 L. The term oliguria refers to a urine volume less than 600 mL/day, and polyuria refers to quantities above 3 L. These definitions are derived from the calculations such as we did in our examples, and are dependent on the assumption of a normal diet.

Oliguria is typically a hallmark of renal failure. In other words, oliguria defines the urine volume needed to excrete the daily amount of body waste. If someone needs to excrete 600 mOsm/day, and the kidney does so in the most concentrated form, then they will still need 600 mL/day in order to do so (600 mOsm/1,000 mOsm/L = 0.6 L). Any urine volume less than that would be insufficient to rid the body of waste (urea and excess sodium), and thus indicates renal failure.

Polyuria develops when an excess of either solute or water is being excreted. Simply measuring the urine osmolality often indicates whether the diuresis is predominantly due to excess solute or water. For instance, if an individual makes 10 L of urine per day, and the urine osmolarity is 70 mOsm/L, then that individual is excreting about 700 mOsm of solute in 10 L of water. Since the average dietary intake of solute is about 600 mOsm, this is a relatively normal amount of solute. The dilute urine indicates that the polyuria is predominantly due to excessive water intake.

If, however, the urine is full of solute, it obviously will be more concentrated, and will have a higher osmolality. For instance, a person urinating 10 L/day, with urine osmolality of 500 mOsm/L, is excreting 5,000 mOsm/day! This is tenfold more than a typical dietary intake, and indicates a solute diuresis.

Both water and solute diuresis may be normal or abnormal. For instance, if an individual drinks many liters of water per day, then the normal response is to excrete many liters of dilute urine per day. However, if an individual develops diabetes insipidus, with a consequent inability to concentrate her urine, then the water diuresis would be abnormal, and she would have to drink frequently in order to keep up with the water loss.

PUTTING IT TOGETHER

Four patients come to the doctor's office, all with the exact same serum sodium value of 120 meq/L. You check a measured osmolality in all patients, and confirm that they are hypo-osmolar. In order to evaluate these patients, you order a battery of tests to complement your history and physical exam. The tests results are shown in *Table 8-1*. Can you come up with a diagnosis for each patient? How would you treat each patient? Try to do the analysis before looking at the discussion that follows.

Note: "Normal" or expected urine sodium and urine osmolarity values vary depending on the amount of water and solute being ingested each day.

All the patients have low serum sodium values and low serum osmolality. Thus, the problem is not from a shift of water from the cell into the plasma, as might be seen with hyperglycemia or mannitol administration. In those patients, although the serum sodium is low (reflecting water shift), the total measured osmolality by freezing point depression is appropriately elevated, reflecting the presence of the additional particles. Thus, all of our patients have hyponatremia and hypo-osmolality.

TABLE 8-1 FOUR CLINICAL EXAMPLES OF HYPONATREMIA

	PATIENT A	PATIENT B	PATIENT C	PATIENT D
History	Vomiting	Shortness of breath	Lung cancer	Always thirsty
BP (mm Hg)	90/40	90/40	120/80	120/80
Exam	Skin tenting	Edema	Normal	Normal
Urine Sodium (meq/L)	10	10	80	30
Urine Osmolarity (mOsm/kg)	500	500	500	40

Next, we attempt to understand the mechanisms that led to each individual's water excess. There are only two. Either the patient is drinking too much water, or the kidneys are not getting rid of enough water. There is no other way to develop hyponatremia.

Let us start off with Patient A. She has a high urine osmolality, suggesting that the ADH axis is turned on. Given our familiarity with *Figure 8-3*, we know that with a serum osmolality of 120 meq/L, ADH should be off. Thus, we need to explain why ADH is still being secreted. Since we cannot directly assess the activity of the osmoreceptor, we start off with an assessment of potential non-osmotic stimuli of ADH. Clinically, hemodynamic stimuli are the most important non-osmotic stimuli. Sure enough, in this patient with a history of vomiting, low blood pressure, and skin tenting, volume depletion is suspected. The low urine sodium, reflecting activity of the renin–angiotensin–aldosterone axis, further confirms that the baroreceptors are activated; this activation is also likely stimulating the release of ADH. As we have said, the body will sacrifice concentration for volume; we must maintain perfusion to our critical organs. We conclude that Patient A has hyponatremia from the appropriate baroreceptor release of ADH in the setting of decreased sensed volume (i.e., hemodynamic stimulus of ADH).

How would you treat this patient? The administration of intravenous saline solution, by correcting the volume depletion, would deactivate the baroreceptors and turn off ADH. The patient would then be able to urinate dilute urine, rid herself of the excess water, and re-establish normal osmolality.

Let us look at Patient B. Like Patient A, he has concentrated urine, indicating that ADH is turned on. Like Patient A, he has a low urine sodium concentration, indicating that the renin–angiotensin–aldosterone axis is turned on. Thus, Patients A and B have similar laboratory findings. However, unlike Patient A, Patient B has a history of shortness of breath and, on exam, is found to have low blood pressure and peripheral edema. This suggests a history of congestive heart failure (CHF). He has a low sensed volume, which is causing ADH release.

Let us move to Patient C. Like the previous two patients, his urine is quite concentrated, again suggesting that ADH is being produced. However, unlike the other two patients, his urine sodium is not low, suggesting that the renin–angiotensin–aldosterone axis has not been activated. In addition, his blood pressure and exam are normal, further suggesting that there is no problem with his sensed volume. Thus, the baroreceptors are likely not activated, and we cannot attribute his ADH activity to a hemodynamic/baroreceptor stimulus.

We then begin to think of other causes of unregulated ADH release. As far as we know, he neither complains of nausea, is not on antidepressants, nor has pain. However, he does have a history of lung cancer. We remember that some lung cancers have been associated with SIADH. This is indeed his diagnosis.

The diagnosis of SIADH can only be made if there is no evidence of sensed volume depletion. Thus, a diagnosis of SIADH cannot be made if a patient has very low urine sodium, in which case one cannot determine whether ADH is being released inappropriately, as in the setting of SIADH, or appropriately, as in the setting of volume depletion. The take-home point regarding SIADH is that it is exclusively a water disorder; i.e., a problem with ADH production. There is no abnormality with sodium handling. In other words, the sensors of volume are functioning normally.

Treatment for Patient C consists primarily of fluid restriction. Remember, he has to ingest less water than he urinates (plus insensible losses from sweat and evaporation from the respiratory system), otherwise his osmolality will drop even further.

Finally, we address Patient D. Unlike the other three examples, his urine is not concentrated; it is quite dilute with urinary osmolarity of 40 mOsm/kg. Thus, we can correctly assume that his ADH axis is inactive. Remembering *Figure 8-3*, we expect that at a serum sodium value of 120 meq/L (correlating with an osmolality of around 240 mOsm/kg), the osmoreceptor would completely extinguish ADH production. Thus, this patient's ADH axis is responding completely appropriately. What is abnormal is his thirst mechanism. For a variety of reasons, including underlying psychiatric illnesses or psychiatric medications, some patients develop an increased desire for water. It is unclear whether this is driven by a more sensitive perception of thirst than normal, or whether it is related to behavioral and/or psychiatric impulses. Nevertheless, these patients drink excessive amounts of water. In fact, they drink more water than their kidneys are able to excrete, despite the downregulation of ADH and the formation of maximally dilute urine. This condition is called psychogenic polydipsia. This patient has no problems with his sodium-handling system (renin–angiotensin–aldosterone). Thus, his exam and urinary sodium are normal. He only has a water-excess disorder.

Use Animated Figure 8-2 (Hyponatremia) to review the diagnoses for these four patient cases. As you select each diagnosis, you can see the status of the osmoreceptors, the baroreceptors, and the level of ADH (elevated or suppressed), along with the exam and lab findings such as urine sodium and urine osmolality.

Summary Points

- The concentration of the body fluid is sensed by the unique cells within the brain, called the osmoreceptor.
- Because the interstitial, intravascular, and intracellular fluid compartments are fully permeable to water, the concentration in each is the same.
- Changes in fluid concentration stimulate the osmoreceptor to activate ADH release and produce the sensation of thirst, both of which lead to water retention; water retention is activated before thirst.
- Non-osmotic stimuli, such as volume depletion, can also stimulate ADH release and thirst.
- Disorders of serum sodium or osmolality are disorders of water regulation.
- Water retention leads to changes in cellular size, manifesting as neurologic symptoms when brain cells are affected; the clinical effects of water retention on the brain are typically seen long before any clinically apparent changes in total body fluid volume can be detected.
- Osmolality is most accurately measured by freezing point depression, but can also be approximated by calculations derived from the routine chemistry panel (standard blood test used in clinical medicine).
- The major components of osmolality are electrolytes, glucose, and urea.
- Ingested alcohols can alter serum osmolality.
- Water excess manifests as hyponatremia, and water deficiency as hypernatremia.
- Water disorders are due to abnormalities in either ADH release or thirst.
- Oliguria is defined relative to the amount of urine needed to excrete the daily amount of waste, i.e., the minimum volume of urine needed to eliminate the solutes ingested. Urine volume in the oliguric range indicates renal failure.
- Polyuria is defined by large urine volumes, and is due to the need to excrete large amounts of solute or water.

Answers TO THOUGHT QUESTIONS

8-1. On first glance, the patient appears to be hyponatremic. However, when the total osmolality is calculated (2 Na + BUN/2.8 + gluc/18), we find that the total osmolality of the patient is actually 291 mOsm/kg, which is in the high range of normal. What accounts for this apparent inconsistency between the measured hyponatremia and the increase in total plasma osmolality?

When insulin is absent (such as in Type I diabetics), glucose cannot be transported across cell membranes, and acts as an impermeable solute. Water flows from regions of low osmolality to regions of high osmolality. Consequently, water moves out of the cell and into the extracellular space (interstitial and vascular compartments), which dilutes the sodium in the plasma and reduces the measured serum sodium. The total number of particles in solution, however, is still markedly increased. Thus, although hyponatremia may be observed, the patient's plasma is actually hyperosmolar.

A clinically useful correction factor has been developed to adjust the measured serum sodium for the degree of hyperglycemia; this adjustment tells you what the serum sodium would be if all of the "excess" glucose in the blood were to move into the cells (a process that would cause water to move from the extracellular to the intracellular compartment), which occurs when you begin to administer insulin to the diabetic patient. Every 100 mg/dL increase above the normal value of 100 mg/dL in serum glucose pulls enough water out of the cell into the plasma to decrease the sodium concentration by 1.6 meq/L.

8-2. In this example, the patient who is placed on diuretics will have a net loss of sodium particles. Understanding why this will *not* lead to hyponatremia is fundamental to the understanding of renal physiology. First, diuretics usually interfere with the kidney's concentrating ability, so that urine is "isosthenuric," or equal to serum concentration. Consequently, diuretic use will lead to the loss of isotonic fluid, having the same concentration as serum. The volume of body fluid will change, but the concentration will not.

This is not to say that diuretics are not common causes of hyponatremia, for in fact they can be. However, the hyponatremia in this situation is not due to the loss of sodium; instead the problem is due to compensatory retention of water. If the volume loss associated with diuretic use is severe, then there could be non-osmotic stimulation of ADH release (the body will sacrifice concentration for volume), interfering with the kidney's ability to excrete water. In this setting, much of the water that the patient drinks will be retained, and hyponatremia and hypo-osmolality will ensue.

8-3. This patient presents with a common complaint of polyuria (frequent urination due to a large volume of urine) and polydipsia (increased thirst). She has dilute urine; thus, you know her ADH axis is not on. There are two possible explanations. One is that she is simply drinking too much water, a disorder termed psychogenic polydipsia that is most often seen in people with underlying psychiatric diagnoses. In this disorder, the patient is making appropriate large volumes of dilute urine in order to keep up with her water intake.

The other possible explanation is that the lithium has induced a state of nephrogenic diabetes insipidus, a condition in which the tubules cannot respond to circulating ADH. In this setting, her kidneys are excreting inappropriately dilute urine, and she is relying on her thirst mechanism to protect her serum osmolality (i.e., the elimination of dilute urine will lead to an elevation of serum sodium, which will trigger thirst).

In psychogenic polydipsia, the osmoreceptors are responding normally to water excess by decreasing ADH production, allowing a water diuresis. In diabetes insipidus the ADH axis is inactive. How can you distinguish between the two?

The distinguishing difference between the two conditions relates to the serum concentration. Psychogenic polydipsia is a disorder of hyponatremia. Thus, the turning off of thirst and ADH is appropriate, as the body attempts to rid itself of excess water. Diabetes insipidus is a disorder of hypernatremia. With elevated serum sodium levels, the ADH axis should be fully activated, and the urine should be concentrated. Since the urine remains inappropriately dilute despite a hypertonic serum, whether there is ADH underproduction or tubular resistance to ADH, simply measuring the patient's serum sodium should help resolve the mechanism underlying our findings. If the sodium is elevated, the diagnosis is diabetes insipidus; if it is low, the diagnosis is likely psychogenic polydipsia. It should be noted that these conditions may overlap. In other words, patients with diabetes insipidus become so accustomed to habitual water drinking that they may actually drink too much, and develop a situation similar to psychogenic polydipsia.

8-4. The question focuses on the capacity of the kidneys to eliminate water. In states of water excess, the normal response of the body is to reduce the secretion of ADH in order to achieve maximally dilute urine. Most individuals can dilute urine down to an osmolality of about 40 mOsm/kg. At this osmolality, the amount of urine volume would then be determined by the amount of solute that needs to be excreted to maintain homeostasis. On an average diet of about 600 mOsm/day, the person will be able to excrete (600 mOsm/40 mOsm/L) 15 L urine. Therefore, he will be able to drink 15 L water. If he drinks more than that, however, he will exceed his maximal water excretion capacity, and will develop water retention, which will be manifested as hyponatremia. If his dietary intake were more than the average, e.g., 1,000 mOsm of solute per day, then he would be able to excrete 25 L/day, and thus drink that amount before developing hyponatremia.

Review Questions

DIRECTIONS: *Each of the numbered items or incomplete statements in this section is followed by answers or by completions of the statement. Select the ONE lettered answer or completion that is BEST in each case.*

1. You are taking care of a patient who is on dialysis because of renal failure. He undergoes dialysis three times a week to remove excess fluid and toxic waste. He does not make any urine. What happens to his serum sodium between each dialysis session?

    A. It increases.
    B. It decreases.
    C. It does not change.

2. A young man with a history of psychiatric illness, on many medications, complains of being thirsty and urinating all the time. He has a normal serum sodium of 137 meq/L, but is found to make over 5 L of urine per day. What are the possible diagnoses?

    A. Diabetes mellitus
    B. Diabetes insipidus
    C. Psychogenic polydipsia
    D. All of the above

3. A patient is brought into the Emergency Department and is found to have very low serum sodium at 110 meq/L; he subsequently is observed to have a seizure. How would you treat him?

    A. Give him a diuretic
    B. Do not let him drink any water
    C. Give him hypertonic fluid (i.e., fluid that has a concentration of sodium three times that of normal body fluid).

4. A patient with a long-standing history of SIADH is able to keep his serum sodium in the normal range by restricting his water intake to no more than 2 L/day. He develops a mild upset stomach after eating raw fish, and does not eat anything for two days. He continues, however, on his 2 L fluid intake. What will happen to his serum sodium?

    A. It will decrease.
    B. It will increase.
    C. It will remain the same.

Maintaining the Serum pH
Acid–Base Balance

chapter **9**

CHAPTER OUTLINE

LEARNING OBJECTIVES

By the end of this chapter, you should be able to:

- describe how the body handles a daily acid load with little change in body pH.
- define what makes a "buffer."
- describe the two bicarbonate pools within our bodies.
- delineate carbonic from noncarbonic acids.
- describe the pathway of CO_2 excretion.
- define the Henderson–Hasselbalch equation.
- define acidosis and alkalosis.
- explain renal handling of filtered bicarbonate.
- describe how the kidney generates new bicarbonate.
- explain the importance of urinary pH in net acid excretion.
- define the serum anion gap.
- define the metabolic states associated with production acidoses.
- describe the relationship of the serum bicarbonate concentration to the anion gap in
  production acidoses.

Introduction to the Acid–Base Status of the Body

The human body is exquisitely sensitive to the changes in serum pH. The normal serum pH is typically 7.4, and changes beyond a narrow range (6.8 to 7.8) are not compatible with life; proteins unravel, enzymatic activity ceases, and the most basic cellular functions are thrown into disarray. Consequently, the body has developed a tightly regulated system to defend against the changes in serum pH. For normal individuals, the serum pH barely changes, despite a wide range of acid and base challenges.

Although we use pH more frequently than hydrogen concentration to describe human physiology, a brief reminder of this relationship is important. The pH is defined as the negative logarithm (to base 10) of the free hydrogen ion concentration. Thus, a serum pH of 7.4, which is in the middle of the normal range for humans, correlates to a serum-free hydrogen concentration of 0.000000039 meq of hydrogen per liter of body fluid. Since this is a logarithmic scale, increasing the concentration to 0.00000039 (moving the decimal point by one), correlates to a serum pH of 6.4, which would mean inevitable death to any individual!

Every day, the human body is challenged with large acid loads. Acid arises from cellular metabolism, which produces about 15,000 hydrogen equivalents per day of organic or carbon-based acids, which are metabolized to **carbonic acid**. Metabolism of food (primarily protein) releases inorganic acids (e.g., sulfate/sulfuric acid from the degradation of cysteine and methionine) at a rate of 70 meq of acid per day. To sustain life, the body must be able to handle all of this acid produced each day without sustaining any change in serum pH, as illustrated in *Figure 9-1*. How this is achieved is the focus of this chapter.

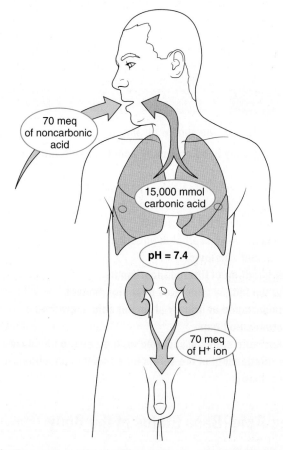

70 meq
of noncarbonic
acid

15,000 mmol
carbonic acid

pH = 7.4

70 meq
of H$^+$ ion

FIGURE 9-1 Net acid production must equal net acid excretion in order to maintain acid balance.
Approximately 15,000 mmol of carbon dioxide, an acid equivalent, is produced daily by cellular metabolism. Given its gaseous nature, it is rapidly excreted by the lungs. Metabolism of an average diet leads to 70 meq of noncarbonic acids that are nonvolatile. These acids must be excreted by the kidneys in order to maintain acid balance. The excretion of both carbonic and noncarbonic acids occurs with almost no change in the serum concentration of hydrogen ions (i.e., serum pH is maintained in a very narrow range.)

EDITOR'S INTEGRATION

The 15,000 hydrogen equivalents produced each day as a consequence of cellular metabolism are eliminated via lungs in the form of carbon dioxide (a product of the dissociation of carbonic acid). Consequently, carbonic acid is often termed a "volatile acid." In contrast, the acid resulting from metabolism of protein and eliminated by the kidney is called "fixed acid." If you stop breathing, your pH drops in a matter of minutes. If you develop kidney failure, it may take several days before the build-up of acid becomes life-threatening. It is important to remember that the respiratory system plays a critical role in maintenance of a normal pH (see *Respiratory Physiology: A Clinical Approach*, Chapter 7, for additional information on this aspect of respiratory physiology).

BUFFERS

The body must excrete acid loads, originating from cell metabolism and from digestion of dietary protein, to maintain steady-state acid balance. As we will learn, the lungs excrete most of the carbonic acid produced by cell metabolism, whereas the noncarbonic acids from dietary sources are excreted by the kidneys. However, while these respiratory and renal processes of excretion are ongoing, the body must "absorb" the added hydrogen ions without sustaining a change in pH. This is achieved by the use of buffers, which are typically weak acids or bases that can mitigate changes in the concentration of free hydrogen by absorbing a hydrogen ion.

As a brief review, remember that pH is determined by the amount of *free* hydrogen ions in a solution. Acids exist in equilibrium with their dissociated ions, as written below:

$$HX \rightarrow H^+ + X^-$$

If HX is a strong acid, the molecule will dissociate, i.e., nearly all of the protons will be free in solution, and will not be bound to the anion, X. If HX is a very weak acid, the reaction will be shifted to the far left, with few free hydrogen ions in solution. In both of these situations, the addition or removal of hydrogen ions will have a large effect on the concentration of free hydrogen ions. If the acid is relatively weak, however, with equal amounts of the acid HX and the free anion X^-, then adding or removing hydrogen ions will have a relatively small effect on the free hydrogen concentration because the reaction will shift in compensation. For example, if a proton is added to the solution, it will bind to the anion to form HX, thereby reducing the concentration of H^+.

This concept is known in chemistry as the Le Chatelier–Braun principle, and basically states that if a chemical system at equilibrium experiences a change in concentration, then the equilibrium shifts to partially counteract the imposed change. Thus, the ability of an acid to "accept" or "donate" a hydrogen ion, thereby mitigating (or buffering) a change in pH, depends on the relationship of the strength of that acid to the solution into which it is placed.

The strength of a particular acid is described by its acid dissociation constant which, when represented in its logarithmic form, **pK_a**, simply describes the pH at which the acid is in equilibrium with its conjugate base. Thus, for the above reaction, equilibrium exists when the HX and X^- concentrations are equally balanced. Every acid has its own pK_a.

In order to understand the buffering capacity of a particular acid, however, the pK_a must be interpreted in context of the solution's pH. For example, the pK_a of formic acid is 3.75.

$$\text{Formic acid} \leftrightarrow H^+ + \text{formate}^-$$

If formic acid is placed into a solution with a pH of 3.75, then formic acid and its conjugate base, formate, will be present at equal concentrations. The addition of further hydrogen would be buffered by the formate. If, however, that same formic acid was placed into a solution with a pH of 1, the formic acid would seem relatively basic, instantaneously accepting many hydrogen ions, which would shift the reaction to the left. With virtually all of the formate anion already binding protons, there is no formate available to bind more protons, and the system has little or no buffering capacity. Conversely, if it were placed into a solution with a pH of 10, then nearly all of the formic acid/formate anion in the solution would be in the form of formate anion, and, unless sufficient protons were added to change the pH of the solution, virtually no formate anions would bind protons, and the solution would have little buffering capacity. On this basis, added protons would change the pH (which relates to the concentration of free protons) dramatically.

In summary, the ability of an acid to buffer a solution, protecting it from changes in free hydrogen concentration despite the addition of free hydrogen, depends on the pK_a of the acid in relation to the solution. The most efficient buffers are those whose pK_a values are similar to the pH of the solution they are buffering. In humans, the most effective buffers are those with pK_a values close to 7.4.

There are many buffering systems in the human body, including carbonic acid, phosphoric acid, uric acid, sulfuric acid, as well as cellular proteins. They are all in equilibrium, and function together to protect the serum pH against the deluge of constant daily acid production. Because of the ability of the lungs to excrete carbon dioxide, the CO_2/HCO_3^- buffering system is by far the most important in regulating pH.

THE BICARBONATE POOL

The bicarbonate anion, as a potential proton acceptor, is the most important base in the body. Upon binding with hydrogen, carbonic acid is formed, which rapidly dissociates into carbon dioxide and water. The net effect is neutralization of the added acid. The pK_a of the bicarbonate system is 6.1, relatively close to normal serum pH. Thus, bicarbonate is able to respond to fluctuations in H^+ production, preventing changes in serum pH. This reaction is stated below.

$$HCO_3^- + H^+ \leftrightarrow H_2CO_3 \leftrightarrow CO_2 + H_2O$$

There are two main pools of bicarbonate in the body. The first is the dissolved bicarbonate within the total body water. As an anion, bicarbonate typically circulates as a sodium bicarbonate salt. The exact volume of distribution of bicarbonate is unknown, but has been estimated to be approximately half of the total body water. In other words, an individual of 70-kg weight, with a total body water of 45 L, has a volume of distribution of bicarbonate of approximately 22.5 L. This means that if a person were to eat 22.5 meq of bicarbonate, his/her serum bicarbonate would increase by approximately 1 meq/L.

However, this formula is a gross estimation, and marked variability exists as to the size of the body's bicarbonate stores. Much of this uncertainty relates to the second body bicarbonate pool, namely, the skeleton. As a solid structure, the skeleton is composed of a vast amount of mineralized ions, including calcium, phosphate, and carbonate. The vast majority of total body carbonate is found within the skeletal system, and it has been estimated that approximately 25,000 meq of bicarbonate exist within the skeleton.

Unlike the serum bicarbonate pool, however, skeletal bicarbonate is in a solid, mineralized form. It cannot act as an efficient buffer to rapid fluctuations in body hydrogen content. However, over longer periods of time, bone can be an important buffer to acid. Under conditions of chronic acid gain, bicarbonate begins to leach out of bone to protect the serum bicarbonate pool. This acid leak is associated with demineralization of the bone, and with loss of other important minerals such as calcium and phosphorus. Over the long term, this process may lead to marked weakening of the skeletal system, and such individuals may suffer recurrent bone fractures.

Thus, the two bicarbonate pools have differing roles. The aqueous bicarbonate pool acts as a ready buffer against sudden fluctuations in serum pH. The solid, mineralized pool provides a larger store of bicarbonate that can be accessed on a more chronic basis, albeit at the cost of bone demineralization.

CO₂ PRODUCTION

As we have discussed earlier, the addition of free hydrogen ions is buffered by bicarbonate. However, in our bodies, the reverse reaction is also occurring on a constant basis. The metabolism of carbohydrates within cells continuously produces CO_2. By combining with water, carbonic acid forms, which then rapidly dissociates to bicarbonate and a hydrogen ion.

$$CO_2 + H_2O \leftrightarrow H_2CO_3 \leftrightarrow HCO_3^- + H^+$$

In the absence of a catalyst, the left-hand portion of this reaction occurs very slowly. The forward reaction ($CO_2 + H_2O \rightarrow H_2CO_3$) occurs at a rate of $0.039\ s^{-1}$, whereas the reverse reaction ($H_2CO_3 \rightarrow CO_2 + H_2O$) occurs at $23\ s^{-1}$. Carbon dioxide, a byproduct of cellular metabolism, is produced constantly.

It is estimated that approximately 15,000 mmol of CO_2 is produced per day within the body's cells. As a gas, this CO_2 diffuses across cell membranes into the surrounding interstitium and the serum. For a normal individual, the partial pressure of carbon dioxide in arterial blood (since it's ultimately in equilibrium with gas in the alveolus, we express the concentration of CO_2 in solution as a partial pressure), is approximately 40 mm Hg. This gas dissolves into solution, and the concentration of dissolved CO_2 can be defined by the simple formula.

$$CO_2\ (mmol/L) = 0.03 \times \text{Partial Pressure of } CO_2\ (mm\ Hg)$$

Thus, for most individuals, the serum CO_2 concentration is 1.2 mmol/L. Even though the forward reaction, which results in the formation of carbonic acid, is very slow, some carbonic acid does form in the serum because of the high concentration of CO_2 and its constant generation from ongoing cellular metabolism. Carbonic acid is a relatively strong acid (pK_a of 3.5), and thus rapidly dissociates into its free hydrogen ion and bicarbonate. In this way, carbon dioxide gas is a potential acid.

Given the tremendous amount of CO_2 produced daily, one might wonder why severe acidosis does not develop. The answer resides in the extraordinary capacity of the lung to exhale gaseous CO_2. As long as the lungs and the rest of the respiratory system (e.g., the ventilatory muscles and the respiratory controller) are functioning normally, whatever CO_2 is formed by cellular metabolism is rapidly exhaled by the lungs; no net gain of acid occurs.

EDITOR'S INTEGRATION

The respiratory controller in the brainstem receives messages from chemoreceptors in the carotid body and at the base of the brain; these receptors monitor pCO_2 and pH in the arterial blood. When pCO_2 rises or pH falls, signals are sent from the chemoreceptors to the respiratory control center, and ventilation increases to enhance carbon dioxide (and acid) elimination.

The challenge for the body is to shuttle the CO_2 from tissue to the lungs without causing an acidosis in transit. Red blood cells, armed with the enzyme carbonic anhydrase, play a critical role in this shuttling process. Carbonic anhydrase is an enzyme that catalyzes the formation of carbonic acid from CO_2 and water. Plasma does not have carbonic anhydrase, yet red blood cells do. Thus, red blood cells act as a CO_2 "sink." CO_2 diffuses into red cells, and because of the presence of carbonic anhydrase, is rapidly converted into carbonic acid. In turn, more and more CO_2 then diffuses into the red cell, fueling carbonic acid formation.

Within the red cell, carbonic acid rapidly dissociates into hydrogen ion and its conjugate base, bicarbonate. The bicarbonate anion exits the cell via an abundant Cl^-/HCO_3^- exchanger, whereas the hydrogen ion is buffered by hemoglobin, preventing the development of intracellular acidosis. Once the red cell reaches the lung, however, the reaction reverses as CO_2 is rapidly exhaled, so that whatever CO_2 is produced in the tissues is exhaled in the lungs. The net effect is the stable concentration of CO_2, H_2CO_3, and H^+ in the blood. The red blood cell has simply shuttled CO_2 from tissue to lung.

BODY pH—A BALANCE OF THE BICARBONATE BUFFER AND CO_2

Because of the huge amount of CO_2 produced daily, and its potential to form carbonic acid, CO_2 levels within the serum play an important role in the amount of free hydrogen within the blood. In addition, the serum bicarbonate as the most important buffer for noncarbonic acids, plays an equally important role. The relationship between these two factors is best described by the **Henderson–Hasselbalch** equation. In simple terms, the Henderson–Hasselbalch equation defines the amount of free hydrogen that will exist for any acid–base system. In other words, if the concentrations of the acid and the conjugate base are known, along with the pK_a of the system, the pH can be predicted. For the carbonic acid system, the equation is as follows:

$$pH = pK_a + \log\frac{[base]}{[acid]}$$
$$pH = 6.1 + \log([HCO_3^-]/0.03(pCO_2))$$

This equation is one of the most important in all of renal physiology, as it describes how the body pH, which is a measure of free hydrogen ions, is related to both the CO_2 concentration and the serum bicarbonate concentration. The lungs are responsible for CO_2 excretion. As we will learn in this chapter, the kidneys are responsible for maintaining the serum bicarbonate concentration. Thus, the Henderson–Hasselbalch equation describes the relationship between the lungs and kidneys with respect to their roles in acid–base regulation, and predicts the resulting pH.

Use Animated Figure 9-1 (Henderson–Hasselbalch Equation) to vary the HCO_3^- and/ or pCO_2 and observe how the blood pH changes. In this figure, we introduce the "balance" analogy, depicting the interplay between HCO_3^-, pCO_2, and pH. In reality, a change in one of the parameters in this diagram would lead to compensatory processes, as we discuss below.

Normal arterial blood pH is approximately 7.40; although, as with all "normal" physiological values, there is a range of normal, in this case between 7.35 and 7.45. When the pH is below 7.35, we say **acidemia** is present (the blood pH is more acid than normal); when the pH is greater than 7.45, we note the presence of **alkalemia** (the blood pH is more alkaline than normal). Often, these terms are used interchangeably with acidosis and alkalosis, which refer to the process that contributed to the respective blood pH change. It is important, however, to keep the terms distinct; there can be multiple processes (-oses) present at the same time in a particular patient, but only one serum pH (normal, acid*emia*, or alkal*emia*) at any given moment.

Since pH is determined by the relationship between the numerator and the denominator of the Henderson–Hasselbalch equation, the serum bicarbonate or pCO_2 in isolation cannot predict the pH. They must always be interpreted together. For example, if a patient is found to have a serum bicarbonate of 15 meq/L (normal 25 meq/L), it is impossible to know if he/she is alkalemic or acidemic without directly measuring the serum pH. The patient could be breathing very rapidly and deeply (increased ventilation), removing large volumes of carbon dioxide from the blood, and reducing the partial pressure of CO_2 to 20 mm Hg. Solving the Henderson–Hasselbalch equation gives a pH of 7.5, clearly alkalemic. Since the denominator has fallen more than the numerator, the pH has risen. In this case, the primary problem is due to overbreathing (i.e., hyperventilation), and the patient has a respiratory alkalosis. In order to protect the serum pH, the kidneys excrete bicarbonate, allowing the numerator to move in the same direction as the denominator. This is known as metabolic compensation, a process that can take 48 to 72 hours to occur.

Return to Animated Figure 9-1 (Henderson–Hasselbalch Equation) and use the controls to set the serum bicarbonate to 15 meq/L and the pCO_2 to 40 mm Hg (normal). In isolation (i.e., if there were no change in pCO_2), this would lead to acidemia. Now also set the pCO_2 to 20 mm Hg. This set of values places the blood pH at 7.5, in the alkalemic range. Clearly, as mentioned above, serum bicarbonate and pCO_2 must be taken together to determine the blood pH. In this case, the patient has a respiratory alkalosis with metabolic compensation. The patient's respiratory condition is the primary problem.

Conversely, if the patient's primary problem was loss of bicarbonate, an acidosis would be present. A bicarbonate level of 15 meq/L with no change in serum CO_2 levels (normal being 40 mm Hg) would lead to a pH of 7.20, as outlined in the Animated Figure example earlier, clearly very acidemic. However, to regulate serum pH, the normal response of the respiratory system would be to compensate, by increasing the ventilation and removing the CO_2. In this scenario, the denominator should move in the same direction as the numerator. If enough CO_2 were eliminated from the blood via increased ventilation to reach a serum partial pressure of 35 mm Hg, the resulting pH would be 7.25. If the CO_2 reaches 30 mm Hg, the resulting pH would be 7.32. In contrast to renal compensation for a respiratory acidosis, which can take several days to achieve, the compensation provided by the respiratory system for a renal acid–base disturbance can occur with seconds to minutes.

Once again, return to Animated Figure 9-1 (Henderson–Hasselbalch Equation) and use the controls to set the serum bicarbonate to 15 meq/L and the pCO_2 to 40 mm Hg (normal). As noted, this would lead to acidemia. Now set the pCO_2 to 35 mm Hg, keeping bicarbonate at 15. You can also try setting the pCO_2 to 30 mm Hg. Either of these values places the blood pH below 7.35, still in the acidemic range. Here, the serum bicarbonate is the same as in the previous example, but the patient is acidemic rather than alkalemic. In this case, the patient has a metabolic acidosis with respiratory compensation. The metabolic condition leading to the decrease in serum bicarbonate is the primary problem.

Just how much the respiratory system can compensate for a renal or metabolic acidosis, i.e., decreasing serum bicarbonate, has been well studied, and is best described by the **Winter's formula.**

$$PaCO_2 = 1.5 \times [HCO_3^-] + 8$$

This formula was obtained by measuring the degree to which normal people usually respond to a reduction in serum bicarbonate. It describes how the respiratory system responds to a primary loss of serum bicarbonate. It is important to note that with rare exceptions, compensatory mechanisms do not bring the pH completely back to 7.40, and will not cause the pH to go beyond 7.40 in the opposite direction of the primary disturbance.

Animated Figure 9-2 (Winter's Formula) depicts the familiar balance, this time shown for a metabolic acidosis with respiratory compensation as described by Winter's formula. You can vary the bicarbonate concentration (the primary disorder) and see the approximate level of compensation that the respiratory system would achieve, as well as the resulting blood pH.

EDITOR'S INTEGRATION

It is important to think of the compensation of the body to a metabolic acidosis (drop in serum bicarbonate) as being achieved by the respiratory system, not just the lungs. The compensatory process requires intact chemoreceptors, central control mechanisms in the medulla, peripheral nerves that connect the brain to the ventilatory muscles, and a stable chest wall, along with normal alveoli and pulmonary capillaries. This integrated system is described in *Respiratory Physiology: A Clinical Approach.*

? **THOUGHT QUESTION 9-1** **A young man comes into the emergency room for dehydration, and is administered 4 L normal saline. Since the amount of fluid in his body increases (and, consequently, his serum bicarbonate concentration decreases), will he develop an acidosis?**

Maintaining the Serum Bicarbonate Level

ACID LOADS IN NORMAL INDIVIDUALS

Healthy individuals are constantly subject to the production of acid within their bodies. As we noted above, cell metabolism produces approximately 15,000 mmol of CO_2 per day, which are shuttled in red blood cells and excreted by the lungs. Thus, as long as the lungs are functional, carbonic acid is not retained.

EDITOR'S INTEGRATION

The number of molecules of CO_2 produced by cellular metabolism varies based on the fuel being used for energy. More molecules of CO_2 are produced per gram of carbohydrate consumed, for example, than for protein or fat. These differences are reflected in the respiratory quotient (RQ), which is the ratio of molecules of CO_2 produced to molecules of oxygen consumed during aerobic metabolism. In the average American diet, RQ = 0.8. If one eats only carbohydrates, RQ = 1.0; in a diet solely comprising protein, RQ = 0.8; and in a diet consisting of fat, RQ = 0.7. A patient with limited pulmonary reserve, i.e., with a lung disease that limits the ability to increase ventilation, may have difficulty clearing carbonic acid if he/she is placed on a diet consisting solely of carbohydrates, because of the increased quantity of CO_2 that results.

However, other acids are constantly being formed on a daily basis. Known as noncarbonic acids, which include acids such as sulfuric acid and phosphoric acid, they are derived from the metabolism of ingested proteins. In an average American diet, individuals eat enough protein to generate approximately 70 meq of noncarbonic acid daily. A vegetarian diet may have less. The addition of these diet-derived noncarbonic acids presents the body with several challenges. Let us represent the acids as H^+X^-, with X^- representing the respective anion (phosphate, sulfate, oxalate, etc.), since the body handles each in a similar fashion.

When added to the system, the bicarbonate pool buffers the new acid, as described by the following reaction.

$$H^+X^- + Na^+HCO_3^- \leftrightarrow H_2CO_3 + Na^+X^-$$

Of course, since we are not charged beings, the bicarbonate anion is balanced by a sodium cation to maintain electroneutrality. The hydrogen ion of the acid is instantaneously buffered with bicarbonate, briefly forming H_2CO_3, which in turn is immediately converted to water and CO_2, the latter of which is exhaled by the lung. The net effect of the reaction will be a loss of a HCO_3^- anion, and the production of a sodium salt, Na^+X^-.

As noted earlier, the average diet results in the addition of 70 meq of noncarbonic acid to the body. One may begin to see the problem, as illustrated in *Figure 9-2*.

After the addition of one meq of H^+X^-, one meq of HCO_3^- will be consumed and one of Na^+X^- will be formed. After the addition of a second meq of H^+X^-, two meq of HCO_3^- ions will be consumed and two meq of Na^+X^- salts will be formed. Since the bicarbonate pool is limited (and starting with a normal serum bicarbonate level of 25 meq/L), one can see that the bicarbonate stores will be consumed over time. In addition, as each reaction occurs, more and more Na^+X^- salts will accumulate. To maintain homeostasis, the body must accomplish two things. First, it must return the serum bicarbonate stores to normal. And second, it must somehow find a way to rid itself of the accumulating salts. Both of these important processes occur in the kidney.

TUBULAR BICARBONATE RECLAMATION

The first step in returning serum bicarbonate stores to normal is preventing bicarbonate loss in urine. Since bicarbonate is a small charged particle, it is freely filtered across the glomerulus. On a daily basis, normal individuals filter almost 4,500 meq of bicarbonate. This number is simply the product of the GFR and the serum bicarbonate concentration (assuming normal GFR [125 cc/min or 180 L/day] and a normal serum bicarbonate level [25 meq/L], one calculates 4,500 meq of bicarbonate are filtered per day).

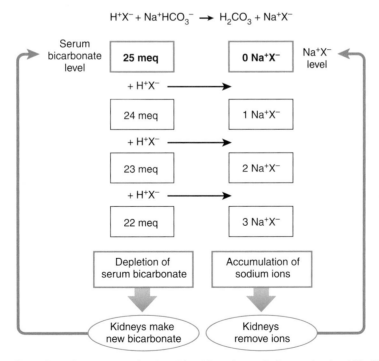

$$H^+X^- + Na^+HCO_3^- \rightarrow H_2CO_3 + Na^+X^-$$

FIGURE 9-2 The effect of producing noncarbonic acid. With each mmol of noncarbonic acid buffered, the serum bicarbonate falls and a sodium anion accumulates (the figure assumes 1 meq/L of H^+ added for 1 meq/L of bicarbonate lost). Thus, in order to prevent depletion of the serum bicarbonate stores and accumulation of sodium anions, the kidney makes new bicarbonate and filters out the sodium anions.

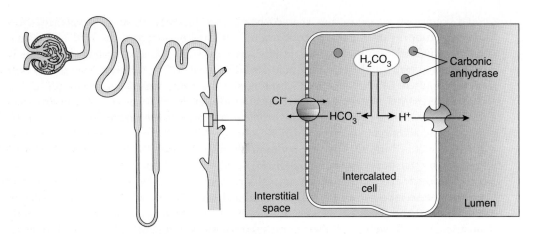

FIGURE 9-3 **Distal hydrogen secretion.** In the presence of intracellular carbonic anhydrase, carbonic acid is cata-lyzed into hydrogen ion and bicarbonate. Hydrogen ATPases are present on the apical membrane of the intercalated cell of the collecting duct. They secrete the hydrogen ions into the lumen. Bicarbonate is returned to the systemic cir-culation via a bicarbonate chloride transporter.

In order to prevent rapid loss of the bicarbonate buffering pool, all filtered bicarbon-ate must be reabsorbed. In Chapter 5, we reviewed the molecular mechanism respon-sible for reabsorption of bicarbonate. The NHE in the proximal tubule, by extruding a hydrogen ion in exchange for a sodium ion in the presence of carbonic anhydrase, facili-tates the reclamation of filtered bicarbonate. Approximately 85% of filtered bicarbonate is reabsorbed in the proximal tubule. Thus, although the pH of the filtrate at the begin-ning of the proximal tubule is the same as serum (7.4), the pH falls to around 6.8 at the end of the proximal tubule as bicarbonate is reabsorbed (and hydrogen ion secreted).

The remaining 15% is reclaimed by mechanisms in the more distal segments of the tubule. In the apical membrane of the intercalated cell of the collecting duct, Hydrogen ATPases secrete hydrogen ions, consuming an ATP in the process. This allows for further reclamation of filtered bicarbonate. These Hydrogen ATPases are stimulated by the hor-mone aldosterone. This process is illustrated in *Figure 9-3*.

Tubular bicarbonate reclamation prevents loss of filtered bicarbonate, but it will not com-pensate for the bicarbonate consumed by the acid generated by metabolism of dietary pro-tein. Thus, in order to maintain serum bicarbonate stores in the face of acid production, the kidneys must have the capacity to generate new bicarbonate anions in addition to avid tubular reabsorption of filtered bicarbonate. This occurs by the excretion of a hydrogen ion into the urine, and the return to the body of a "new" molecule of bicarbonate, replenishing the stores used to buffer the daily net acid load. This process is discussed in the next section.

GENERATING NEW BICARBONATE

In order to stay in acid–base balance, we must excrete the same amount of hydrogen ions that we consume per day. The excretion of hydrogen ions in the renal tubule allows us to produce new bicarbonate, which replaces the bicarbonate consumed by the produc-tion of noncarbonic acid. Carbon dioxide in the renal tubular cells, in the presence of carbonic anhydrase and water, forms carbonic acid. As we discussed earlier, carbonic acid then dissociates into H^+ and HCO_3^-; the hydrogen ion is secreted into the tubule and the bicarbonate ion crosses the basal membrane into the interstitial fluid. The next result is the creation of a bicarbonate ion.

Although the NHE and Hydrogen ATPases allow for acid secretion, this process of hydrogen ion secretion alone cannot handle the approximately 70 meq of hydrogen that must be eliminated each day as a consequence of the food we eat. Unlike the gastric epithelium, which can tolerate a pH of 1 due to its protective mucosal barrier, the renal tubular epithelium is relatively naked, and consequently cannot tolerate a pH of less than 4.5. It must have a mechanism to buffer the pH of the urine as bicarbonate is reclaimed and hydrogen ions are secreted. Along the proximal tubule, the pH falls to around 6.8, correlating to a free hydrogen concentration of 0.00000015 meq/L. Distal acidification can decrease the pH to approximately 4.5, which correlates with a free hydrogen concentration of 0.00003 meq/L. If we can only generate urine with an H^+ concentration of 0.00003 meq/L, we will either need to make about 2 million liters of urine per day, or we need a better method of excreting hydrogen ions beyond simple acidification!

To eliminate enough acid to maintain net acid balance and not destroy the tubular epithelium, more than simple hydrogen excretion is needed. In the next section, we describe the two major mechanisms whereby the kidney can secrete hydrogen; as we noted earlier, each hydrogen ion secreted leads to the generation of new bicarbonate molecule that is returned to the body.

Ammoniagenesis

In a chemical reaction unique to the kidney, proximal tubule cells are able to utilize a widely abundant amino acid to produce bicarbonate. This process, termed **ammoniagenesis**, allows the excretion of additional hydrogen ions and the generation of a new bicarbonate ion.

Glutamine is the most abundant naturally occurring nonessential amino acid, and can be found within a wide array of dietary sources. Given its abundance, and its ability to be synthesized, it provides an unending substrate for renal ammoniagenesis. Proximal tubule cells absorb glutamine from peritubular capillaries and, in a complex reaction, convert glutamine into ammonium (NH_4^+) and alphaketoglutarate. The subsequent metabolism of alphaketoglutarate results in the generation of two bicarbonate ions, which are returned to the systemic circulation. The NH_4^+ ion is transported across the apical membrane via the NHE, and is eventually eliminated in the urine. The net effect is the production of new bicarbonate ions. This process is illustrated in *Figure 9-4*.

In order for this reaction to continue, NH_4^+ must be excreted in the urine. One might expect that NH_4^+, because it is lipid insoluble and cannot cross the tubular epithelium without specific protein transporters, would travel with the tubular fluid and not be reabsorbed. However, NH_4^+ is in equilibrium with ammonia, as defined by the following reaction.

$$NH_3 + H^+ \leftrightarrow NH_4^+$$

Unlike NH_4^+, NH_3 is lipid soluble and crosses the tubular epithelium. Thus, the potential loss of NH_3, which would drive the above reaction to the left and lead to a free hydrogen ion with subsequent lowering of the pH of tubular fluid, has the potential to greatly undermine the acid-carrying capacity of this system.

The relationship of NH_3 to NH_4^+ is defined by its pK_a of 9. The relative amount of diffusible NH_3 is determined by the pH along the tubule. In the more proximal parts of the tubule, where the pH ranges between 6 and 7, there is relatively more NH_3 than in the more acidic distal parts, where the pH is typically less than 5.5. Since NH_3 is lipid soluble, the more proximal parts of the tubule could potentially lose NH_3 into the interstitium and back into the body, undermining acid excretion. This is less of a problem in the highly acidic distal aspects where the reaction is shifted to the right.

In order to prevent the dissolution of NH_3 from the earlier parts of the tubule, a countercurrent system exists, as seen in *Figure 9-4*. In a manner similar to the countercurrent exchange of the urinary concentration system (see Chapter 5), the interstitial concentration of NH_3 is kept high by medullary recycling. NH_4^+ is produced in the proximal tubule, in a process that generates new bicarbonate. The NH_4^+, at equilibrium with its soluble

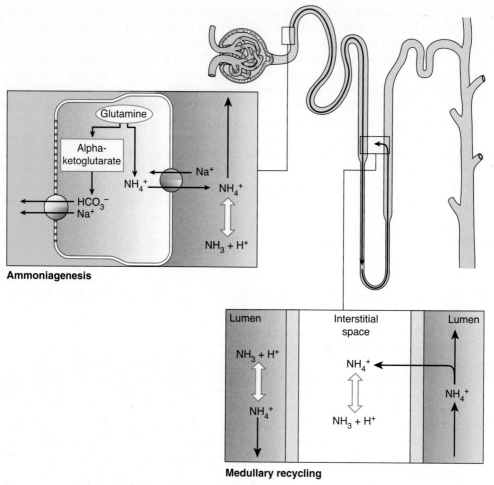

Ammoniagenesis

Medullary recycling

FIGURE 9-4 Ammoniagenesis and medullary recycling. Proximal tubule cells convert the amino acid glutamine into NH_4^+ and alphaketoglutarate. Alphaketoglutarate is metabolized into two bicarbonate ions, which are then transported out of the cell into the interstitium via a bicarbonate chloride transporter, leading to new bicarbonate formation. The NH_4^+ exits the cell to the tubule's lumen via the NHE (introduced in Chapter 5). NH_4^+ is in equilibrium with NH_3; given its charge, the former is not permeable across the tubular cell's apical membrane, whereas the later is. In order to prevent the leak of NH_3 out of the tubule, a process of medullary recycling occurs. NH_4^+ in the tubular fluid is absorbed back into the interstitium in the thick ascending tubule, after which it dissociates into NH_3 and a hydrogen ion. This leads to a high interstitial concentration of NH_3, and prevents diffusion of NH_3 out of the tubule.

conjugate base NH_3, flows through the hairpin loop of the Limb of Henle. In the ascending limb, NH_4^+ is reclaimed via the NK2Cl cotransporter. Upon entering the less acid tubular epithelial cells, NH_3 is formed and enters into the medullary interstitium, only to be returned to the descending limb. This countercurrent recycling maintains a high interstitial concentration of NH_3. Since the movement of NH_3 from the tubule depends on both the tubular permeability and the differences in concentration gradient between the lumen and the interstitium, the high interstitial concentration limits NH_3 loss from the tubule.

Ammoniagenesis is a very complex process, and, as such, is very sensitive to the changes of renal function. Even mild kidney dysfunction, as might occur with underperfusion from volume depletion, can greatly curtail the process. On the other hand, ammoniagenesis also has the potential to greatly increase the body's ability to excrete acid. Because of the efficiency of medullary recycling, and the unlimited supply of glutamine, ammoniagenesis can be upregulated to excrete as much as 600 to 700 meq of hydrogen ions (in the form of NH_4^+) per day.

Titratable Acids

Just like their role in the serum, buffers play a critical role in facilitating acid excretion in the urine. By acting as a hydrogen sink (i.e., binding to H^+ so that protons can be eliminated without altering the pH of the fluid—remember, pH reflects the concentration of *free* hydrogen ions in solution), they allow the excretion of relatively large amount of hydrogen ions without damaging the tubular epithelium. In the serum, the most important buffer system utilizes the bicarbonate anion. As we have just learned, however, almost all filtered bicarbonate is reabsorbed by the tubules and, consequently, is not available to act as a buffer in the urine. Instead, other urinary buffers come into play to facilitate hydrogen excretion.

The phosphoric acid system is one of the most important urinary buffers. Phosphate can pick up three potential hydrogens in forming phosphoric acid, and is a relatively strong acid, with a pK_a as shown below for each phase of the dissociation.

$$pK_a \quad 2.14 \quad\quad 6.80 \quad\quad\quad 12.4$$
$$H_3PO_4 \rightarrow H_2PO_4^- \rightarrow HPO_4^{2-} \rightarrow PO_4^{3-}$$

The anion after the first dissociation of hydrogen, $H_2PO_4^-$, is called dihydrogen phosphate; HPO_4^{2-} is called monohydrogen phosphate, and the anion without any hydrogen ions is simple termed phosphate. When measuring a serum phosphorus level, all of the different structures are included. However, at a serum pH of 7.4 (relatively alkaline to $H_2PO_4^-$, but notably acidic in relation to PO_4^{3-}), most serum phosphate is in the monohydrogen form, HPO_4^{2-}.

As a small ion, phosphate is freely filtered across the glomerulus. Since the tubule fluid at its inception has a pH similar to serum (7.4), almost all the phosphate is in the monohydrogen form. In order for phosphate to accept additional hydrogen ions, the urine must become more acidic, at least to a pH below the pK_a between the dihydrogen and monohydrogen forms. In other words, the phosphate system only becomes effective as a buffer when the urine can be acidified to a pH less than 6.8. Thus, although the phosphate system can be a useful buffer, acidification of the urine to a pH significantly less than serum is critical for the reaction to ensue.

There is a second limitation of the phosphate-buffering system. The amount of phosphate in the body is fixed, depending purely on the diet and the balance of filtered to reabsorbed phosphate. Tubular reclamation of phosphate is controlled by a whole host of factors independent of pH. Thus, the amount of phosphate available to serve as a buffer is dependent on factors unrelated to the acid–base status of the individual.

Other filtratable anions, including citrate and sulfate, can act as buffers. However, like phosphate, they are in limited quantity and, since they have lower pK_a values, are generally less effective as buffers. Collectively, all these different filtered anions are known as "**titratable acids**." The term comes from the way in which the buffering capacity of these anions is measured. As noted previously, the phosphate concentration in urine includes all different forms (mono, dihydrogen, etc.) of the molecule; consequently, the concentration is not an accurate assessment of the hydrogen-carrying capacity of the system. Instead, the amount of hydrogen buffered by all the various forms of the anion is measured by simply adding sufficient alkali to an individual's urine to raise the pH to 7.4. When the urine pH reaches 7.4, signaling the removal of all the buffered hydrogen ions relative to serum, one can quantify how much secreted hydrogen has been secreted and buffered by filtered ions.

On average, about one-third of the daily hydrogen excreted is ultimately eliminated in the urine via titratable acids. Failure to reach a urine pH below 5.5, however, will render most of the potential buffers useless, and greatly undermines net acid excretion. Because there is a fixed quantity of these acids in the urine, there is a fixed potential for either increasing or decreasing the amount of excreted hydrogen. Thus, even with acidification of the urine, and utilizing all the filtered buffers, there is still limited capacity to excrete hydrogen ions. In the setting of increased acid loads, the fixed amount of titratable acids is unable to achieve the necessary goal of acid excretion to sustain a normal pH in the blood.

FILTERING OUT EXCESS ANIONS

We have discussed how the kidney makes new bicarbonate and how excess hydrogen ions are excreted in the urine without damaging the tubular epithelium. Let us move on to the second important task, removing the sodium salt that occurs as the anion of the acid is buffered, as illustrated by the equation on page 163. For dietary acids, this anion is primarily phosphate or sulfate.

Before we discuss how the body rids itself of this anion, we should discuss how to clinically assess for the presence of such anions. This is perhaps most simply done by drawing a chart with all the positive charged particles on one side, and all the negatively charged particles on the other. Of course, since we are not electrically charged beings, all the positive and negative charges in our bodies must sum up to equal zero; all the positives must equal all the negatives. This is relationship is illustrated in *Figure 9-5*.

When we send a patient's blood to the lab, only several common ions are measured; namely, sodium, potassium, chloride, and bicarbonate. The presence of other anions or cations must be inferred from changes in these measurable ions. For most individuals, the dietary acid anions, namely, sulfates and phosphates, accumulate and are associated with a decline in bicarbonate anion as buffering occurs. Thus, although the total amount of cations always equals the total amount of anions, if you were to look only at the *commonly measured* ions, there would be relatively more sodium and potassium ions than the sum of chloride and bicarbonate ions because of the presence of other anions, such as phosphate and sulfate (albumin, a common protein in the blood, is also negatively charged and contributes significantly to the unmeasured anions in the blood). The presence of these unmeasured anions contributes to what is termed the "**anion gap**," which simply refers to the anions that are not measured in routine laboratory tests.

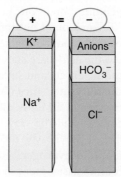

$$(Na^+ + K^+) - (HCO_3^- + Chloride^-) = Anion\ Gap$$

FIGURE 9-5 **Serum anion gap.** In our blood, all the positive charges must balance out all the negative charges. Routine laboratory tests do not assess all of the anions; consequently, there is a difference between the measurable cations and measurable anions. This is termed the anion gap, and refers to the presence of anions that are not routinely measured by clinical laboratories.

The anion gap is defined by the following formula.

$$(Na^+ + K^+) - (HCO_3^- + Chloride^-) = Anion\ Gap$$

Although potassium is commonly measured as part of the standard electrolyte blood test, the body regulates the level of potassium very closely; a normal range is between 3.6 and 4.4 meq/L. Consequently, changes in serum potassium do not significantly affect the anion gap and the calculation is most often made without including that cation. Using this approach, the normal upper limit of the anion gap is 12; these "missing" anions are due to the protein, albumin, and circulating phosphates and sulfates.

As we have discussed, the average American eats about 70 meq of acid (as metabolized from dietary protein), and produces 70 meq of new anions each day. How do we maintain a normal anion gap under these conditions? The answer is that the kidney removes these newly produced anions. This is accomplished by simple filtration across the glomerulus. As discussed earlier, these filtered anions become important proton acceptors in the urine, buffering against pH changes. Thus, the filtration of these anions is critical for the generation of new bicarbonate, which is connected to the elimination of hydrogen ions as described previously. It should be noted that many of these filtered anions are reabsorbed across the tubules. Nevertheless, anion filtration is important in net hydrogen ion excretion.

In summary, in response to the daily acid load associated with eating, the kidneys must excrete hydrogen into the urine, thereby replenishing the consumed bicarbonate buffer stores. In addition, the kidneys must filter the formed sodium salts, typically sodium phosphate or sodium sulfate, that are produced by the buffering process in the blood. In most individuals, these two renal processes occur in synchrony. However, hydrogen excretion, particularly the ammoniagenesis component, is much more fragile than the process of filtration of anions, and can sometimes be severely damaged while the process of filtration remains relatively intact.

ACID BALANCE IN THOSE WITH IMPAIRED RENAL FUNCTION

Each day, in order to stay in balance, the kidneys must excrete the same amount of hydrogen as one consumes from the diet. For people with various types of kidney diseases, handling this continuous acid load can be problematic, and acid retention is one of the hallmarks of renal failure. Remembering that healthy kidneys both filter the anion salt as well as excrete a hydrogen ion, there are two potential types of acid disturbances in those with kidney disease: those that are associated with a normal anion gap, and those in which the anion gap is increased.

As we mentioned, ammoniagenesis is a very complex cellular process, and is easily impaired by even mild renal injury. Thus, in mild kidney disease, the kidneys' ability to excrete hydrogen is impaired, and net hydrogen balance becomes positive. Clinically, detecting net hydrogen balance can be quite difficult. Because of the large buffering capacity of bone, individuals can be in net positive acid balance, yet not sustain any decrement in the serum bicarbonate concentration. This occurs at the expense of bone health; since skeletal bicarbonate is stored as calcium carbonate, utilization of the bicarbonate to buffer protons leads to loss of calcium and gradual bone demineralization.

Eventually, with more progressive kidney disease, the capacity of bone to buffer acid is exhausted and the serum bicarbonate begins to fall. The serum chloride concentration will increase to maintain electroneutrality. However, because the filtering capacity of the kidneys is relatively hardy, anions are still excreted and there is no increase of the normal serum anion gap. At this point, the patient will have an acidemia, as evidenced by low serum bicarbonate and a low pH, yet a normal anion gap. Clinically, this condition is characterized as a "non-anion gap" acidosis, referring to the fact that the acidosis occurs without anion retention within the serum.

With time, as an individual's renal function progressively deteriorates, both the acid-excreting capacity and the glomerular filtration capacity decrease. Consequently, the ensuing acidosis is associated with an increase in the anion gap, and the condition is characterized as an anion gap acidosis. The acidosis is due to the inability to excrete sufficient amounts of hydrogen to compensate for dietary intake, whereas the increased gap is due to the inability to filter sodium sulfate and sodium phosphate. Usually, the filtering capacity of the kidney (i.e., the ability to eliminate the molecular products of metabolism, as assessed via the GFR) is retained until the glomerular filtration rate is severely reduced. Thus, an anion gap acidosis due to renal failure usually only occurs in those with markedly impaired renal function.

In Animated Figure 9-3 (Acid Balance in Impaired Renal Function), you can view the process by which acid conditions evolve as detailed earlier. Choose the state of mildly impaired renal function in the diagram and note how the pH of the blood and the anion gap remain normal for some time due to bone buffering. Then choose the condition in which bone buffering has been exhausted and observe how the pH falls, but a normal anion gap is maintained due to the increase in chloride concentration. Finally, choose the state in which renal function is severely impaired; in this condition, you can see that the anion gap increases as the capacity to rid the body of excess anions is compromised.

As we will learn in the next section, there are many other types of anion gap acidoses that occur independently of changes in renal function and are often due to ingested acids and abnormal metabolism in the body associated with conditions such as diabetes mellitus and hypoxemia.

In this section, we have described acid accumulation associated with impaired renal function as determined by the GFR, since this is the standard method of assessing how well the kidneys work. However, there are certain conditions in which impaired renal acid excretion develops despite a normal GFR. These disorders are described as primary tubular disorders in which isolated deficiencies in renal bicarbonate absorption or hydrogen excretion lead to an acidosis; they are clinically known as "**renal tubular acidoses (RTAs).**" Since the GFR remains intact, there will not be an associated increase of the anion gap. Thus, these disorders are non-anion gap acidoses. Whereas similar in this respect to the condition seen in early renal failure, the RTAs differ in that GFR in an RTA is preserved.

RENAL TUBULAR ACIDOSIS

As we have noted previously, the tubules must reclaim all filtered bicarbonate and excrete hydrogen ions (to match dietary acid intake) in order to prevent acidosis from developing. A breakdown in either one of these processes leads to acid accumulation.

There are several types of RTAs, categorized according to the location of the tubular defect that leads to the acidosis. Each one leads to a unique and predictable phenotype. A proximal RTA occurs when there is an abnormality in the proximal reclamation of filtered bicarbonate, likely due to a defect in the NHE in the proximal tubule. This leads to a quantitative defect in the proximal tubule's absorptive capacity of filtered bicarbonate. Whereas most individuals can reclaim all filtered bicarbonate (approximately 4,500 meq/day), the patients with a proximal tubule acidosis can absorb notably less. Thus, these patients lose bicarbonate in the urine, and the urine pH rises. With this loss of bicarbonate, the serum bicarbonate falls, and an acidemia ensues. As this process continues, the serum bicarbonate concentration falls, the total filtered bicarbonate falls, and a new equilibrium is reached when the amount of filtered bicarbonate becomes low enough that the defective proximal tubule is able to reclaim all of the now reduced filtered bicarbonate. The urine pH drops accordingly. Typically, the serum bicarbonate in patients with proximal RTAs does not fall below 15 meq/L.

In contrast to the proximal tubular acidosis, defects in the distal tubule are associated with a problem in excretion of protons. There are two types of distal RTAs. In the first type, patients have a profound abnormality with the distal Hydrogen ATPase, and they are unable to acidify their urine at all. Their ability to utilize ammonium and titratable acids as buffers is limited, and the net acid excretion is greatly undermined. These patients develop profound acidemia, sometimes with serum bicarbonates less than 10 meq/L. Because this condition is also associated in some individuals with potassium wasting, the defect is termed "hypokalemic distal RTA."

In the second type of distal RTA, patients develop hyperkalemia. As mentioned previously, aldosterone activates the distal Hydrogen ATPase and stimulates hydrogen excretion. Thus, the lack of aldosterone can lead to an inability to excrete hydrogen and potassium, which results in a "hyperkalemic distal RTA." In addition, the resulting hyperkalemia interferes with ammoniagenesis, which reduces the amount of buffer available for hydrogen excretion. Since the Hydrogen ATPase is relatively intact (just not being stimulated appropriately in the absence of aldosterone), and there are aldosterone-independent mechanisms stimulating hydrogen excretion, the overall degree of acidosis is usually mild. Serum bicarbonate usually does not fall below 15 meq/L in patients with this condition.

? **THOUGHT QUESTION 9-2** **Predict the urine pH in a patient with a proximal tubular acidosis, a hypokalemic distal tubular acidosis, and a hyperkalemic RTA. Explain your answer.**

States of Acid Excess—Production Acidoses

Because of the constant intake of dietary acids, individuals with impaired kidney function can develop acidemia. However, there are other conditions in which increased acid production, or loss of body bicarbonate, can lead to acidemia in the setting of normal renal function.

Let us return to the equation below.

$$H^+X^- + Na^+HCO_3^- \leftrightarrow H_2CO_3 + Na^+X^-$$

To this point, we have discussed the addition of approximately 70 meq of phosphoric and sulfuric acids (breakdown products of protein) per day to the body. The serum bicarbonate buffers the added acid, forming carbonic acid, which is converted into CO_2 and water, and a sodium salt (as represented by Na^+X^-) is left. In healthy individuals, the lost bicarbonate is regenerated as hydrogen ions are excreted in the urine, and the Na^+X^- salt is filtered and excreted in the urine.

What happens, however, if much larger amounts of acid are suddenly added to the body? In this setting, bicarbonate would fall and Na^+X^- salt would form. If the amount of acid added to the body were large enough to overwhelm the kidney's acid-excreting ability and its filtration ability, acidemia would ensue accompanied by accumulation of Na^+X^- salts, which would be evidenced by an increase in the size of the anion gap.

This is exactly what happens in **production acidoses**, conditions in which the body suddenly begins to make large amounts of acid, which overwhelm the kidney's hydrogen-excretion and salt-filtration capacity. The net effect is the development of an anion gap acidosis.

KETOACIDOSIS

The healthy body typically relies on carbohydrate metabolism as its energy source. However, under certain conditions, the body shifts away from carbohydrates to the metabolism of amino acids and fatty acids, forming ketones as an alternative energy source. Ketosis most often occurs in diabetics, due to the relative deficiency of insulin, but is also seen in states of fasting and in alcoholics who are malnourished.

The two common ketones produced in humans are acetoacetic acid, which breaks down into acetone, and beta-hydroxybutyrate. Both substances are acids, with pK_a values of 3.5 and 4.7, respectively. In serum, they fully dissociate, producing a free hydrogen and an anion.

In returning to the equation discussed earlier, if ketones are represented as H^+X^-, the addition of many H^+X^- will rapidly shift the equation to the far right. Consequently, the sodium bicarbonate levels fall, carbonic acid is created and immediately metabolized into CO_2 and water, and sodium salts form. These salts are made up of the conjugate base of the ketone such as sodium acetate (from acetoacetate) or sodium butyrate (from beta-hydroxybutyrate).

In patients with ketoacid production, the degree to which acidosis develops and the anion gap increases is ultimately determined by the balance between acid production and renal excretion. If the ketone production is small, as after a short fasting period, then the kidneys should be able to compensate, and no perturbation will develop. Starvation and alcohol ketoacidosis are usually associated with moderate ketone production; although the kidneys cannot fully compensate, the acidosis and the increase in the anion gap are relatively mild. In contrast, in individuals with Type I diabetes, which is characterized by a deficiency of insulin, the body may make hundreds of ketones per day and the shift to ketosis can be profound and severe. This sudden increase of acid production can result in a marked acidemia as well as a pronounced increase in the anion gap.

If well-functioning kidneys can upregulate ammonia production and excrete 500 to 700 meq of hydrogen per day, why do patients with diabetic ketoacidosis, who make about the same amount of ketoacids per day, develop acidemia? The answer to this dilemma lies in the definition of "well-functioning" kidneys. In patients with diabetic ketoacidosis, the kidney's ability to make ammonium and filter anions dwindles dramatically due to profound volume depletion, which reduces the GFR and impairs ammoniagenesis. Volume depletion may be due to vomiting, a common symptom in these patients, as well as the increase in salt and water losses associated with the osmotic diuresis that accompanies glucose in the urine. In addition, the sudden increase of ketones in the urine act as a relatively nonreabsorbable anion; the ketone salt is filtered across the glomerulus and exceeds the ability of the tubule to reabsorb it, which leads to loss of the salt in the urine.

The loss of filtered ketones in the urine has additional ramifications for the acid–base balance of the patient. The filtered ketone anions, as conjugate bases, have the potential to accept a hydrogen. Once insulin levels are restored, usually by exogenous administration of the hormone, the liver can metabolize the ketone anions back into bicarbonate. Thus, filtering the anions into the urine is akin to losing a potential base.

Treatment for diabetic ketoacidosis includes administration of large amounts of intravenous fluid, which improves the kidney's ability to excrete hydrogen, as well as administration of intravenous alkali in severe cases to replace the lost ketone anion.

Clinically, the diagnosis of ketoacidosis is suspected based on the patient's history of diabetes and symptoms, and confirmed by the presence of ketones in the urine and/or serum. The most commonly used assay for measuring ketones is a urine "dipstick" analysis. This test utilizes a nitroprusside reagent, which cannot detect the presence of beta-hydroxybutyrate, although it can sensitively detect acetone and acetoacetate.

THOUGHT QUESTION 9-3 Two patients with Type I (deficiency of insulin) diabetes come into the emergency room with pneumonia, and each is discovered to have a profound anion gap acidosis due to diabetic ketoacidosis. Both have a serum pH of 7.15, with a serum bicarbonate of 10, and an anion gap of 26. The first patient also has long standing renal failure, and has been on dialysis for 5 years. He makes no urine. The second has no history of kidney problems. Based on your knowledge of the physiology of these conditions, how would the management of each of these patients differ with respect to fluids and their acid–base status?

LACTIC ACIDOSIS

Lactic acidosis occurs in settings of tissue hypoxia, at which point cells must shift from oxidative metabolism and the Krebs cycle to anaerobic metabolism and the Cori cycle; the latter results in the production of lactic acid. Lactic acidosis is most commonly seen in disease states such as sepsis (severe infection) or pronounced hypotension. In addition, it can also be a marker of cellular death, such as might be found with bowel ischemia.

ALCOHOL INGESTION

There are many different types of alcohol, and the ingestion of each can lead to a production acidosis. Ethanol (C_2H_5OH, molecular weight 46) is the standard alcohol included in beer, wine, and liquor. Methanol (CH_3OH, molecular weight 32) is used in antifreeze and solvents. Ethylene glycol ($HOCH_2CH_2OH$, molecular weight 62) has a very low freezing point and has thus gained widespread use in deicers, antifreeze, and air conditioning systems. Both methanol and ethylene glycol are toxic and a single ingestion can be fatal. However, given their sweet taste, they are sometimes used as a cheaper alternative to ethanol by individuals with a strong alcohol addiction, or by those intentionally trying to hurt themselves.

Ethanol is metabolized in the liver by two oxidation reactions. It is first converted into acetaldehyde by the enzyme alcohol dehydrogenase. Acetaldehyde is in turn converted into acetate, using the enzyme aldehyde dehydrogenase. In both of these steps, electrons are transferred to the energy carrier NAD^+, resulting in a marked increase of cytosolic NADH. The abundance of NADH can shift the liver away from glucose production toward other types of energy production, including ketones. Particularly in those with chronic, heavy alcohol ingestion, this shift away from gluconeogenesis toward ketosis can lead to profound hypoglycemia, which can induce or exacerbate the behavioral manifestations of alcohol ingestion, i.e., further impair brain function. In addition, the production of ketones can lead to severe acidosis and the development of an increased anion gap. Unlike diabetics, however, alcohol ketoacidosis is typically associated with normal or low sugar levels, which can be a useful distinguishing factor in the clinical setting. And unlike diabetics, the treatment of alcohol ketoacidosis typically does not involve insulin administration.

The detection of alcohol ketoacidosis can sometimes be tricky. In the metabolism of ketones, acetoacetate has two final pathways. It can be spontaneously converted into acetone, or, in the presence of the reduced NADH, it can be shuttled toward beta-hydroxybutyrate formation. Since the metabolism of alcohol produces NADH, the predominant ketone is beta-hydroxybutyrate. However, as mentioned earlier, the urinary screening test for ketones detects acetoacetate and acetone, but not beta-hydroxybutyrate. Thus, the urine dipstick does not always identify alcohol ketoacidosis, and if clinically suspected, a serum ketone analysis, which does detect all three forms, is warranted.

Surreptitious alcohol ingestion may be detected via the **osmolar gap.** An osmolar gap refers to a difference between the calculated and measured osmolality (we defined how to measure and calculate osmolality in Chapter 8). Alcohols also are "particles" and contribute to serum osmolality, yet they are not part of the equation we use to assess serum osmolarity (**calculated osmolality**). They are detected, however, on a specific test of serum osmolality that uses freezing point depression to actually measure all particles within serum (**measured osmolality**). Thus, in alcohol ingestion, the measured osmolarity is often higher than the calculated osmolality, i.e., there is an "osmolar gap." Thus, if one directly measures the serum osmolality and compares that value to the calculated number, one can detect the presence of unmeasured particles. An osmolar gap greater than 10 suggests the presence of an unmeasured particle.

Recognizing ethylene glycol and methanol ingestion is an important challenge to health care workers; an undiagnosed ingestion can be rapidly fatal, yet brisk treatment can prevent injury. Ethylene glycol is metabolized into glycolic acid and oxalic acid in a reaction catalyzed by alcohol dehydrogenase. Both are relatively strong acids with pK_a values less than 4. The acids donate hydrogen ions, causing an acidosis, and generate anions (glycolate and oxalate, respectively), which accumulate in the serum and cause an increase in the anion gap. These metabolic products are profoundly toxic, leading to an array of neurological, cardiovascular, and renal symptoms.

Methanol is metabolized into formaldehyde and then into formic acid. Its ingestion initially manifests as an osmolar gap, but as the parent compound is metabolized, the osmolar gap closes because an acidosis develops and the serum anion gap increases. Formic acid is particularly toxic to the brain, and can lead to blindness, coma, and death.

Although the majority of patients with anion gap acidoses have either lactic acidosis or ketoacidosis, it is important to recognize the metabolic disturbances that indicate alcohol ingestion. Ethanol is associated with an osmolar gap, but is metabolized to carbon dioxide and water with no acid formation. Ethylene glycol and methanol initially form an osmolar gap, but when metabolized lead to a large anion gap acidosis. Immediate intervention to prevent the production of the toxic acid byproducts can be lifesaving.

PUTTING IT TOGETHER

A young man comes into the emergency room with 4 days of watery diarrhea. His blood pressure is low. He is found to have a serum pH of 7.2, with a bicarbonate level of 16, consistent with a metabolic acidosis. His anion gap is normal. His creatinine, a marker of his glomerular filtration rate, is slightly increased, most likely due to volume depletion with his large stool loss. Is his acidosis due only to his loss of bicarbonate in the stool, or are there other factors involved? How do you begin to think about this problem? What is your analysis?

With several days of diarrhea, this patient has clearly had bicarbonate loss associated with increased bowel movements. The bicarbonate concentration of stool differs based on the type of gastrointestinal illness. Typically, the bicarbonate concentrations of most types of stool range from 15 to 30 meq/L. As we have discussed, most individuals with normal kidney function can upregulate ammoniagenesis, secreting up to 500 to 700 meq of hydrogen per day. If this man was able to excrete 600 meq of hydrogen in his urine (thus returning 600 meq of bicarbonate to his serum), he should be able to tolerate 20 L stool loss per day (assuming 30 meq of bicarbonate/L of stool). Cleary, the diarrhea cannot be that bad since cardiovascular collapse would ensue with such huge volume losses.

The normal anion gap eliminates lactic acidosis, which might occur if perfusion to tissue were compromised by the volume losses associated with the diarrhea, as a consideration. Similarly, ingestion of alcohols and moderate to severe renal failure can be excluded from further consideration.

The solution to this seeming paradox is found in the effect of the patient's volume status on his ability to eliminate protons. Because he is volume depleted, his ability to produce ammonia is greatly curtailed. As we have said, ammoniagenesis is a relatively fragile renal mechanism. Under conditions of volume depletion, the kidneys lose the ability to make ammonium, and acid excretion falls dramatically. If this man had presented to the emergency room on the first day of his illness, and had sufficient intravenous fluid to prevent volume depletion, it is likely that his ammonium excretion would have increased sufficiently to match his bicarbonate losses, and acidosis would not have ensued.

Summary Points

- On an average American diet, approximately 70 meq of noncarbonic acid is generated daily.
- Approximately 15,000 mmol of carbonic acid is generated by cellular metabolism, and rapidly transported to the lung, where they are eliminated as CO_2 via ventilation.
- The noncarbonic acids are buffered primarily by aqueous bicarbonate.
- The buffering of noncarbonic acids generates sodium salts, which are represented by the serum anion gap.
- The kidneys are responsible for filtering the sodium salts resulting from the buffering of noncarbonic acids, as well as regenerating new bicarbonate ions to compensate for those consumed in the buffering process.
- In order to generate a new bicarbonate ion, a hydrogen ion must be excreted into the urine.
- The urine pH cannot be lower than 4.5.
- Ammonia and titratable acids serve as useful urinary buffers, which allow the excretion of large amounts of hydrogen ions within the urine with little change in the urine pH.
- Titratable acids require urinary acidification in order to be useful buffers.
- Ammoniagenesis is a very efficient mechanism for hydrogen excretion.
- The anion gap refers to the accumulation of dietary-derived anions (weak bases such as sulfates and phosphates) that are not measured on routine laboratory analyses.
- The body excretes dietary-derived anions by filtration across the glomerulus.
- The anion gap increases during a production acidosis (e.g., lactic acidosis) or in renal failure (i.e., the GFR is reduced and the kidneys are unable to filter the dietary acid load).
- In early kidney disease, a non-anion gap acidosis develops (largely due to reduced ability to secrete hydrogen ions via ammoniagenesis). As the filtration capacity of the disease kidneys worsens, however, an anion gap acidosis develops.
- Acidosis due to an isolated defect in tubular handling of hydrogen with preserved filtration function is termed "renal tubular acidosis." It is a non-anion gap acidosis.
- Acidosis associated with diarrhea is due to loss of bicarbonate-rich stool and is characterized as a non-anion gap acidosis.
- Production acidosis refers to a condition in which the production of acid exceeds that which is expected from dietary metabolism. The associated conjugate base of the acid forms an unmeasured anion; thus, these conditions are associated with an "anion gap acidosis."
- Ketoacidosis and lactic acidosis are the most common types of production acidoses.
- Metabolism of certain alcohols can lead to life-threatening problems associated with anion gap acidosis and an increased osmolar gap.

Answers TO THOUGHT QUESTIONS

9-1. In patients given large amounts of intravenous fluids, the serum bicarbonate may fall, potentially reducing the concentration of available buffer. However, the concentration of dissolved carbon dioxide will fall too, so that the relative ratio of acid to base in the Henderson–Hasselbalch equation will not change, and the pH will not be altered. In addition, although the serum bicarbonate level may decrease, there are many other buffering systems in the body (including intracellular proteins and the skeleton), protecting the body from changes in pH. Thus, although fluid administration may cause serum bicarbonate levels to decrease, thus suggesting a "dilution acidosis," there is usually very little actual change in the serum pH.

9-2. In proximal RTAs, proximal bicarbonate wasting occurs when the filtered load exceeds the reabsorptive capacity. As long as the serum bicarbonate is greater than 15 meq/L, there will be bicarbonaturia, and the urine pH with be greater than 5.5. If, however, the bicarbonate level is low enough so that the filtered amount is so small that the abnormal tubule can reclaim all the filtered bicarbonate, the urine will once again become acidic (remember, in these patients the distal acidification mechanisms are intact).

In the hypokalemic (or normokalemic) distal RTA, little hydrogen can be excreted. Thus, distal acidification is impaired, and the urine pH is greater than 5.5. In the hyperkalemic distal RTA, however, the defect is milder and some hydrogen excretion occurs. In addition, because the hyperkalemia interferes with ammoniagenesis, there is a shortage of an important urinary buffer. Thus, the urine pH falls relatively easily. Such patients usually have acidic urines (pH < 5.5).

In summary, the urine pH may or may not be elevated in proximal RTAs due to the amount of bicarbonaturia. The urine pH is usually greater than 5.5 in hypokalemic distal RTA due to the complete inability to excrete hydrogen. Because the defect is milder in the hyperkalemic distal RTA and there is often a deficiency in the ammonia buffer, the urine pH is usually acidic in this condition.

9-3. Both patients have developed an anion gap acidosis due to the production of ketones. They both, therefore, need insulin, in order to correct their relative insulin deficiency (the pneumonia, as with most infections, reduces the sensitivity of cells to insulin, thereby exacerbating any absolute reduction in insulin levels and contributing to the development of ketoacidosis).

The overall volume status of each patient, however, is likely quite different. The patient with a history of normal kidney function will probably be very volume depleted. First, the high glucose levels associated with diabetic ketoacidosis (DKA) will increase the amount of glucose in the urine, which will then exceed the ability of the tubule to reabsorb glucose and lead to an osmotic diuresis with loss of salt and water. Second, the ketone anions, upon being filtered through the kidney, are lost via the urine and carry sodium and water with them. In addition, because the ketone anion might have been metabolized to bicarbonate by the liver once insulin was administered, its presence in the urine means loss of a potential base. Thus, along with insulin, this patient will require intravenous saline and may need bicarbonate supplementation.

The dialysis-dependent patient makes no urine. There can be no osmotic diuresis. Furthermore, although ketones and its conjugate base are being formed, they are not being filtered; instead, they are retained within the patient's body. Thus, this patient will not have volume depletion. As the patient's pneumonia is treated with antibiotics, and as insulin is administered, the patient will shift back toward carbohydrate metabolism, and the retained ketones will be metabolized back into bicarbonate. Treatment for the dialysis patient will consist primarily of insulin, with little need for intravenous saline and much lower need for bicarbonate replacement.

Review Questions

DIRECTIONS: *Each of the numbered items or incomplete statements in this section is followed by answers or by completions of the statement. Select the ONE lettered answer or completion that is BEST in each case.*

1. A biologist is diagnosed with chronic kidney disease. On his routine diet, he gener-
    ates about 70 meq of acid per day. He measures his daily excretion of acid, and finds
    that on most days, he only excretes about 50 meq of acid. Despite being in daily
    net acid gain, his serum bicarbonate level remains unchanged at 24 meq/L. What
    accounts for the stability of his serum bicarbonate despite net acid gain?

    A. His lungs compensate by breathing out more carbonic acid.
    B. He excretes acid via his stool.
    C. He buffers the acid excess with skeletal bicarbonate.
    D. He does not absorb all the acid from his diet.

2. A patient's urine pH is noted to decrease from 7 to 6 on two consecutive urine
    samples. What does this mean about net acid excretion?

    A. The lower urine pH indicates that more acid is being excreted.
    B. The lower urine pH indicates that less acid is being excreted.
    C. The lower urine pH does not indicate changes in net acid excretion.

3. A dialysis patient (assume no intrinsic kidney function) is admitted to the hospital
    for abdominal pain. On the first day, her serum bicarbonate is 24 meq/L. The next
    day, her serum bicarbonate is 14 meq/L with a serum pH of 7.10. Which statement
    is true?

    A. The acidosis occurs because she is not able to excrete the normal dietary load of
        acid.
    B. The acidosis occurs because she is producing new acid.
    C. The acidosis occurs because she has a respiratory problem.

Metabolic Alkalosis
The Other Side of the Renal Acid–Base Story

chapter **10**

CHAPTER OUTLINE

INTRODUCTION
PROTECTING AGAINST ALKALOSIS
• The importance of GFR
TUBULAR HANDLING OF BICARBONATE
ASSESSING VOLUME STATUS IN ALKALOSIS
METABOLIC ALKALOSIS DUE TO GASTRIC
   ACID LOSS

METABOLIC ALKALOSIS DUE TO DISTAL
   TUBULE SECRETION
PUTTING IT TOGETHER
SUMMARY POINTS

LEARNING OBJECTIVES

By the end of this chapter, you should be able to:

- **define alkalosis.**
- **distinguish a primary increase of serum bicarbonate from that which is part of the kidney's compensation for a respiratory related increase of CO_2.**
- **explain bicarbonate handling within the kidney.**
- **describe the renal capacity to excrete bicarbonate.**
- **describe the mechanisms that lead to renal bicarbonate reclamation.**
- **explain the roles of the GFR and the tubular bicarbonate in the generation of metabolic alkalosis.**
- **describe the role of the proximal and distal tubules in generating and maintaining an alkalosis.**

Introduction

In Chapter 9, you learned how the large pool of bicarbonate provides the first line of protection against the constant acid onslaught that our bodies face on a daily basis. Bicarbonate, either in an aqueous (serum) or a mineral (bone) form, plays a critical role in the stabilization of the serum pH. Whereas the amount of free hydrogen ions in the plasma is amazingly small, at approximately 0.000000039 meq/L, the serum concentration

179

of bicarbonate is typically 24 to 26 meq/L, almost 615 million times more concentrated! This bicarbonate concentration allows for the tight buffering against changes in the body pH.

Although this pool of bicarbonate provides critical protection against acid loads, the concentration of serum bicarbonate can, at times, become inappropriately elevated. We use the term "inappropriate" to distinguish this process from an increase of serum bicarbonate that reflects an appropriate response to increasing serum CO_2 levels, as reflected by the partial pressure of CO_2 (i.e., the pCO_2), in the blood. If the lungs are not functioning properly, CO_2 levels rise in the serum; carbonic acid forms, which leads to a drop in pH (a process termed respiratory acidosis). The appropriate response of the kidneys is to excrete acid in the distal renal tubule, which leads (as we described in Chapter 9) to the generation of a bicarbonate that is reabsorbed into the blood. Consequently, one sees the serum bicarbonate rise in parallel to the rise in pCO_2; the rising bicarbonate level is a byproduct of the kidney's elimination of acid. *Inappropriate* increases of bicarbonate refer to those conditions in which the serum bicarbonate increase occurs independently of a respiratory acidosis and, instead, leads to alkalinization of the blood. This process is called **metabolic alkalosis**.

The great majority of the time, despite periodic ingestion or production of bicarbonate, our bicarbonate levels remain normal. Due to several physiologic mechanisms, we are well protected against the formation of alkalosis. Under certain conditions, however, our protective mechanisms against alkalosis become overwhelmed. We shall tackle the physiology of metabolic alkalosis in this chapter.

Protecting Against Alkalosis

The kidneys have a remarkable capacity to rid the body of excess bicarbonate. Early physiology experiments in dogs elucidated the process of renal bicarbonate excretion. Dogs, initially made acidemic, received infusions of sodium bicarbonate. When the serum bicarbonate was less than normal (around 25 meq/L), no infused bicarbonate was lost in the urine; urinary bicarbonate excretion was zero. As expected, the infused bicarbonate was correcting the acidemia. However, once the serum bicarbonate rose above 25 meq/L, indicating alkalemia, the kidneys began to excrete massive amounts of bicarbonate. The more bicarbonate that was infused, the more bicarbonate was filtered and ultimately eliminated in the urine.

The tremendous ability of the kidneys to rid the body of excess bicarbonate is predictable. Like the other small, charged particles within serum (e.g., sodium, potassium), bicarbonate is freely filtered across the glomerulus. Thus, the amount of filtered bicarbonate is simply the product of GFR and the serum concentration of bicarbonate. For individuals with a normal GFR (125 mL/min or 180 L/day) and a normal serum bicarbonate level (25 meq/L), almost 4,500 meq of bicarbonate are filtered per day. One can see that the GFR is an important determinant of bicarbonate handling.

Obviously, filtered bicarbonate must be reclaimed by the tubules; otherwise, overwhelming acidosis would ensue. Typically, since most individuals are under an acid challenge from their normal diets, the tubules absorb almost 100% of filtered bicarbonate. Approximately 85% of the filtered bicarbonate is reclaimed by the NHE in the proximal tubule. The remaining 15% is reclaimed more distally, using the Hydrogen ATPase in the collecting duct. The fate of bicarbonate under normal daily conditions is illustrated in *Figure 10-1*.

However, under certain conditions, the tubules can reduce their bicarbonate reclamation quite dramatically, thereby allowing the filtered bicarbonate to pass out of the body in the urine. Although there is some uncertainty about the exact numbers, it is generally

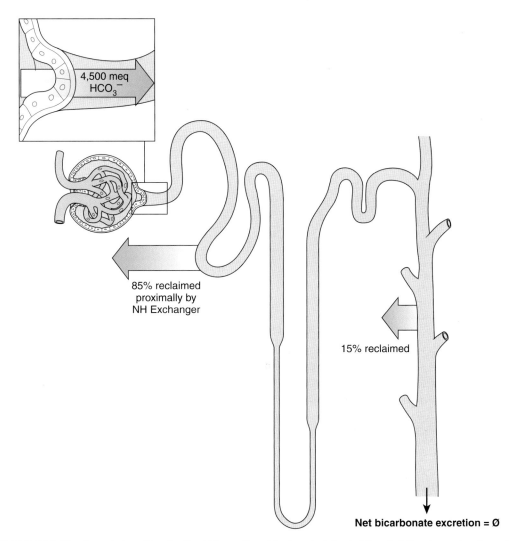

FIGURE 10-1 Bicarbonate handling by the kidney. Since bicarbonate is freely filtered at the glomerulus, the net amount of bicarbonate filtered daily by the kidney is simply the product of the GFR and the serum bicarbonate concentration. On average, we filter approximately 4,500 meq of bicarbonate ions daily. Since the average diet provides an acid load, the kidney reclaims all filtered bicarbonates, and none is lost in the urine. Most of this reclamation occurs in the proximal tubule, with only about 15% occurring more distally.

thought that the kidneys can reduce tubular bicarbonate reclamation to about 65%. In other words, under conditions of maximal bicarbonate excretion, the kidneys can excrete about 35% of a filtered load.

Consequently, individuals with normal kidney function could probably eat close to 1,500 meq of bicarbonate without going into net positive bicarbonate balance. To put that into perspective, a single teaspoon of baking soda, which is sodium bicarbonate, has 50 meq of bicarbonate. Someone would have to eat over 30 teaspoons of baking soda before becoming alkalemic.

Given the tremendous ability of the kidney to rid the body of excess bicarbonate, one must wonder how conditions of bicarbonate excess can ever develop. As we shall learn, changes in the way the kidney handles bicarbonate may greatly undermine its natural excretory capacity. Understanding why the kidney maintains the state of bicarbonate absorption, rather than allowing excretion of the bicarbonate excess, is the key to under-standing all metabolic alkaloses.

THE IMPORTANCE OF THE GFR

Since the amount of bicarbonate filtered depends on the GFR, net bicarbonate excretion does relate to the GFR. In patients who are on dialysis and make no urine, and thus have no filtration, there is obviously no excretion of bicarbonate. For most other people, the GFR plays a relatively small role in net bicarbonate excretion. Simple mathematics explains why.

A 90% reduction of the GFR, from 125 mL/min (180 L/day) to 12.5 mL/min (18 L/day), will reduce net bicarbonate filtration from 4,500 meq to 450 meq/day. Assuming a maximal tubular excretion rate (approximately 35% of filtered load excreted), about 150 meq of this bicarbonate could be excreted. This is a lot of bicarbonate, much more than most people could ever eat. Despite a huge decrease in GFR, the kidneys are still able to excrete relatively large amounts of bicarbonate compared to what is likely to be added to the body; thus, alka-losis is not seen as a consequence of impaired glomerular function. It follows that issues with tubular reclamation rather than decreased glomerular filtration of bicarbonate are the likely explanatory mechanisms for metabolic alkalosis. Therefore, the most fundamental question in understanding alkalosis is: Why do the tubules persistently absorb filtered bicarbonate in certain conditions?

 THOUGHT QUESTION 10-1 **A dialysis patient, with a long history of stomach ulcers, self-medicates with a homemade antacid, consisting of a teaspoon of baking soda daily (50 meq of sodium bicarbonate). How many meq of bicarbonate can his kidneys excrete daily? How would you expect his serum bicarbonate levels to change in the days between his dialysis sessions?**

Tubular Handling of Bicarbonate

Let us briefly review the mechanisms that protect against acidosis (as described in Chapter 9), since it is these same mechanisms that can lead to states of bicarbonate excess. In other words, the mechanisms that usually function to regenerate bicarbonate in the setting of dietary acid ingestion are the same mechanisms that, under certain conditions, can actu-ally lead to bicarbonate excess. In the proximal tubule, the NHE excretes one H^+ ion into the lumen in exchange for a reclaimed Na^+ ion, allowing for bicarbonate reclamation (recall that the proton combines with bicarbonate in the lumen to form carbonic acid, which dissociates to CO_2 and water in the presence of carbonic anhydrase; the CO_2 then diffuses into the tubular epithelial cell where the process is reversed and a bicarbonate is formed). New bicarbonate ions (in contrast to reclamation of filtered bicarbonate) are gen-erated as a byproduct of acid excretion; the protons secreted into the lumen are buffered by ammonia and titratable acids. These two processes, bicarbonate reclamation and bicar-bonate generation, determine the body's serum bicarbonate level. The body's acid base status regulates these processes. As expected, in the presence of acidemia (or bicarbonate deficit), the body should reclaim all filtered bicarbonate and generate new bicarbonate to correct the bicarbonate deficit.

However, there are other important regulators of the tubular bicarbonate handling that are pH independent. Understanding these "other" non-pH driven mechanisms is the essence of this chapter.

Let us begin with a review of the proximal NHE. As we have learned in Chapter 5, this important protein plays a fundamental role in the trans-tubular movement of many solutes; it reclaims the great majority of filtered sodium, bicarbonate, and many organic ions, along with facilitating the secretion of ammonium ions. Thus, it is not surprising that more than just acid–base status can regulate this protein.

The process of translating this important protein from its nuclear DNA, which is followed by protein synthesis, modification, and eventual shuttling to the apical membrane, is biologically complex, and each step is a potential site for regulation. One of the most important regulatory pathways relates to the ability of sensed volume depletion to stimulate the expression of the proximal tubule NHE. Since stimulation of the NHE leads to sodium reclamation (and given the presence of aquaporins, water will follow), isotonic volume expansion occurs. As sodium is reclaimed, a hydrogen ion is excreted, resulting in the reclamation of filtered bicarbonate. Thus, in the setting of sensed volume depletion, tubular bicarbonate reclamation is activated. This important mechanism is the basis for understanding why the tubules avidly retain bicarbonate in the context of a volume depleted state despite an excess of serum bicarbonate. It can be summarized by the observation, "The kidney will sacrifice acid–base status for volume." In other words, despite alkalemia, if the kidney senses volume depletion, it will stimulate avid sodium reabsorption. A byproduct of this process is bicarbonate reclamation. In the great majority of cases of alkalosis, activation of the NHE, and the resulting avid proximal tubular reclamation of filtered bicarbonate, is the mechanism that prevents the body from ridding itself of excess bicarbonate.

It should be noted that even though avid proximal tubule bicarbonate retention prevents the body from ridding itself of excess bicarbonate, it does not cause the initial alkalosis. In other words, proximal tubular reclamation may maintain an already established alkalosis, but is unlikely to cause it—recall that under normal conditions, we reabsorb virtually all of the filtered bicarbonate. Typically, the process of generating the initial alkalotic state is due to loss of acid, usually from the gastrointestinal tract. Vomiting is the most common cause; the proton pump in the stomach that produces acid leads to the generation of bicarbonate that is absorbed into the interstitial fluid, a process very similar to the one present in the distal tubule.

Bicarbonate handling in the distal tubule can also lead to alkalosis. In Chapter 9, we discussed the mechanisms of hydrogen secretion within the collecting duct. The intercalated cells have H ATPases within the apical membrane. In addition, under certain conditions, an HK exchanger can contribute to hydrogen secretion. These proteins provide pathways for continued hydrogen excretion, which can lead to an alkalosis if unchecked. Remember, for each hydrogen ion that is secreted into the lumen and excreted in the urine, a bicarbonate ion is generated and absorbed into the body.

What are the pH independent mechanisms that would drive these pumps to secrete hydrogen, thereby generating bicarbonate, when the body is already alkalemic? The most important pH independent mechanism is the hormone aldosterone. Aldosterone stimulates the Na/K ATPase along the basolateral side of the intercalated cells, generating an electrochemical gradient, which leads to the excretion of hydrogen ions. Aldosterone also increases the expression of the H ATPase. Thus, in settings of excessive aldosterone production, usually seen as a response to sensed volume depletion and activation of the renin–angiotensin–aldosterone axis, increased collecting duct secretion of hydrogen can cause an alkalosis. The importance of sensed volume in mediating tubular bicarbonate handling is illustrated in *Figure 10-2*.

In addition to sensed volume, there are other non-pH stimuli. Electrolyte abnormalities can affect the activity of these hydrogen pumps. Severely low potassium

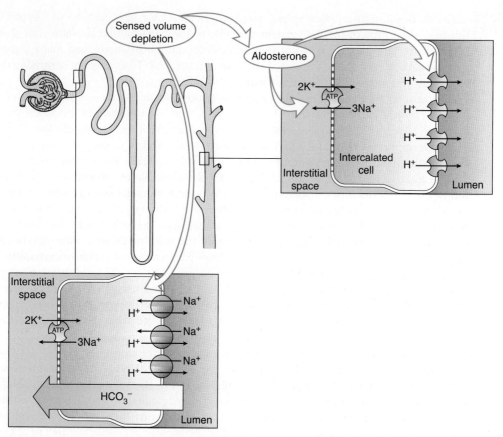

FIGURE 10-2 Aldosterone and bicarbonate handling in the kidney. The body's sensed volume is a very important regulator of tubular bicarbonate handling. In the setting of sensed volume depletion, the activity of both the NH exchanger in the proximal tubule and the H ATPase in the collecting duct are increased, leading to hydrogen secretion. In the proximal tubule, hydrogen secretion leads to bicarbonate absorption; in the distal tubule, hydrogen secretion leads to the creation of new bicarbonate. Sensed volume depletion is a more powerful stimulus than pH (the body will tolerate alkalemia rather than volume depletion), so these mechanisms may perpetuate alkalemia.

levels (K <2 meq/L) can stimulate apical membrane HK exchangers in the collecting duct, causing the absorption of potassium in exchange for hydrogen excretion. Consequently, profound hypokalemia can cause a metabolic alkalosis. Less severe changes in the serum potassium are less likely to affect hydrogen excretion and, consequently, are less likely to be the sole cause of an alkalosis. In addition, there are conditions in which aldosterone is secreted independently of the renin–angiotensin axis (aldosterone producing tumors). In this setting, patients are usually sodium avid and volume overloaded. However, because the aldosterone increases the H ATPase activity, alkalosis often develops.

In summary, there are two major areas of tubular bicarbonate handling, the proximal and distal tubules. Although these sites typically alter their hydrogen handling in response to acid–base homeostasis, there are several conditions in which the usual pH driven regulatory mechanisms are superseded, which may lead to alkalemia. Sensed volume depletion can cause unabated proximal tubular bicarbonate reclamation. Increased aldosterone production, and less frequently, hypokalemia, can induce distal hydrogen wasting, thereby causing and maintaining an alkalemia. Almost all cases of alkalosis can be explained by one of these two mechanisms.

Assessing Volume Status in Alkalosis

As described above, the sensed volume status of an individual plays a critical role in maintaining an alkalosis. The process used to assess the volume status of a patient in the setting of alkalosis is similar to what one uses in all patients; one focuses on baseline and orthostatic blood pressures, changes in body weight, elevation of the jugular venous pulse, edema, and skin turgor. In addition, one can assess the urine electrolytes. The normal response to sensed volume depletion is activation of the renin–angiotensin–aldosterone system, which is usually detected clinically by a low urine sodium level. In most patients, urine sodium less than 10 meq/L suggests volume depletion with consequent activation of the RAA system. In alkalotic patients, however, the urine sodium may not be a good marker of volume status or of the RAA system activity.

In patients with volume depletion and alkalemia, despite the overall tubular bicarbonate avidity, small amounts of the filtered bicarbonate may make it through the tubule and into the urine. Such a small amount is insufficient to correct the overall alkalemia of the individual, but is enough to increase the pH of the urine. As this negatively charged anion flows down the tubule, it will pull with it a positively charged particle, most frequently sodium. Thus, the bicarbonate acts as a non-reabsorbable anion, artificially increasing urine sodium. Even in those with volume depletion, and consequent activation of the RAA system, the urine sodium concentration may be high.

A better marker of the RAA system in individuals with metabolic alkaloses is urinary chloride. Since chloride has a negative charge, and will not be affected by a bicarbonate anion, chloride functions as a relatively good sense of the perceived volume status of an individual. Thus, a low urine chloride suggests volume depletion in an individual with metabolic alkalosis. A high urine chloride suggests volume expansion, and points to one of the other mechanisms.

Metabolic Alkalosis due to Gastric Acid Loss

As we noted before, avid absorption of filtered bicarbonate by the proximal tubule may prevent an alkalosis from resolving, but it will not initiate the alkalosis. There must be some initiating event that generated the initial alkalotic state.

The great majority of such scenarios occur from gastric fluid loss. Gastric fluid typically contains anywhere between 60 to 140 meq of H^+/L. Frequently, hospitalized patients receive nasogastric tubes that can drain many liters of gastric content, inducing marked alkalemia. Gastric fluid is isotonic, meaning that the osmolality, due primarily to Na and Cl, is the same as what is seen in blood. The loss of this isotonic hydrogen rich fluid leads to two conditions; alkalosis and volume depletion. In contrast, most colonic losses (e.g., diarrhea) are bicarbonate rich, thereby inducing acidosis.

Unless corrected, volume depletion resulting from vomiting will sustain the alkalosis. In these settings, the urine chloride is typically low, as the tubules are salt avid. The urine sodium may or may not be low; the level depends on the degree of bicarbonate tubular avidity as noted above. If the volume depletion is mild, then some bicarbonate may escape tubular reclamation. This small amount will not be enough to correct the alkalemia. However, it will be enough to raise the urine pH and, because of its negative charge, carry with it a positive charged sodium ion. As the volume depletion intensifies, almost no bicarbonate will escape tubular reclamation. At that point, both the urine chloride and the urine sodium will be low.

Use Animated Figure 10-1 (Metabolic Alkalosis from Vomiting) to view the steps that lead to generation and maintenance of a metabolic alkalosis from vomiting.

Metabolic Alkalosis due to Distal Tubule Secretion

Unlike proximal bicarbonate absorption, distal tubular hydrogen secretion can both generate and maintain an alkalosis, and can occur in settings of either volume depletion or volume overload. Since hydrogen secretion can lead to a net loss of hydrogen, it is possible to generate a state of bicarbonate excess. The maintenance of such a generated alkalosis is determined by continued distal hydrogen secretion.

Diuretic use is a relatively frequent cause of alkalemia. Diuretics, particularly those that affect the thick ascending limb or distal convoluted tubule, block sodium reclamation. They have no direct effect on proximal tubule handling of bicarbonate or distal tubule hydrogen secretion. Thus, their administration leads to loss of sodium and chloride, without any direct effect on bicarbonate levels. With chronic use, however, volume depletion can develop, leading to an increase of proximal tubular bicarbonate reclamation. In addition, volume depletion leads to activation of the RAA system, thereby increasing apical H ATPase and basolateral Na/K ATPase expression in the collecting duct. Because the diuretics are blocking sodium absorption in the thick ascending limb or distal convoluted tubule, there is continued delivery of sodium to the collecting duct, despite volume depletion. This combination of increased H ATPase and Na/K ATPase activity, along with increased distal delivery of sodium, enhances the efficiency of hydrogen excretion. This is the mechanism by which diuretics can cause and maintain an alkalemia.

There are several conditions in which aldosterone, rather than being produced normally in response to activation of the renin–angiotensin system, is autonomously produced. These states lead to volume expansion, as the tubules retain sodium independently and cannot be turned off. In a similar manner, there is continued, unregulated secretion of hydrogen ions, which can both generate and maintain an alkalosis. In these cases, patients have volume overload and alkalosis, and frequently have high blood pressure, along with hypokalemia, due to the accompanying potassium loss in the tubule.

? **THOUGHT QUESTION 10-3** Two friends, Harold and Bob, meet for dinner at the nearby pub. Harold has a history of gastric ulcers, and is on a proton pump inhibitor, which prevents gastric cells from secreting hydrogen into the stomach lumen. Bob is totally healthy, and takes no medications.

If you measured their serum and urine pH after their meals, what would you expect them to be at 1 hr and 6 hr post-meal?

PUTTING IT TOGETHER

A young man develops food poisoning after eating at a church BBQ, and has terrible stomach cramps and vomiting. The next day, he goes to visit his primary care physician, but has difficulty staying for the whole visit as he is continuously vomiting. Because he is otherwise healthy, and likely has a viral illness, the physician recommends that he eat salty chicken broth, and return to see him in three days. The virus runs its course, and the vomiting stops after 48 hr, but the patient remains nauseous and cannot keep anything down. He returns for his repeat visit.

The physician collects blood and urine at both visits. The blood pressure and blood chemistries are noted below, along with his urine pH. Can you explain his urine pH at each visit? In addition, what would you predict his urine sodium and chloride to be at each visit? How do you analyze this problem? (Review and complete *Table 10.1*)

This young man develops severe vomiting from a viral illness. The loss of hydrogen ion in this emesis will lead to an excess of serum bicarbonate; as the gastric epithelium secretes a proton into the lumen of the stomach, a bicarbonate ion enters the interstitial fluid and ultimately into the blood. It is not unusual for individuals to make bicarbonate ions due to secretion of hydrogen ions as part of the digestive process. However, most individuals rapidly filter the bicarbonate in the glomerular capillaries and, by limiting tubular reclamation, develop rapid post-prandial bicarbonaturia; consequently, they never develop alkalemia. In this unfortunate patient, however, his vomiting has led to volume depletion, due to the loss of accompanying solute and fluid in the emesis. At first visit, his blood pressure is already low, and he has developed a metabolic alkalosis as evidenced by a pH of 7.44 and elevated serum bicarbonate.

Although his volume depletion is relatively mild at the first visit to the doctor, it is sufficient to stimulate proximal tubular Na^+ and bicarbonate reabsorption. Most of what is filtered is reclaimed, preventing the correction of his alkalemia. As we learned, the kidney will sacrifice acid/base status in an effort to restore the body's overall volume of fluid. In this protective mode, the kidneys retain enough bicarbonate to maintain the alkalemia. However, because the volume depletion is still relatively mild, some filtered bicarbonate escapes proximal reclamation, and makes it into the urine, as evidenced by a high urine pH. Since the negatively charged bicarbonate will necessitate a positively charged sodium to follow, the urine sodium may be elevated to a level one would not expect in a volume depleted state and, therefore, is not a good marker of the RAA system activity at this time. The negatively charged urine chloride, since it is unaffected by the bicarbonate anion, is a better marker of

TABLE 10-1 PHYSIOLOGICAL CONSEQUENCES OF PROLONGED VOMITING		
	VISIT 1 (24 HOURS)	VISIT 2 (72 HOURS)
Blood pressure	108/60	94/60
Serum pH	7.44	7.5
Serum HCO_3	29	31
Urine pH	8	5
Urine chloride	?	?
Urine sodium	?	?

overall volume status. At first visit, the patient's urine chloride was found to be 10 meq/L, confirming activation of the RAA system due to volume depletion. His urine sodium was 30 meq/L.

Over the next two days, the patient's vomiting gradually ceases, yet he is unable to take enough chicken broth to correct his volume depletion. Thus, proximal bicarbonate reclamation remains fully activated. The patient's volume depletion has become so profound, as evidenced by a notably low blood pressure, that almost all sodium and bicarbonate are being reclaimed in an attempt to restore body volume. Consequently, his urine pH has returned to a lower range. This "paradoxical aciduria" occurs for two reasons. First, almost all filtered bicarbonate is reclaimed. Second, since hypokalemia is a frequent complication of vomiting, distal tubule hydrogen secretion increases. Hypokalemia stimulates the expression of the apical HK exchanger. At this stage, because of complete proximal tubule bicarbonate reclamation, there is no bicarbonaturia to induce a negative charge in the tubule that would pull sodium along with it through the tubule; consequently, both the urine sodium and chloride concentrations will be very low (i.e., <10 meq/L).

Summary Points

- There is a large pool of circulating bicarbonate that protects against acidosis.
- Under normal conditions, the kidney filters excess bicarbonate, preventing an increase of the serum bicarbonate.
- Under certain conditions, the kidneys reclaim bicarbonate despite an increase of serum pH, a condition known as metabolic alkalosis.
- In some situations, such as vomiting, a loss of acid causes a net generation of bicarbonate in the tubule; this "new" bicarbonate enters the serum. In other situations, the kidneys themselves are responsible for a loss of hydrogen, leading to increasing serum bicarbonate levels. In both scenarios, however, the kidneys are responsible for maintaining this alkalosis by overly active bicarbonate reclamation or bicarbonate generation.
- The RAA system plays an important role in stimulating renal bicarbonate reclamation. Because RAA system activation is a normal response to volume depletion, states of volume depletion are a frequent reason why metabolic alkaloses are maintained.
- Autonomous production of aldosterone can lead to volume expansion and alkalosis.
- Because the transporters in the distal tubule handle hydrogen and potassium ions simultaneously, abnormalities of potassium often accompany metabolic alkalosis.

Answers TO THOUGHT QUESTIONS

10-1. This patient is eating many meq of bicarbonate per day. Since he is on dialysis, he likely has no kidney function and his GFR is near zero. Thus, he cannot filter any bicarbonate, and whatever he eats remains in his body.

The second question is a bit more difficult. Remember, the kidneys are also responsible for excreting hydrogen ions in times of acidosis. Thus, depending on how much protein the patient eats, which determines how much potential acid he is eating, he might still be in positive acid balance. For instance, if he eats a high protein diet, protein metabolism might generate 100 meq of acid, leaving a net positive acid gain. In this setting, his serum bicarbonate would fall slowly each day as it is consumed by buffering the acid. If he eats a low protein diet, however, generating only 35 meq of acid per day, then he would be in net positive alkali balance, and his serum bicarbonate would increase slowly each day.

10-2. Because of the patient's congestive heart failure, his body is likely sensing volume depletion (despite being volume overloaded). This sensed volume depletion could stimulate activity of the H/K ATPases in the collecting duct and the NH exchangers in the proximal tubule, leading to hydrogen loss (thus generating the alkalosis) and avid proximal tubule bicarbonate reclamation (leading to maintenance of the alkalosis), respectively. In addition, because the loop diuretic can lead to potassium loss and hypokalemia, additional hydrogen may be lost from the collecting duct.

10-3. Bob's stomach functions normally. Thus, as part of digestion, his gastric cells secrete hydrogen into the lumen and, at the same time, bicarbonate is added to the serum. This may transiently increase the serum bicarbonate level minimally, and respiratory compensation will protect the pH and keep it near normal. Thus, very little change in serum pH is expected. Furthermore, since Bob's kidney function is normal, the transient increase of bicarbonate will soon be addressed by filtration by the kidney and excretion in the urine, elevating the urine pH to the alkali range (typically 6.5 to 7) for 3 to 4 hr after a meal.

EDITOR'S INTEGRATION

As food moves from the stomach to the small intestine, the process of digestion requires activity of a range of enzymes that do not function in an acid environment. To neutralize the acidic material coming from the stomach, the pancreas secretes bicarbonate, which travels down the pancreatic ducts and enters the lumen of the small bowel. This is another source of bicarbonate loss from the body.

Harold's stomach does not make hydrochloric acid, and thus little bicarbonate is secreted into the serum. Consequently, the serum pH remains normal, and the urine pH will be unaffected, and will remain acidic.

At 6 hr after the meal, both Harold and Bob will have a normal serum pH, and an acidic urine pH. Remember that most American diets provide a source of acid. This may initially seem confusing. The alkaline tide emanating from the stomach represents a transient production of alkali associated with gastric secretion; the kidneys rapidly filter bicarbonate leaving no net change in acid–base status. However, since the ingested protein will soon be metabolized resulting in the production of non-carbonic acid, including sulfuric and phosphoric acids, the net effect of eating is an acid load. The kidney is responsible for responding to this constant acid onslaught, and does so by secreting hydrogen ions into the urine in the distal tubule, thereby generating new bicarbonate in the serum. Thus, outside of the few hours after meals, the typical urine pH for most individuals is acidic.

Review Questions

DIRECTIONS: *Each of the numbered items or incomplete statements in this section is followed by answers or by completions of the statement. Select the ONE lettered answer or completion that is BEST in each case.*

1. A 60-year-old man presents to his primary care physician for evaluation of new onset hypertension. He reports a 5 lb weight gain over the past two months. His blood pressure is high at 180/90 mm Hg, and he is noted to have edema in the lower extremities. His labs are notable for a bicarbonate level of 40 meq/L and serum potassium of 2 meq/L. His serum pH is 7.49. What do you think is the reason for his high bicarbonate level?

    A. He is eating too much baking soda.
    B. His kidneys are unable to secrete bicarbonate ion because of sensed volume depletion.
    C. He has an aldosterone producing tumor.

2. A young man develops profuse vomiting over the course of 2 days after eating sushi that he had left unrefrigerated. He presents to his local emergency room, where he is found to be hypotensive, with a blood pressure of 94/62. His serum bicarbonate is 37 meq/L and his blood pH is 7.50. What is the best treatment to correct his blood pH?

    A. Administration of acid
    B. Administration of intravenous fluid
    C. Administration of a diuretic that blocks proximal tubule bicarbonate reclamation

3. An elderly woman develops congestive heart failure after suffering a heart attack. She gains 20 lbs of fluid due to sodium retention, and becomes quite short of breath. Her doctor prescribes a strong diuretic called furosemide, which leads to naturesis and a loss of 5 lbs. One week after starting the diuretic, her labs show that her bicarbonate level has increased from 25 meq/L to 29 meq/L, with a serum pH of 7.47, and normal serum potassium. Why has she become alkalemic?

    A. She is eating too much baking soda.
    B. Her kidneys are unable to secrete bicarbonate ion because of sensed volume depletion.
    C. She has an aldosterone producing tumor.

4. How would you treat the elderly patient in Question 3?

    A. Administration of acid
    B. Administration of intravenous fluid
    C. Administration of a diuretic that blocks proximal tubule bicarbonate reclamation

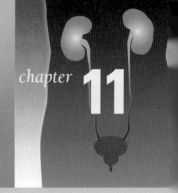

chapter 11

Integration Chapter
The Case of the Marathon Runner

What goes wrong, how does he compensate, and how do we help him recover?

CHAPTER OUTLINE

INTRODUCTION
THE CASE OF THE MARATHON RUNNER
FINAL THOUGHTS

LEARNING OBJECTIVES

By the end of this chapter, you should be able to:

- **describe how fluids in body compartments respond to abrupt changes in intake and loss of fluid.**
- **delineate how the body makes use of multiple physiologic processes to protect circulating volume.**
- **describe how glomerular filtration is regulated in response to abrupt changes in volume status.**
- **detail how tubular transport is regulated in response to abrupt changes in volume status.**
- **explain how the regulation of serum osmolality is maintained during large changes in water intake and excretion.**

Introduction

You have learned how the kidney performs a range of functions from clearing the blood of potentially toxic products of metabolism, to excreting or conserving vital electrolytes, depending on the needs of the body, to playing a role in the preservation of blood pressure, to allowing us to live in a water constrained world. A general theme of physiological processes is to restore the body to near optimal homeostatic conditions when the environment or disease disrupts our equilibrium.

In this chapter, we will use the example of a marathon runner to integrate many of the concepts you have learned throughout this book. Running a 26-mile race, particularly under hot and humid conditions, poses a number of physiological challenges to the body. After providing a short case summary, we will pose a sequence of thought questions for you to ponder. Please give them serious consideration before proceeding to the discussion of the answers. If necessary, go back to previous chapters to refresh your memory of key principles. In this way you will consolidate your knowledge and strengthen your ability to apply what you have learned to solve clinical problems.

The Case of the Marathon Runner

A 25-year-old accountant plans to run the Boston Marathon. Anticipating a very hot day, he drinks large quantities of water and sports drinks for the full day before the race, and "carb" loads the night before with a large pasta meal. On race day he forgets his packets of salt and sugar supplements, but remembers to take the non-steroidal anti-inflammatory drug (ibuprofen) to prevent the knee pain he always gets after about 10 miles of running.

During the race, mindful of the heat and his profuse sweating, he drinks one or two cups of water at the water stations at each mile. He runs at a 10 min/mile pace for the first 20 miles. He feels reasonably well until he reaches the top of the major long hill on the course at which point he begins to feel a bit dizzy; he is now at mile 22.

The sun is out on this windless day and temperatures reach 80°F on the course. He notes that, unlike his long-distance training runs, he has not needed to void during nearly 4 hr he has been running. Knowing that he has only 4 miles to go, he pushes hard through the next 3 miles, but collapses 1 mile before the finish line. Paramedics move him to a medical tent. He is unconscious. His pulse is 140 and very weak. Blood pressure is 80 mm Hg systolic; he is panting, with a respiratory rate of 32 breaths/min. His forehead and fingers feel warm and his face is flushed.

The Boston Marathon medical staff is equipped to measure plasma sodium concentration on an emergency basis and a reading comes back at 120 meq/L (hyponatremic). An IV is placed in the unconscious accountant's arm and normal saline is infused at a rapid rate. He is rushed to a nearby emergency room, where blood work reveals: Hematocrit 50 (normal 39 to 44); Sodium, 121 meq/L, Potassium, 3.9 meq/L, Chloride, 85 meq/L, Bicarbonate, 18 meq/L, serum osmolality 238 mOsm/kg. A Foley catheter is placed in his bladder. He has 50 mL of urine, which is dark, and has an osmolality of 980 mOsm/kg, and sodium concentration of 9 meq/L (see *Table 11-1* for normal values of these blood tests).

Before we explain in detail what has happened, try to answer the following **Thought Questions** about the body's response to the stresses of the long-distance run, using what you have learned throughout your study of renal physiology.

TABLE 11-1 NORMAL BLOOD TEST VALUES	
Sodium	136–144 meq/L
Potassium	3.5–5.0 meq/L
Chloride	98–106 meq/L
Bicarbonate	22–28 meq/L
Serum osm	285–295 mOsm/kg

? THOUGHT QUESTIONS

11-1. What has happened to his total body salt and water content?

11-2. What has happened to the volume in his intracellular space, his interstitial space, and his circulatory space?

11-3. How has his body responded physiologically to his condition as he has been running? How is he trying to compensate and restore homeostatic conditions?

11-4. During his run, despite taking in a great deal of water, he has made no urine. Why has this happened? What has happened to his glomerular filtration rate? How have the afferent and efferent arterioles adapted during the run? How have his tubules altered his salt reabsorption in response to his condition as he was running?

11-5. What has happened to his thirst mechanism and his production and release of ADH? How has this affected water handling in his renal tubules? Why has his serum sodium dropped to 120? What are the risks of this drop?

Answers TO THOUGHT QUESTIONS 11-1, 11-2, 11-3, 11-4, 11-5

11-1 and 11-2. Total body salt and water and its distribution in his body compartments. As he started to run in the heat, he experienced rapid loss of water through evaporation of sweat and the increased ventilation required to supply oxygen to his muscles. He has lost salt through his perspiration. While running, he drank only water and took in no supplements, so he lost salt without replenishing it.

Because of the heat, his thermoregulatory reflexes assured that he would remain peripherally vasodilated (blood vessels in the skin dilate to bring blood and heat to the surface of the body, which enhances his loss of fluid and salt through perspiration, the primary means by which the body dissipates heat during exercise). Reduced interstitial hydrostatic pressure favored flux of salt and water out of his intravascular space; since red cells were held in the intravascular space, his hematocrit rose.

The net effect of his exercise and exposure is a loss of significant amounts of salt and water from the interstitial and intravascular compartments, leading to a low blood pressure and elevated heart rate (the dilation of the vasculature, as noted above, also contributes to a decreased blood pressure). Through his copious water intake, he actually replaced this lost fluid (his body weight when initially measured turned out to be the same as his pre-race weight), but did not do so with equal proportions of salt and water. Instead, he drank water alone, so that his total amount of salt is decreased, and the ratio of salt to water has decreased as well (i.e., the concentration of sodium in the body is reduced as evidenced by his hyponatremia).

Use Animated Figure 11-1 (Water Balance) to try out this scenario: First administer 8,500 cc of water (the equivalent of 1 to 2 cups per mile over 25 miles) and observe how the water distributes across body fluid compartments, leading to hyponatremia. Then choose a fluid output of 8,500 cc with a composition of 70 meq/L Na^+ and 12 meq/L K^+ (approximating sweat at a heavy rate of about 2 L/hr) and run the fluid out. You are left with hyponatremia and a depletion of extracellular (intravascular plus interstitial) fluid volume. Enough of this fluid shift (extracellular to intracellular) has come from the intravascular space that it results in the hemodynamic parameters mentioned. We discuss this further in the next thought question.

The cardiovascular and respiratory systems are also "activated" by a series of stimuli to support the body's needs during exercise. The sympathetic nervous system is activated, in part by the anticipation of exercise and competing in the race and in part by the drop in blood pressure that accompanies the dilation of the blood vessels in the active muscle groups. As a result of the release of norepinephrine from neurons and epinephrine from the adrenal gland, the heart rate and cardiac muscle contractility increase and the amount of blood pumped each minute may go up by as much as 500%. The rate and depth of breathing also increase as the respiratory system must adapt to the increasing need for oxygen and the higher production of carbon dioxide as energy is generated from cellular metabolism. See *Respiratory Physiology: A Clinical Approach*, for a full description of how the cardiovascular and respiratory systems integrate to support the body during exercise.

11-3. **Activation of salt-retaining pathways.** Loss of intravascular volume reduced the rate of blood return to the heart (preload), causing a fall in forward cardiac output and a fall in blood pressure in the aortic arch and carotids. Sensing the fall in blood pressure, baroreceptors in these vessels started firing, leading to increased sympathetic nerve activity, and increased circulating catecholamines. Reduced blood pressure, increased sympathetic nerve activity and circulating catecholamines caused constriction of his afferent arterioles, reducing renal perfusion pressure. Initially, simultaneous, vigorous constriction of his efferent arterioles maintains some glomerular filtration. However, as his afferent vasoconstriction intensifies, the hydrostatic pressure in the glomerular capillary bed falls to levels too low to permit adequate filtration. As filtration drops, the resulting fall in tubular fluid flow stimulates the juxtaglomerular apparatus to release renin, which leads to formation of angiotensin II. High levels of catecholamines and angiotensin II stimulate the adrenal cortex to produce aldosterone. These forces culminate in sodium reclamation.

11-4. **Renal response to initial salt-retaining processes.** As noted above, as his renal perfusion pressure is falling, initial efferent vasoconstriction may have preserved glomerular filtration. Since he had taken a non-steroidal anti-inflammatory drug, however, release of vasodilatory prostaglandins in the afferent arteriole may have been blocked. Consequently, he constricted **both** his afferent and efferent arterioles in response to reduced renal perfusion pressure, leading to a fall in GFR. As his GFR is falling, the high levels of catecholamines, sympathetic nerve activity, and angiotensin II stimulate avid salt reabsorption in the proximal tubule. Aldosterone markedly stimulates salt reabsorption in the distal nephron, including his thick ascending limb, distal convoluted tubule, and collecting duct. On this basis, his urine sodium is low. The combined effects of these effects on glomeruli and tubules sharply reduce his urine output.

11-5. **Thirst mechanism and water handling.** Because of a severe decrease in sensed body volume, concentration independent stimulation of thirst and ADH release occurs. This encourages more water intake. In addition, pathways other than sensed body volume may lead to elevated levels of ADH release during exercise despite the dropping serum osmolarity (1), which can contribute to hyponatremia. As aquaporins are inserted into the collecting duct, renal water retention is kept high. Free water retention by the kidneys, as well as his thirst and large free water intake, lead to a rapid decline in his serum osmolality (he is replacing the loss of Na and water with water alone). Because the osmolality of his brain cells is higher than that of plasma, water moves from the extracellular to the intracellular compartment; his brain begins to swell, which leads to altered neurological status and loss of consciousness.

Observe the change in size of the intracellular compartment in Animated Figure 11-1 after you have simulated the water intake and sweat loss; an increase in the intracellular volume is a danger, as mentioned above, given the brain's location in a rigid fixed-volume container, the cranium.

? **THOUGHT QUESTION 11-6** What should we do now to help this patient? What kind of fluid and electrolytes should he receive? Predict the impact your treatment will have on his fluid compartments, his volume regulatory responses, and his glomerular and tubular function.

Answer TO THOUGHT QUESTION 11-6

11-6. Our marathon runner is still unconscious, and the emergency room staff place a second, large bore IV catheter and administer normal saline with 20 meq KCl, initially as two 1-L boluses in an hour, and then as a steady infusion at 500 mL/hr. After 2 hr he begins to make urine and he wakes up. Blood pressure is now 125/80 mm Hg, pulse is 58 beats/min, and respiratory rate is 18 breaths/min. Urine output begins to match IV fluid input and his rate of infusion is tapered. Repeat blood work, taken after some urine output, reveals: a hematocrit of 44, sodium of 134 meq/L, potassium of 4.2 meq/L, chloride of 105 meq/L, bicarbonate of 15 meq/L, serum osmolality of 278 mOsm/kg, urine osmolality of 285 mOsm/kg, and urine sodium of 95 meq/L.

Return to Animated Figure 11-1, starting from the hyponatremic state where we previously left off. Now start administering normal saline with 20 meq KCl and observe the changes in extracellular fluid sodium concentration. Then introduce some urine output (for example, with 30 meq/L Na^+ and 20 meq/L K^+) and see how that affects the extracellular fluid sodium concentration.

As treatment proceeds, you should be asking yourself additional **Thought Questions:**

? **THOUGHT QUESTIONS**

11-7. As we administered volume (i.e., isotonic saline solution), how has it distributed in his body fluid compartments?

11-8. How have his volume regulatory and water regulatory processes responded? What has happened in his glomeruli and tubules?

11-9. Why have his serum chemistries changed?

Answers TO THOUGHT QUESTIONS 11-7, 11-8, 11-9

11-7. Effect of saline on his body fluid compartments. Saline enters his veins, expanding his intravascular space and interstitial space. Since saline is relatively hypertonic to the patient's current osmolality, water will shift out of the brain cells, and the swelling will decrease.

Choose and administer 1,000 cc of normal saline in Animated Figure 11-1 when the tank is in the initial hyponatremic state and notice how much fluid shifts out of the intracellular space. Normal saline is only mildly hypertonic relative to the patient's sodium concentration, and a significant amount of normal saline is needed to effect a decrease in intracellular volume.

11-8. Volume regulatory and renal responses to saline. Increased salt and water entering his vein promptly increases his preload, stretching first his right atrium and then, as his right ventricular output rises in response to increased preload, stretching his left atrium, leading to increased left ventricular preload and increased cardiac output.

EDITOR'S INTEGRATION

Recall from cardiovascular physiology that preload refers to the volume of a contracting muscular chamber (such as the atrium or ventricle). As the volume increases, the length of individual myocytes increases, which may enhance actin–myosin overlap and the force of contraction in keeping with the Frank–Starling principle. See *Cardiovascular Physiology: A Clinical Approach,* for a more complete discussion of this concept.

Right and then left atrial stretch provokes release of atrial natriuretic peptide (ANP). ANP itself shuts off sympathetic nerve output, renin release and aldosterone production. It also augments GFR (by dilating renal afferent arterioles) and blocks tubular reabsorption of sodium in the proximal tubule and collecting duct.

Increased cardiac output raises blood pressure and stretches baroreceptors, which turn off previously activated signals that had been stimulating the hypothalamus; consequently, we now see deactivation of the sympathetic nervous system, and reduced levels of circulating catecholamines. Increased blood pressure and increased renal perfusion augment GFR, leading to increased tubular fluid flow past the juxtaglomerular apparatus. This increased flow shuts off renin release, leading to a rapid fall in angiotensin, thereby halting aldosterone release.

The fall in sympathetic nerve activity, along with reduced circulating levels of catecholamines and angiotensin, and increased ANP, reduces proximal tubule absorption of salt. The fall in aldosterone reduces salt reabsorption in the collecting duct. Increased GFR and reduced tubular salt reabsorption lead to increased urine volumes. In addition, as body volume is replaced, stimuli for ADH release are removed, as discussed below, leading to dilute urine.

11-9. **Effect of saline on serum chemistries.** Restoration of sensed body volume removes the volume mediated stimuli for ADH and thirst, thereby reducing water reabsorption and ingestion and allowing the kidneys to excrete water (i.e., make dilute urine). In the absence of ADH, collecting duct cells remove aquaporins from their apical membranes, rendering this portion of the tubule relatively water impermeable again. On this basis, urine osmolality falls to 50 to 100 mOsm/kg, allowing rapid excretion of water and normalization of his serum sodium and osmolality.

> **?**   THOUGHT QUESTION 11-10   **How do we decide how much saline to administer to the runner?**

Answer TO THOUGHT QUESTION 11-10

11-10. Because the kidney is exquisitely sensitive to volume status and the balance of salt-retentive and salt-wasting hormones, monitoring urine output will tell us promptly when he has received adequate fluid resuscitation sufficient to normalize preload and cardiac output. We can also measure urine sodium, and watch it rise from a level below 10 to values above 50.

Final Thoughts

You are now armed with the knowledge and reasoning abilities to attack some of the most challenging issues in clinical medicine. As you move forward in your training, there will be a temptation to jump to an answer based on recognizing a few pieces of a case puzzle; we urge you to resist this temptation. Rather, reason through the case history and physical exam findings, analyze the data utilizing the physiological mechanisms you have learned, and create a scientific story that explains the patient's picture. With this approach, you are on your way to becoming a great doctor.

REFERENCE

1. Rosner MH, Kirven J. Exercise—associated hyponatremia. *Clin J Am Soc Nephrol.* 2007;2:151–161.

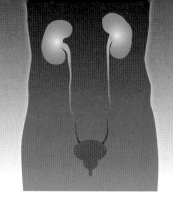

Answers to Review Questions

CHAPTER 1

1-1. **The correct answer is A.** As the amount of urea in the blood increases from metabolism of protein, more urea is filtered through the glomerular capillary because the concentration gradient between the blood and the renal tubular space has increased; urea is a small molecule that easily passes through the endothelial lining. The amount of urea in the urine will also increase. Filtration of urea would only decrease if blood flow through or the pressure within the glomerular capillary has decreased. Absorption of urea from the tubule is increased only in conditions in which total body water is diminished.

1-2. **The correct answer is B.** Since Bob has ingested salt tablets prior to the run, he begins with a greater amount of Na in his system than does John. Thus, he will filter more Na throughout the run. Both runners will be trying to accommodate for the Na losses in the sweat by absorbing as much Na as possible from the renal tubule.

CHAPTER 2

2-1. **The correct answer is B.** The size of the cells is determined by osmotic forces. The NaK ATPases provide a net outward osmotic force across the cell membrane with respect to the major ions in the intracellular and the extracellular fluid since 3 Na ions move into the fluid surrounding the cell in exchange for 2 K ions; this outward force is balanced by the net inward force provided by intracellular proteins (this is the oncotic force, which is the term used for the osmotic force created by proteins). If the NaK ATPases are poisoned, the inward oncotic force is unbalanced, leading to cell swelling and death.

2-2. **The correct answer is E.** Diarrhea is usually isotonic, meaning that both Na and water are lost in similar concentrations to that of the body; consequently, there is no change in the osmolarity of the extracellular fluid and, thus, no movement of water into or out of cells (remember, movement of water into and out of the cells is dependent on osmotic forces). This Na and water loss will be reflected by a decrease in the sizes of the intravascular and the interstitial space, which are in equilibrium with each other. As salt and water leave the interstitial space into the intestinal lumen, hydrostatic pressure in the interstitial space decreases. The result is movement of salt and water from the vascular space into the interstitial space.

2-3. **The correct answer is B.** The blood pressure is determined, in part, by the volume of fluid within the vasculature. The vascular space is in equilibrium with the interstitial space; the volume of the two spaces is the consequence of the balance between the hydrostatic and oncotic forces in each space. Because of the loss of intravascular protein, the inward oncotic force in the blood vessel decreases, leading to a shift of fluid out of the vessel into the interstitium. Consequently, the young woman's blood pressure should be lower than her normal level.

2-4.   **The correct answer is E.** As discussed in the chapter, the pulmonary vasculature is different from the capillaries in the rest of the body, in that it is relatively leaky to albumin. Thus, it does not rely on an inward oncotic force to maintain equilibrium with the interstitial space; rather, the pulmonary capillaries have a very low hydrostatic pressure, which prevents much loss of fluid to the interstitium. The loss of serum albumin will, therefore, not cause pulmonary edema. Pleural effusions, however, occur due to the extravasation of fluid out of thoracic blood vessels that perfuse the pleural tissue. These vessels are similar to systemic blood vessels, and rely on inward oncotic pressure to balance the hydrostatic pressure of the vessel and prevent excessive loss of fluid to the interstitium. This patient is likely to develop edema (swelling) in her soft tissues, and she is likely to have pleural effusions, but not pulmonary edema.

CHAPTER 3

3-1.   **The correct answer is D.** There are several factors that make the tubule susceptible to injury due to lack of oxygen (and, hence, a low blood pressure, which correlates with oxygen delivery to the tissue). First, the unique structure of the kidney's vascular supply, which includes a glomerular capillary followed "in series" by the tubular capillary, means that much of the vascular volume is lost via filtration in the glomerulus before it reaches the tubule. Second, because the efferent arteriole constricts to maintain glomerular pressure and filtration, the flow of blood leaving the glomerulus to the tubular arteriole and capillary is further reduced. Finally, since the tubule is responsible for reabsorbing so many liters of filtrate, it has a high demand for oxygen, further potentiating its risk of ischemia, i.e., with a high demand for oxygen, it is poorly tolerant of conditions that limit supply. The endothelial cells that line the vessels always are awash in oxygen and rarely are damaged due to low blood pressure. Similarly, the podocyte and the basement membrane of the glomerulus are sustained by the maintenance of blood flow to the glomerulus by constriction of the efferent arteriole.

3-2.   **The correct answer is B.** This woman has developed a "nephritis," defined from a histopathological perspective as inflammation in the kidney. In her situation, the antigen–antibody complexes settle on the "inside" of the body, not passing across the basement membrane and epithelial cell/podocyte into the urinary space. Since they are "inside", these complexes are seen by circulating macrophages, lymphocytes, and other scavenger inflammatory cells, which respond by stimulating local inflammation (thus, there are inflammatory cells in the urine). As more and more inflammatory cells respond, the capillary loops become clogged with cells and debris, and lose their ability to filter. Hence, renal failure (inability to filter) and hypertension (due to volume overload since the kidney cannot excrete excess salt and water) ensue. Although such patients may have small amounts of protein in the urine, they are usually not sufficient enough to cause a decrease in the serum albumin.

3-3.   **The correct answer is B.** Unlike the patient in question 2, in whom inflammation involved the mesangium and capillary loops (on the inside of the basement membrane), this patient has developed a specific insult to the podocyte. Because the podocyte is responsible for structural support of the glomerular tuft, its damage disrupts the unique relationship between the filtration slits and the basement membrane, and allows the loss of large amounts of protein from the filtering blood into the urine. Because the podocyte is on the "outside" of the body, separated from the capillary by the basement membrane, damage to the podocyte is not seen by the same marauding inflammatory cells as in question 2. Thus, inflammation does not develop, and usually, the capillary loops remain open, and filtration occurs normally (hence, no evidence of renal failure and normal excretion of salt and water, which prevents the development of hypertension).

3-4. **The correct answer is C.** Since this medication damages the tubule, and not the glomerulus (specifically the podocyte), proteinuria is not likely to occur. Because the tubule is responsible for reclaiming filtered particle and water, tubular damage can lead to their loss, resulting in low serum phosphorus and high serum sodium. If the tubular damage is severe enough, leading to sloughing off of the tubular epithelial cells and consequent tubular blockage, then filtration to that tubule will cease, and renal failure will ensue.

CHAPTER 4

4-1. **The correct answer is A.** Because the NSAIDS will preferentially lead to constriction of the afferent arteriole, renal plasma flow decreases, leading to decreased pressure within the glomerulus. This, in turn, will cause a decrease in the GFR. Since less creatinine-filled fluid is filtered, and the total amount of creatinine produced by muscle is unchanged, the patient's serum concentration of creatinine will increase. The creatinine will rise until the patient's system achieves a new steady state at which time the amount filtered and excreted once again equals the amount produced each day (recall that as the serum concentration of creatinine increases, the diffusion gradient across the glomerular capillary increases and more creatinine can be eliminated per milliliter of blood that is filtered).

4-2. **The correct answer is A.** Because these medicines lead to a dilation of the efferent arteriole, the pressure within the glomerulus decreases. Since the GFR is dependent on the hydrostatic pressure in the glomerular capillary, the GFR will decrease as well. Consequently, less creatinine is filtered, and the serum concentration will rise. In conditions of low blood pressure, e.g., an acute bleeding episode, this effect on the efferent arteriole becomes even more problematic. For patients with sustained hypertension, however, this decrease in glomerular pressure is therapeutic, as it can protect the kidney from renal damage that occurs from prolonged elevated pressures.

4-3. **The correct answer is A.** Both these medicines will reduce intraglomerular pressure, leading to a decrease in the GFR. However, in addition, these medications in combination can cause marked hypoperfusion to the renal tubules, leading to cell ischemia and prolonged renal failure. ACE inhibitors, in addition to their effect on the renal vasculature, also cause dilation of the systemic arterioles. Thus, the ability of the body to compensate (i.e., try to maintain a normal blood pressure) for the loss of body volume by constricting systemic arterioles is compromised (recall that angiotensin II is a potent vasoconstrictor and the ACE inhibitor prevents the formation of angiotensin II).

4-4. **The correct answer is C.** Tubular secretion will increase the amount of creatinine that is excreted in the urine, independently of how much is filtered across the glomerulus. Thus, in the setting of taking such medications, the amount of creatinine in the urine will reflect how much is filtered as well as how much is secreted across the tubule, and will be an overestimation of the true GFR (review the equation we use for measuring GFR if you are still confused about this question).

CHAPTER 5

5-1. **The correct answer is C.** In the proximal tubule, there is dramatic reclamation of sodium, primarily through the NH exchangers. However, there are also many aquaporin channels, so that water reclamation accompanies the sodium reclamation. Thus, although the total amount of sodium decreases along the length of the tubule, the concentration stays the same.

5-2. **The correct answer is A.** In the beginning sections of the proximal tubule, NH exchangers direct the reclamation of sodium ions along with bicarbonate ions. Aquaporins allow water to flow. Chloride ions initially remain within the lumen, and thus, their concentration increases. Toward the later parts of the proximal tubule, where paracellular chloride movement can occur, this relatively high chloride concentration facilitates chloride reclamation down its concentration gradient.

5-3. **The correct answer is C.** Magnesium. The K channels on the apical membrane of the thick ascending limb allow potassium recycling across the apical membrane, as sodium is reclaimed from the lumen, into the cell, and then over the basolateral membrane via the Na/K Atpase. Because so many more sodium ions are reclaimed daily than potassium ions, potassium recycling must occur in order to keep the NK2Cl channel working. Because of this potassium recycling, a positive charge develops within the tubule lumen, which drives movement of other positively charged ions, such as magnesium and calcium, out of the lumen into the cell. If the potassium is not recycled into the lumen of the tubule, the charge in the tubule will be less positive, and the driving force to reabsorb other cations will diminish. All of the other choices for answers are anions, and their absorption is not related to this mechanism.

5-4. **The correct answer is D.** The ENaC is an ion channel that only allows the movement of sodium. Sodium moves alone from the lumen into the intercalated cell of the collecting duct. The movement of a single positive ion generates a negative charge within the lumen. This lumen negativity facilitates potassium secretion. In all other sections of the tubule, sodium is moved in co-transport with an anion, bicarbonate in the proximal tubule or chloride in the thick ascending limb and distal convoluted tubule, so that lumen negativity does not develop. This makes sense, since the earlier sections of the tubule are charged with reclamation of such large amounts of filtrate (and hence sodium ions), and any lumen negativity would hinder further sodium reclamation. However, in the collecting duct, relatively few sodium ions remain to be reclaimed (60% reabsorbed in the proximal tubule and more in the thick ascending limb of the Loop of Henle), and only fine-tuning of sodium balance is occurring. The collecting duct plays an important role in potassium secretion; thus, having a positive lumen charge is necessary.

5-5. **The correct answer is B.** Aldosterone stimulates the Na/K ATPases on the basolateral membrane of principal cells in the collecting duct, thereby facilitating the net movement of sodium from the tubule lumen. The consequent lumen negativity facilitates potassium secretion. In the setting of a medication that blocks aldosterone, potassium secretion will be impaired, and serum levels will increase.

CHAPTER 6

6-1. **The correct answer is B.** This patient's primary problem is damage to the heart muscle and impaired contraction of the ventricle, which lead to reduced blood flow to vital organs. His baroreceptors detect low blood pressure and the volume sensors detect low volume, both of which lead to sodium retention and total body volume expansion. Sometimes, this compensatory fluid retention can improve heart function. However, in this case, the fluid retention is making the patient short of breath due to pulmonary edema (leakage of fluid from pulmonary capillaries into the interstitium of the lung due to increased hydrostatic pressures in the pulmonary circulation), and is clearly pathologic. The goal of treatment is to restore a more normal volume status by administering diuretics. As a better volume status is achieved, the patient's lungs will clear of fluid, and his overall hemodynamics will improve (better oxygenation with less liquid in the lung will enhance cardiac function and less filling of the ventricle may also improve the contractile function of the heart), leading to improvement of his renal function as well. If we were to administer normal saline, we would further expand the extracellular fluid compartment leading to worse edema.

6-2. **The correct answer is B.** This is somewhat of a tricky question. The natriuretic peptides facilitate natriuresis, or loss of sodium. So, if they functioned in isolation, indeed this woman would lose sodium (and experience a decrease in body volume). However, the natriuretic peptides are just one of the several response mechanisms used by the body to adjust body fluid volume. The sympathetic nervous system and the RAA system are more powerful than the natriuretic peptides, and are stimulated by the reduced sensed volume due to the low output from the heart. In this woman with congestive heart failure, the net effect would be sodium retention, leading continued to volume gain.

6-3. **The correct answer is D.** The two keys to this question are that (1) this is a healthy college student and (2) it asks about *permanent* changes. After eating sodium, the student's sodium concentration will increase imperceptibly. This will immediately initiate thirst, so that the student will drink enough fluid to return his body's fluid concentration to normal. Since the thirst mechanism is triggered by the osmoreceptors, water ingestion will be matched to keep the serum Na normal, i.e., the body volume will increase in an isotonic manner. This increased extracellular (and, hence intravascular) fluid will then stimulate his volume sensors to excrete sodium. His osmoreceptors will excrete just enough water to match sodium loss with water loss (again with no change in concentration). The net effect is that the student excretes exactly what he eats, so that neither the body volume of fluid nor concentration of Na will change.

6-4. **The correct answer is B.** Unlike the healthy college student above, this man has a history of high blood pressure. In individuals with high blood pressure, the body handling of sodium is abnormal. Often, such individuals have a slight, but clinically important, disposition to retain sodium, leading to volume expansion, and high blood pressure. Thus, when the man eats a diet high in sodium, his body does not excrete all the sodium, but retains a small portion. The body's regulation of concentration is normal, so that he will retain just enough ingested water to maintain a normal fluid concentration. The net effect is that his body volume will increase, but the concentration will not change.

CHAPTER 7

7-1. **The correct answer is C.** Urea recycling plays an important role in the generation of the interstitial gradient, and thus, the eventual concentration of the urine. Urea is a soluble nitrogenous breakdown product of proteins. Thus, individuals on very low protein diet, such as Mike, will have a paucity of filtered urea, and will not be able to generate a urea concentration gradient. Early experiments suggest that very low protein diets reduce the concentrating capacity of urine by about one-third. Individuals on low protein diets usually can concentrate only to 700 to 800 mOsm/kg, whereas those on normal or high protein diets can concentrate up to 1,200 mOsm/kg. This illustrates the clinical importance of urea in the concentration mechanism.

7-2. **The correct answer is B.** The generation of an interstitial gradient plays a critical role in the ability to make concentrated urine, and thus conserve water (the term dehydration in medicine refers to water loss rather than sodium loss, which is termed "volume depletion"). The initiating step in this process occurs in the thick ascending limb. The extrusion of sodium from the basolateral aspect of the cell membrane creates an electrochemical gradient favoring sodium movement out of the tubule lumen into the cell. This occurs through the NK2Cl channel, which is blocked by furosemide. Thus, the woman on furosemide will have difficulty concentrating her urine, and will be at risk for dehydration. Conversely, since hydrochlorothiazide works at the distal convoluted tubule, its use will not interrupt the interstitial gradient, and the women taking it will have no problem concentrating her urine.

7-3. **The correct answer is A.** Because this man drinks so much water, his kidneys appropriately excrete many liters of very dilute urine. Passing large quantities of very dilute urine through the kidney interferes with the establishment of the medullary gradient necessary for creating concentrated urine. This effect is called "medullary washout"; consequently, in the immediate period after stopping water intake, his maximal urinary concentration will be less than normal.

CHAPTER 8

8-1. **The correct answer is B.** Between each session, the dialysis patient continues to eat and drink. Most often, her water intake far exceeds than which is lost due to insensible losses (evaporation from the lungs and sweat from the skin is approximately 600 cc/day), and thus her serum sodium will decrease since we usually ingest more water proportionate to sodium intake. At each dialysis session, that excess water is removed, restoring the serum sodium concentration to the normal range.

8-2. **The correct answer is D.** Each of the above diagnoses is plausible. If the patient has diabetes mellitus, his high sugars induce a hyperosmolar state (with a normal serum sodium), and a glucose-driven or osmotic diuresis (accounting for the polyuria). If the patient has an inability to concentrate his urine (as can be seen with diabetes insipidus), his urine output will be large and dilute, and if the patient is drinking a lot due to psychogenic polydipsia, his urine output will be large too. Classically, patients with diabetes insipidus have high serum concentrations (i.e., hypernatremia) due to excessive water loss. However, since they rely on their thirst mechanism to protect their body concentration, such patients may develop conditional water drinking (i.e., they become "conditioned" to drink a large volume of liquid), and can actually present with normal, or even low serum sodium.

8-3. **The correct answer is C.** The patient is seizing because his brain cells are swelling with water. It is an emergency to limit this swelling. Although limiting his access to water would gradually correct his serum sodium (and brain swelling), irreversible damage could occur before this process is complete. Giving a diuretic would remove sodium and water in roughly equal proportions (i.e., isotonic), so that his body concentration likely would not change much. Instead, by giving a hypertonic fluid, his serum concentration will rise, pulling fluid out of the brain cells, and preventing further neurologic damage.

8-4. **The correct answer is A.** Because the patient has SIADH, his urine concentration is fixed due to the constant release of ADH. The amount of urine that he makes, and thus, the amount of water he excretes each day (which also determines how much he can drink per day) is determined by how much solute he excretes. Now that he is not eating, his solute excretion will fall, and he will, therefore, make less urine (albeit at the same concentration). Consequently, if he drinks the same amount of water as he did before his stomach problem, he will become progressively hyponatremic.

CHAPTER 9

9-1. **The correct answer is C.** Because his kidneys are failing, they cannot excrete enough acid to balance out his daily acid intake, leading to acid retention. The large bicarbonate pool of the skeleton is utilized to buffer this acid load, so that the serum bicarbonate level will not initially change. This leads to bone demineralization, however. With time, the bone will not be able to keep up with continuous acid load, and the patient's bicarbonate will eventually begin to decrease.

9-2. **The correct answer is C.** Urine pH simply refers to the amount of free hydrogen ions in the urine. Free hydrogen ion concentration is always extremely low; otherwise, degradation of the renal tubular epithelium would occur. In order to excrete a significant amount of acid, important buffers (e.g., ammonia, phosphate, sulfate) must be in the urine. They allow acid excretion without changes in pH. It should be noted, however, that for the predominant urinary buffers to work efficiently, the urinary pH should be less than or equal to 5.

9-3. **The correct answer is B.** The patient's serum bicarbonate has fallen precipitously from 24 to 14 meq/L in 24 hr. This is due to the production of a large amount of new acid, presumably from lactic acidosis due to bowel tissue than its not getting sufficient oxygen. Although it is true that dialysis patients cannot excrete their normal dietary acid loads, this is usually only in the 70 meq/day range, leading to a decrease of 1 to 2 meq/L of serum bicarbonate per day. Patients with respiratory acidosis (low ventilation levels leading to accumulation of carbonic acid) have elevated levels of bicarbonate as the carbonic acid dissociates into bicarbonate and a proton. Remember, bicarbonate does not serve as an effective buffer for H^+ in respiratory acidosis.

CHAPTER 10

10-1. **The correct answer is C.** This patient has new onset of hypertension due to his volume overload, a consequence of sodium retention in the setting of an aldosterone producing tumor. The aldosterone also stimulates intercalated cell secretion of H^+, leading to bicarbonate generation and reclamation. This is the cause of his alkalemia. There is no indication of sensed volume depletion. High blood pressure, weight gain, and edema all suggest volume overload. As you may recall from our discussion in Chapter 10, one would have to consume very large quantities of baking soda to cause a metabolic alkalosis, and ingestion of baking soda would not cause this degree of hypokalemia (as the blood pH rises, there will be some shift of H^+ ions out of cells in exchange for K^+ moving into cells).

10-2. **The correct answer is B.** By vomiting up acid, the man has developed a profound alkalemia. His kidneys are not excreting the excess bicarbonate because of volume depletion. The appropriate activation of the renin–angiotensin–aldosterone system in the setting of volume depletion causes pH independent avid tubular bicarbonate reclamation (recall effects of RAA system on sodium reclamation and the effects on hydrogen ion excretion and bicarbonate production). By administering saline, and restoring the patient's volume, the renin–angiotensin–aldosterone system will be turned off, and the tubules will be allowed to efficiently filter bicarbonate, restoring the blood pH to normal. Administration of acid (usually HCl) to correct a metabolic acidemia is rarely done in extreme cases. Acetazolamide is a diuretic that will diminish alkalosis, but the primary problem here is volume depletion, which would be exacerbated by use of a diuretic.

10-3. **The correct answer is B.** Because of her congestive heart failure, her pressure and flow receptors sense decreased body volume. Of course, this is not accurate; as she is volume overloaded (still weighing 15 lbs more than previously). However, the sensed volume depletion stimulates distal hydrogen secretion and proximal bicarbonate reclamation, which can generate and maintain an alkalosis, respectively. An aldosterone producing tumor would likely be associated with an abnormally low serum potassium.

10-4. **The correct answer is C.** This patient's primary problem is that her volume sensors are detecting volume depletion, stimulating bicarbonate generation and reclamation; yet she is clearly volume overloaded. Ideally the treatment of choice would be to fix her heart failure, although this is not easily achieved. Instead, a diuretic that blocked tubular reclamation of bicarbonate would be useful. On the one hand, it would reduce her serum bicarbonate concentration, resolving her alkalemia. In addition to blocking bicarbonate reclamation, it also would block sodium reclamation, leading to improvement in the excess total body fluid volume. Administering fluid would only make matters worse, as the problem is with her sensors of volume (i.e., she is already fluid overloaded), and the infusion of acid would not address the underlying problem.

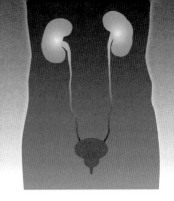

Glossary of Terms

Acidemia: The presence of an acid serum pH compared to normal; usually defined as pH less than 7.35.

Active transport: Process of moving molecules against their electrochemical gradient, directly utilizing the energy provided by NaK ATPases.

Adequacy of clearance: A conceptual term used to describe the amount of fluid cleared through a filtering system, relative to the starting amount of fluid available to be cleared. In terms of normal physiology, it is defined as the amount of fluid cleared completely of urea by the kidneys, divided by the volume of fluid in which urea dissolves (which is equal to total body fluid).

Afferent arteriole: Muscular arteriole that supplies blood to the glomerular capillary; it has the ability to dilate or constrict in response to changes in blood pressure, thereby regulating perfusion (and thus hydrostatic pressure) and filtration across the glomerular capillary as well as blood flow to the medulla of the kidney.

Aldosterone: Steroid hormone produced by the adrenal cortex. Its major effect is to stimulate sodium reclamation by the tubules.

Alkalemia: The presence of an alkaline serum pH compared to normal; usually defined as pH greater than 7.45.

Alkalosis: Refers to a process that decreases the overall hydrogen concentration of the blood (alkalemia); this can occur because of too much bicarbonate in the serum (metabolic alkalosis) or too little carbonic acid (which is derived from carbon dioxide—respiratory alkalosis).

Ammoniagenesis: An important process whereby the proximal tubule cells can utilize an amino acid to generate new bicarbonate ions.

Angiotensin: An important peptide that is produced in an inactive form (angiotensinogen) and, under the influence of renin, is subsequently converted into angiotensin (initially angiotensin I which then is converted into angiotensin II). Angiotensin II has myriad effects, including stimulation of aldosterone release from the adrenal cortex as well as tubular sodium reclamation and arterial vasoconstriction.

Anion gap: Refers to the presence of anions that are not measured by routine chemistry assays of serum electrolytes. The normal anion gap is approximately 12 meq/L, but can increase when the GFR is severely impaired or there is a marked increase of anion production.

Antidiuretic hormone (ADH): A peptide, produced in the hypothalamus and stored in the posterior pituitary, whose release is primarily controlled by the osmoreceptor. It has important effects on the collecting duct, including stimulation of the insertion of water channels into the apical membrane, which is critical for water reclamation; also known as vasopressin.

Apical membrane: Membrane or side of the tubular epithelial cells that abuts the tubule lumen.

Aquaporins: Proteins which are present in a cell membrane and permit the movement of water molecules (but not particles) to pass through the cell membrane.

Atrial natriuretic peptide (ANP): A protein, released from the atria of the heart in response to stretch, which has important natriuretic effects.

Autoregulation: The ability of a blood vessel to regulate its own resistance, usually by an increase of vessel tone, in response to changes of perfusion pressure.

Baroreceptors: Receptors that sense changes in pressure.

Basolateral membrane: Membrane or side of the epithelial cells lining the tubule that abuts the renal interstitium.

Brain natriuretic peptide (BNP): Similar to atrial natriuretic peptides in function, but primarily found in and released from the ventricles (in response to stretch) rather than atria.

Buffer: Weak acid or base that acts to mitigate changes in the pH of a solution.

Calculated osmolality: Determination of the concentration of particles in the blood derived from the sodium, glucose, and urea concentration detected on a routine chemistry assay.

Carbonic acid: Volatile acid derived from the metabolism of carbon dioxide and excreted by the lungs.

Carbonic anhydrase: An enzyme that catalyzes the reaction of carbon dioxide and water to bicarbonate, and a hydrogen ion.

Channel: Membrane proteins that allow a molecule to move down its electrochemical gradient without depending on energy provided by the NaK ATPases (passive transport).

Clearance: The amount of fluid (in liters) that is completely cleared of a particular substance.

Collecting duct: The final section of the renal tubule before it enters into the renal pelvis; impermeable to particles and water in its baseline state. The presence or absence of unique, highly selective, proteins (aquaporins) in the apical membrane of the collecting duct can alter its permeability. These proteins are regulated by an array of hormones produced elsewhere in the body. It is responsible for fine-tuning of the filtrate; responsible for absorption of electrolytes and water, and secretion of acid and some electrolytes (primarily potassium). There is an outer cortical collecting duct and an inner medullary collecting duct.

Cotransporter: Membrane protein that combines the movement of a particle to that of sodium; the sodium moves down its electrochemical gradient, which was initially generated by membrane NaK ATPases, and its movement is linked to the second molecule.

Countercurrent exchange: The process of using a hairpin loop in the vasa recta capillary network to prevent it from washing out the high concentration within the medullary interstitium.

Countercurrent multiplier: The process of combining structural modifications and a hairpin loop in the renal tubule to create a system that can multiply the fixed energy capacity of NaK ATPases in order to build a high concentration gradient in the interstitium.

Distal tubule: Portion of the tubule between the thick ascending limb and the collecting duct, important in electrolyte reclamation.

Edema: An abnormal accumulation of fluid within the skin or within one or more body cavities; signifies excessive interstitial water.

Effector mechanism: The process by which a system reacts to a perceived change, inducing a compensatory response.

Efferent arteriole: Muscular arteriole that drains the glomerular capillary; it has the ability to dilate or constrict, which is a key component of the kidney's regulatory mechanisms to maintain appropriate filtration pressure within the glomerular capillary.

Endocytosis: Process of internalizing protein from the cell membrane into the cell.

Epithelial sodium channel (ENaC): A channel, found in the apical membrane of collecting duct epithelial cells, which allows the movement of sodium down its concentration gradient.

Exchangers: Also called counter-transporters; membrane protein that combines the movement of another particle to that of sodium; the sodium moves down its electrochemical gradient, which was initially generated by membrane NaK ATPases, and its movement is linked in the opposite direction to the second molecule.

Exocytosis: Process whereby a cell can secrete cellular proteins across the cell membrane.

Extracellular space: The space outside of the cells.

Filtration equilibrium: The point at which the hydrostatic force driving filtration out of the glomerular capillary loop is balanced by the inward oncotic force, so that filtration ceases.

Filtration fraction: The portion of the fluid (plasma) delivered to the glomerular capillaries that is subsequently filtered into the tubules. It is defined by the equation: FF = GFR/renal plasma flow.

Filtration slits: Small openings between podocyte finger-like extensions, through which filtrate passes en route from the glomerular capillary to the urinary space.

Fractional excretion of sodium (FENa): The amount of sodium that is excreted in the urine relative to the amount that is filtered across the glomerulus. The FENa gives an estimation of how avidly the tubules are reclaiming sodium.

Free water: A term used to describe the presence of water without any particles.

Glomerular filtration rate (GFR): The rate at which fluid is filtered out of the glomerular capillary across the basement membrane into the renal tubule. It defines the body's ability to excrete metabolic waste.

Glomerulus: The "filtering unit" of the kidneys; a tuft of capillaries across which fluid is filtered out of the serum (cells and protein remain in the blood while water and small particles pass through the endothelium) and into the collecting space of the renal tubule.

Glucosuria: The presence of glucose in the urine.

Henderson–Hasselbalch equation: An important chemistry equation that describes the amount of free hydrogen in solution as determined by the amount of acid and base in a system, in relation to that system's pK_a. It is used to calculate the body's pH, in relation to the amount of carbonic acid and bicarbonate base. Since the respiratory system handles carbonic acid and the kidneys handle bicarbonate, the equation describes how the interplay between the respiratory and the renal function determines body pH.

Hydrostatic force: Pressure exerted by fluid.

Interstitial space: The conceptual body compartment that exists both outside of the blood vessel and outside of the cell.

Intracellular space: The body compartment defined by the collective volume within cells.

Intravascular space: The body compartment defined by the volume of all blood vessels (including arteries, veins, and capillaries).

Juxtaglomerular apparatus (JGA): Collection of cells that sit between the renal tubule and its supplying afferent arteriole; these cells can detect changes in tubule flow and, by orchestrating several response mechanisms, can dilate or constrict the afferent arteriole. Important for regulation of filtration to the associated glomerulus and tubular sodium reclamation.

Loop of Henle: A "U" shaped segment of the renal tubule, comprising the thin and thick descending and ascending limbs, which plays a critical role in the ability to alter the concentration of the urine.

Macula densa: Modified epithelial cell within the juxtaglomerular apparatus (JGA) that can detect filtrate flow within the tubule.

Measured osmolality: Determination of the concentration of particles in fluid that uses freezing point depression; detects the presence of all particles in serum, not just sodium, glucose, and urea.

Myogenic stretch: The capacity of blood vessels to respond to increased vessel stretch, usually due to an increase of perfusion pressure, with a compensatory increase in vessel tone (vasoconstriction).

Nephron: The basic structure of the kidney, composed of a glomerulus and its corresponding renal tubule.

Nocturia: The need to awaken at night to urinate.

Noncarbonic acid: Nonvolatile acids, such as sulfuric and phosphoric acids, often derived from metabolism of dietary protein; handled by the kidney.

Oncotic pressure: Form of osmotic pressure exerted by proteins that cannot cross a semipermeable barrier; most commonly used with respect to protein in blood plasma. Usually exerts force to pull water into the circulatory system.

Orthopnea: Shortness of breath while lying flat.

Osmolality: A measure of fluid concentration defined as the number of particles per kilogram of fluid.

Osmolar gap: A difference between the calculated and the measured osmolality; indicates the presence of unmeasurable particles, such as alcohols.

Osmolarity: Measure of fluid concentration, defined as the number of particles per liter of fluid.

Osmoreceptor: A specialized cell that has the capacity to sense changes in fluid concentration

Osmosis: Movement of water across a selectively permeable membrane into a region of higher solute concentration; movement of water continues until the solute concentrations on the two sides of the membrane are equal.

Osmotic pressure: The pressure that needs to be applied to a solution to prevent the inward flow of water across a semipermeable membrane.

Paracellular: Refers to movement of substances between neighboring cells.

Paroxysmal nocturnal dyspnea: The symptom of awakening at night with shortness of breath, usually a result of increased body volume due to an underlying volume retentive disorder (such as congestive heart failure); reflects redistribution of fluid from the interstitium into the vascular space when the individual assumes the recumbent position (at which time the hydrostatic pressure in the veins diminishes and the Starling forces favor movement of fluid from the interstitium to the vascular space).

Passive transport: Process of moving molecules down their electrical or chemical concentration gradient, and thus, not requiring additional chemical energy.

pK_a: The pH at which an acid is in equilibrium with its conjugate base.

Podocyte: Finger-like epithelial cells that sit upon the basement membrane of the glomerulus, forming the third layer (along with the glomerular capillary and basement membrane) of the glomerulus. There are fine slit-like separations between the podocyte units through which the glomerular filtrate passes. The podocyte provides structural support to the glomerulus.

Polarity: Special organization of a cell, such that each side has a unique structure and function, which is important to the overall cell function.

Production acidosis: Refers to an acidosis that occurs due to the increased production (in contrast to ingestion) of acid.

Protein trafficking: Process of shuttling proteins from nucleus to cell membrane, and back.

Proximal tubule: The first and most abundant part of the renal tubule, responsible for the reclamation of the majority of filtered particles and water.

Pulmonary edema: The presence of fluid within the interstitium and the alveoli of the lungs, often due to increased pulmonary capillary pressure.

Renal blood flow: Amount of blood that flows to the kidneys.

Renal calyx: Cup-like division of the renal pyramids that catches urine as it exits in the collecting ducts within the renal pyramids.

Renal cortex: Outer portion of the renal parenchyma, which contains the glomeruli; the cortex receives blood flow out of proportion to its metabolic needs to allow for filtration through the glomeruli.

Renal medulla: Inner portion of the renal parenchyma, containing the deeper parts of the renal tubule, including the Loop of Henle and the collecting ducts. The medulla receives less blood flow than the cortex and is at greater risk of ischemic injury.

Renal pelvis: Funnel-like dilated section of the ureter that collects all the filtrate as it passes through the collecting ducts.

Renal pyramids: Cone-shaped section of renal parenchyma, containing bundles of collecting ducts; opens into the renal calyx.

Renal tubular acidosis: A collection of disorders of the renal tubules that leads to an acidosis. Can occur due to problems with bicarbonate reclamation or hydrogen secretion. Associated with a normal anion gap.

Renal tubule: A long tube lined with epithelial cells that catches all the filtrate as it passes across the glomerulus, and eventually empties into the collecting system of the renal pelvis (via the collecting duct) to be excreted as urine. Along the way, the tubule reclaims many of the filtered substances.

Renin: Peptide secreted by granular cells in the juxtaglomerular apparatus (JGA) of the kidney in response to decreased tubular flow. Renin production leads to an orchestrated response pathway that results in avid sodium reclamation in the kidney (renin–angiotensin–aldosterone system).

Secondary active transport: Process of moving molecules against their electrochemical gradient that does not depend directly on the NaK ATPases; rather, the molecule is linked to the movement of a second ion, usually sodium, which moves down its concentration gradient generated by the NaK ATPase.

Sodium phosphate transporter: A protein in the apical membrane of proximal epithelial cells that links phosphate movement to that of sodium.

Starling forces: Summary of forces across a capillary wall (balance between hydrostatic and oncotic forces) that determines net fluid movement across the wall.

Steady state: Term used to describe homeostatic balance, i.e., the amount of a substance added to the body (either by ingestion or by metabolism of other molecules or tissue) is equally balanced by the amount that is excreted, so that there is no net gain or loss.

Thick ascending limb: Ascending section of the Loop of Henle; highly impermeable to sodium and water. Important pumps on the apical membranes of cells within the thick ascending limb move sodium ions from the lumen into the interstitium.

Thin descending limb: Thin descending section of the Loop of Henle; this part of the tubule is permeable to sodium and water.

Tight junction complex: Unique collection of proteins that seal the connections between cells (making them impermeable to water), thereby preventing paracellular movement of water and small particles (e.g., ions).

Titratable acid: Filtered anions that act as urinary buffers, accepting a secreted hydrogen ion, thereby protecting the urine from excessive pH changes; their presence in the tubular fluid enables the kidney to excrete more hydrogen ions.

Total body water: The total amount of water found in an individual's body, typically around 60% of total body weight; equal to the sum of the intracellular and the extracellular fluid.

Transcellular: Refers to movement of substances through the cell; requires that the substance be able to pass across the cell membrane.

Transport proteins: Often found within the membrane of a cell, these proteins are responsible for the movement of ions.

Transporter: Transport proteins that are able to move molecules against their concentration gradient.

Tubuloglomerular feedback: The feedback system in which changes in flow in the tubules can influence the glomerular filtration rate (GFR) by inducing changes in afferent arteriole vasoconstriction.

Urea: Amine-containing compound produced by the metabolism of nitrogen-containing substances. Metabolism of high protein-containing foods will increase urea production. Urea is water soluble and thus distributes across total body water. Urea is excreted by the kidneys.

Ureters: Muscular tubes that use a peristalsis movement to propel urine from the collecting duct to the bladder.

Urinary space: The space between the glomerulus and the tubule in which filtered fluid collects before entering the tubule.

Vasa recta: Collection of capillaries that perfuse the renal tubules; they are a capillary loop "in series" with the renal artery; arises from the efferent arteriole after it drains the glomerular capillary.

Volume of distribution: The volume of fluid and/or tissue across which a certain substance is disbursed in the body. For example, some drugs distribute across water only—thus their volume of distribution is equivalent to the amount of water in the body. Other drugs, however, deposit into and can be stored in fat cells; thus, the volume of distribution of that drug can be many times the total body fluid volume.

Winter's formula: An empiric formula derived by studying the respiratory response to metabolic acidosis; used to determine what the serum pCO_2 should be as the serum bicarbonate level decreases.

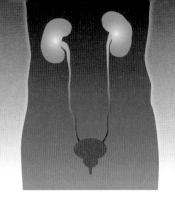

Index

Note: Page numbers followed by "f" denote figures; those followed by "t" denote tables.